Drug Use in Prisoners

Drug Use in Prisoners

Epidemiology, Implications, and Policy Responses

Edited by

Stuart A. Kinner, PhD

NHMRC Senior Research Fellow
Professor of Adolescent and Young Adult Health Equity
Centre for Adolescent Health, Murdoch Children's Research Institute
Honorary Professor, Centre for Mental Health
Melbourne School of Population and Global Health, University of Melbourne
Honorary Professor
Mater Research Institute-UQ, University of Queensland
Brisbane, Queensland, Australia
Adjunct Professor
Griffith Criminology Institute, Griffith University
Brisbane, Queensland, Australia
Honorary Associate Professor
School of Public Health and Preventive Medicine, Monash University
Melbourne, Victoria, Australia
Fellow, Netherlands Institute for the Study of Crime and Law Enforcement
Amsterdam, Netherlands

Josiah D. "Jody" Rich, MD, MPH

Professor of Medicine and Epidemiology
Brown University
Director, The Center for Prison Health and Human Rights
The Miriam Hospital
Providence, Rhode Island, USA

OXFORD
UNIVERSITY PRESS

Oxford University Press is a department of the University of Oxford. It furthers
the University's objective of excellence in research, scholarship, and education
by publishing worldwide. Oxford is a registered trade mark of Oxford University
Press in the UK and certain other countries.

Published in the United States of America by Oxford University Press
198 Madison Avenue, New York, NY 10016, United States of America.

CIP data is on file at the Library of Congress
ISBN 978-0-19-937484-7

9 8 7 6 5 4 3 2 1

Printed by WebCom, Inc., Canada

CONTENTS

PROLOGUE

The world prison population is now approaching 11 million people and continues to grow in the majority of countries. As many as 30 million people pass through prisons each year. In many countries, the so-called war on drugs has resulted in the mass incarceration of drug-involved individuals, who suffer disproportionately from poor physical and mental health, infectious disease, social marginalization, and economic disadvantage. Over the past two decades, a growing body of literature has examined patterns of drug use in people who cycle through prisons, documented some of the health and social implications of this drug use, and most recently begun to evaluate policies and programs designed to respond to these complex health issues. In this volume we bring together experts from 10 countries to review and consider what is known about drug use in prisoners: the epidemiology, the public health and criminal justice implications, and recommendations for evidence-based policy reform. Critically, we use a multidisciplinary approach to explore these issues, taking into account the perspectives of criminologists, human rights lawyers, clinicians, and public health experts.

Chapter 1 explores the relationship between drug use and crime and considers how the "war on drugs" has skewed the prevalence of drug users in custody. Chapter 2 describes the prevalence of drug use in prisons globally, laying the groundwork for more focused discussion of drug use among prisoners in chapters 3, 4, 5, and 11. Other authors consider some of the key health problems experienced by incarcerated drug users, including mental disorders (chapter 10), HIV (chapter 7), hepatitis (chapter 9), and tuberculosis (chapter 8). The contributors also provide an overview of the evidence for supply reduction (chapter 15), demand reduction (chapter 16), and harm reduction (chapter 17) in prison settings, while chapter 12 articulates a human rights approach to drug use in prisoners. Chapter 6 examines patterns of drug use after release from prison, and chapter 13 considers how drug use after release from prison contributes to high rates of reincarceration. Chapter 18 discusses prevention of drug-related deaths in ex-prisoners, and chapter 14 considers some of the broader public health implications of drug use after release from prison. Chapter 19 attempts to summarize some of the key points made in the book, and offers qualified conclusions and recommendations.

Whereas many commentators have focused on illicit drugs, in this book we also consider legal drugs—in particular alcohol and tobacco—given the high prevalence of use of these substances in people who experience incarceration, and their significant contribution to the burden of disease. Where the contributors refer to "drugs," this should typically be understood to include both illicit *and* licit substances. In addition, whereas some countries such as the United States make a distinction between prisons and jails, most do not. Throughout this volume we use the term *prison* to refer to both prisons and jails, and the term *prisoners* to refer to adults held in either prisons or jails, unless otherwise specified. Finally, throughout this volume we try to avoid the term *offender* to refer to people in prison. In our view the pejorative and reductionist nature of this term fails to reflect debate about the appropriateness of drug laws, and ignores the often complex health and social needs of incarcerated people who use drugs.

Although the contributors represent diverse perspectives, there are some important areas of common ground and some recurring themes. One is that among people who cycle through prisons, complex health and social needs are normative and necessitate a multidisciplinary, coordinated response. Another recurring theme is that drug users who experience incarceration are members of our communities—not a discrete population of "offenders"—and that most return to these communities after a relatively short period of time in custody. Consequently, achieving better outcomes for incarcerated people who use drugs matters not only for prisons but also for public health and public safety and, of course, for these vulnerable members of our communities and their families. A final and critical theme that pervades the book is the importance of evidence. In each chapter the contributors provide a careful review of what is known and what is not known, premised on the simple notion that evidence-based policy is effective policy.

This book does not provide all of the answers, but it lays out the evidence and, equally important, identifies some critical knowledge gaps. The contributors pose some challenging questions and offer some possible solutions. We commend this volume to you, and we hope that you find it both informative and challenging.

Stuart A. Kinner, PhD
Josiah D. Rich, MD, MPH

ACKNOWLEDGMENTS

The authors would like to thank Professor Michael Gossop and Professor Jim Byrne for providing external review of some sections of this book. We would also like to thank Manasa Reddy and Cheneal Puljević for editorial assistance. Stuart Kinner is funded by Australian National Health and Medical Research Council (NHMRC) Senior Research Fellowship APP1078168. Jody Rich and this work were partly supported by grants K24DA022112 and P30AI042853 from the US National Institutes of Health (NIH).

CONTRIBUTORS

Zahra Alam-Mehrjerdi, PhD
Program of International Research and
Training, National Drug and Alcohol
Research Centre, University of New
South Wales, Randwick, New South
Wales, Australia

Haider A. Al-Darraji, MBChB, MSc
Centre of Excellence for Research in
AIDS, University of Malaya, Kuala
Lumpur, Malaysia
Centre for International Health,
Department of Preventive and Social
Medicine, University of Otago,
Dunedin, New Zealand

Frederick L. Altice, MD
Centre of Excellence for Research in
AIDS, University of Malaya, Kuala
Lumpur, Malaysia
School of Medicine, Yale University,
New Haven, Connecticut, USA
School of Public Health, Yale University,
New Haven, Connecticut, USA

Dominique de Andrade, PhD
Centre for Youth Substance Abuse
Research, Queensland University of
Technology, Brisbane, Australia
Griffith Criminology Institute
and Menzies Health Institute
Queensland, Griffith University,
Brisbane, Queensland, Australia

Lyuba Azbel, MSc
London School of Tropical Medicine
and Hygiene, London, England, UK

Ingrid A. Binswanger, MD
Institute for Health Research, Kaiser
Permanente, Colorado, USA
Division of General Internal Medicine,
University of Colorado School of
Medicine, Aurora, Colorado, USA

Julie Brummer, MPH
WHO Regional Office for Europe,
Copenhagen, Denmark

Chloé Carpentier, MA, MSc
United Nations Office on Drugs and
Crime, Vienna, Austria

Jennifer Clarke, MD
Medical Program Director, Rhode
Island Department of Corrections,
Providence, Rhode Island, USA
Associate Professor of Medicine, The
Warren Alpert Medical School,
Brown University, Providence, Rhode
Island, USA

Joanne Csete, PhD
Columbia University, Mailman
School of Public Health, New York,
New York, USA

Philip Davis, PhD
United Nations Office on Drugs and
Crime, Vienna, Austria

Kate Dolan, PhD
Program of International Research and
Training, National Drug and Alcohol
Research Centre, University of New
South Wales, Randwick, New South
Wales, Australia

Stefan Enggist, MA
Federal Office of Public Health (FOPH),
Bern, Switzerland

Michael Farrell, PhD
Program of International Research and
Training, National Drug and Alcohol
Research Centre, University of New
South Wales, Randwick, New South
Wales, Australia

Andrea K. Finlay, PhD
Center for Innovation to
Implementation, Menlo Park,
California, USA
National Center on Homelessness
Among Veterans, Department of
Veterans Affairs, Washington DC, USA

Margaret E. Hellard, PhD, FAFPHM
Centre for Population Health, Burnet
Institute, Melbourne, Victoria,
Australia
School of Public Health and Preventive
Medicine, Monash University, Alfred
Hospital, Melbourne, Victoria,
Australia
Alfred Health, Infectious Disease
Department, Alfred Hospital,
Melbourne, Victoria, Australia

Ralf Jürgens, PhD
Global Fund to Fight AIDS, TB and
Malaria, Geneva, Switzerland

Stuart A. Kinner, PhD
Centre for Adolescent Health, Murdoch
Children's Research Institute
Centre for Mental Health, Melbourne
School of Population and Global
Health, University of Melbourne,
Melbourne, Australia
Mater Research Institute- UQ,
University of Queensland,
Brisbane, Queensland, Australia
Griffith Criminology Institute, Griffith
University, Brisbane, Queensland,
Australia
School of Public Health and Preventive
Medicine, Monash University,
Melbourne, Victoria, Australia
Netherlands Institute for the Study of
Crime and Law Enforcement,
Amsterdam, Netherlands

Sarah Larney, PhD
National Drug and Alcohol Research
Centre, University of New South
Wales, Randwick, Australia
Alpert Medical School, Brown
University, Providence, Rhode
Island, USA

Michael Levy, MPH
Hume Health Centre, Alexander
Maconochie Centre, Canberra,
Australia
School of Medicine, Australian National
University, Canberra, Australia

Rick Lines, PhD
Harm Reduction International,
London, England, UK

Ryan McNeil, PhD
British Columbia Centre for Excellence
in HIV/AIDS, Vancouver, Canada
Department of Medicine, Division of
AIDS, University of British Columbia,
Vancouver, British Columbia, Canada

M-J Milloy, PhD
Division of AIDS, Department of
    Medicine, University of British
    Columbia, Vancouver, Canada
BC Centre for Excellence in HIV/AIDS,
    St. Paul's Hospital, Vancouver, British
    Columbia, Canada

Babak Moazen, MSc
Non-Communicable Diseases Research
    Center, Endocrinology and
    Metabolism Population Sciences
    Institute, Tehran University of
    Medical Sciences, Tehran, Iran

Sahar Saeedi Moghaddam, MS
Non-Communicable Diseases Research
    Center, Endocrinology and
    Metabolism Population Sciences
    Institute, Tehran University of
    Medical Sciences, Tehran, Iran

Lars Møller, MD
WHO Regional Office for Europe,
    Copenhagen, Denmark

Linda Montanari, MA
European Monitoring Centre for Drugs
    and Drug Addiction, Lisbon, Portugal

Mary Mun, BSc
New York University, New York,
    New York, USA

Manasa Reddy, MPH
The Center for Prisoner Health and
    Human Rights, The Miriam Hospital,
    Providence, Rhode Island, USA

Josiah D. Rich, MD, MPH
Brown University, Rhode Island, USA
The Center for Prisoner Health and
    Human Rights, The Miriam Hospital,
    Providence, Rhode Island, USA

Luis Royuela, MSc
European Monitoring Centre for Drugs
    and Drug Addiction, Lisbon, Portugal

David Wyatt Seal, PhD
Department of Global Community
    Health and Behavioral Sciences,
    Tulane University School of Public
    Health and Tropical Medicine, New
    Orleans, Louisiana, USA

Will Small, PhD
British Columbia Centre for Excellence
    in HIV/AIDS, Vancouver, Canada
Faculty of Health Sciences, Simon
    Fraser University, Burnaby, British
    Columbia, Canada

Kathryn Snow, MSc
Melbourne School of Population
    and Global Health, University of
    Melbourne, Melbourne, Victoria,
    Australia

Mark Stoové, PhD
Centre for Population Health, Burnet
    Institute, Melbourne, Victoria,
    Australia

Faye S. Taxman, PhD
Center for Advancing Correctional
    Excellence!, Department of
    Criminology, Law and Society,
    George Mason University, Fairfax,
    Virginia, USA

Robert L. Trestman, MD
Virginia Tech/Carilion School of
    Medicine, Carilion Clinic, Roanoke,
    Virginia, USA

Ashbel T. Wall, JD
Rhode Island Department of
    Corrections, Cranston, Rhode
    Island, USA

Rebecca J. Winter, MPH
Centre for Population Health, Burnet
  Institute, Melbourne, Victoria,
  Australia
School of Public Health and Preventive
  Medicine, Monash University,
  Melbourne, Victoria, Australia

Sarah Yancey, MPH, MPS
The Center for Collaborative Systems
  for Security, Safety, and Regional
  Resilience, University of Washington,
  Seattle, Washington, USA

CHAPTER 1

The "Drugs-Crime Nexus"

DOMINIQUE DE ANDRADE, PhD

INTRODUCTION

Although many drug users experience little or no long-term harm related to their drug use, and the vast majority are never subject to sanctions by the criminal justice system, drug misuse remains a significant challenge for both public health and the criminal justice system. For a subset of users, drug use becomes progressively more problematic and compulsive over time. In addition to causing harm for the user, problematic drug use can take a toll on society, putting a strain on families and on health and welfare systems. One significant adverse consequence of substance misuse, particularly in the context of punitive drug policies, is incarceration.[1] This chapter aims to unpack the complex relationship between drugs and crime and the way that drug policy not only frames drug use in society but also plays a defining role in the likelihood of drug users experiencing incarceration, accessing treatment, and in their long-term health outcomes.

DEFINING DRUGS

A drug is defined as "any chemical agent that affects biological function."[2] This includes both illicit drugs and licit drugs such as tobacco, alcohol, and many pharmaceutical drugs. Depending on the drug and its chemical composition, different consumption methods may be used, including intravenous injection, intranasal snorting, inhalation (smoking), and oral consumption.

Drugs can be categorized based on uses, legal status, composition, effect on the body, harm or risk status, or the likelihood that addictive patterns of use will develop. One of the more useful ways of categorizing drugs is based on the effect drugs have on the central nervous system.

Stimulants

Stimulants arouse the central nervous system, speeding up its activity and making the user more alert.[3] Examples include caffeine, nicotine, cocaine, and amphetamines. Caffeine, a legal stimulant naturally found in coffee beans and tea leaves, is withdrawn by adding water. It is also found in an artificial form in some soft drinks and energy drinks. Nicotine, found naturally in the tobacco leaf, is most commonly consumed through the smoking of tobacco. It can also be absorbed through the chewing or sniffing of tobacco (snuff).

Derived from the coca leaf, cocaine in its freebase form is commonly known as "crack" and is smoked. In its other chemical form as hydrochloric salt, it can be either snorted or dissolved in water and injected. Coca leaves can also be chewed. Similar to cocaine in biological effect, amphetamines are synthetically made and can be injected or taken orally. One pure form of amphetamine is synthesized methamphetamine, or "ice," which is commonly smoked due to its resistance to high temperatures, but can also be injected. Unlike ice, methamphetamine hydrochloride cannot be smoked because it breaks down at high temperatures; it is commonly taken orally, intravenously, or by snorting.

Depressants

Depressants relax the central nervous system, slowing down its activity.[3] Examples include alcohol, benzodiazepines, opioids, and volatile substances. Originating from the juice extracts of the opium poppy, opiates have major medicinal uses, particularly as highly effective analgesics (eg, unrefined opium, morphine, and codeine). Morphine is chemically treated to make heroin, which is typically injected but can also be smoked or, in a very pure form, snorted. Crude opium can also be smoked. Morphine and codeine are in most places legally prescribed as painkillers and taken intravenously or orally. The synthetically designed opioids oxycodone and meperidine are used to treat opiate addiction, while methadone, buprenorphine, and the more rarely approved LAAM are used specifically to treat heroin addiction.

Other depressants include barbiturates, used for medicinal purposes (eg, surgical anesthetic), and benzodiazepines (eg, Valium), used to treat anxiety. Due to their pharmacological similarities to alcohol, inhaled solvents (ie, glue sniffing) can also be included in this category.

Hallucinogens

Hallucinogens affect the central nervous system by altering sensory input to the brain.[3] Examples include lysergic acid diethylamide (LSD) and magic mushrooms. Magic mushrooms are a natural hallucinogen while LSD is a synthetic hallucinogen that can be consumed orally or intravenously.

Other

This category consists of psychoactive drugs that do not fit neatly into another category but clearly have mind-altering effects.[3] Examples include ecstasy (MDMA) and cannabis. Ecstasy is synthetically made and similar to amphetamines. Because it increases the activity of particular neurotransmitters, the user experiences more energy and a heightened emotional state. Marijuana leaves come from the cannabis or hemp plant. Tetrahydrocannabinol (THC) is the principal psychoactive element of cannabis, responsible for psychoactive effects. "Skunk" is considered to be a more potent variety of cannabis with higher levels of THC. Marijuana is commonly smoked but can also be taken orally.

DRUG-RELATED CRIME STATISTICS

There is now compelling evidence of a relationship between drug use and criminal behavior. One meta-analysis of the drugs-crime relationship concluded that the likelihood of offending is seven to eight times greater for drug users than for non–drug users.[4] Incarcerated individuals (in federal, state, and local prisons) in the United States are seven times more likely than the general population to have a substance abuse disorder.[5] In 2001, the Drug Use Careers of Offenders (DUCO) study surveyed 2,135 incarcerated men across a number of Australian prisons.[6] Almost two-thirds (62%) of participants reported using illicit drugs regularly in the 6 months prior to their most recent arrest. The two types of drugs most commonly used were cannabis (53%) and amphetamines (31%). A lifetime history of illicit drug use was particularly common among those serving time for property or fraud, and for chronic offenders.[6]

Arrestee drug use monitoring data collected in the United States, Australia, England, and Wales confirms a strong relationship between drug use and offending. Data from the 2013 Arrestee Drug Abuse Monitoring II (ADAM II) program in the United States showed that the majority of sampled arrestees tested positive (via urinalysis) for illicit drugs, with percentages across five major cities ranging from 63% to 83%.[7] Similar findings have emerged from the 2013–2014 Drug Use Monitoring in Australia (DUMA) program, which indicated that 73% of recent arrestees tested positive for at least one illicit drug,[8] and from the New English and Welsh Arrestee Drug Abuse Monitoring (NEW-ADAM) program (which last collected data in 2002), in which 69% of arrestees tested positive for at least one illicit drug.[9]

EXPLANATIONS FOR DRUG-RELATED CRIME

The nature of the relationship between drug use and criminal behavior—often referred to as the "drugs-crime nexus"—is complex. The extensive literature on this relationship suggests that it is to some extent bi-directional. While a number of studies examining individuals' offending trajectories have found criminal behavior to precede drug use,[10,11] there is some evidence that drug use precedes offending.[12,13]

There is also a third notion—that "crime and drug use spring from a set of common causes and then act to continue and intensify each other."[14]

Drug-related crime is first and foremost crime committed in violation of drug (and related) legislation. Drug laws across different countries have a considerable impact on the likelihood and extent of drug user involvement with the criminal justice system. Goldstein's tripartite conceptual framework expands on the legal definition of drug-related crime and identifies three mechanisms that serve as drivers of such crime: economic-compulsive, psychopharmacological, and systemic.[15] Each explanation gives rise to different prevention approaches and challenges in responding to drug-related crime.

The economic-compulsive explanation argues that many chronic drug users cannot support their drug addiction through legitimate means and thus turn to crime to acquire the necessary funds.[15] These "acquisitive crimes" include theft, robbery, burglary, drug sales, prostitution, and other financially motivated crimes and are often committed to fund opiate or stimulant addiction.[14] Data from the Australian DUMA program in 2009 provide some support for the economic-compulsive explanation. Of 114 police detainees who attributed their offense to heroin use, 45% reported committing the offense to obtain money to buy the drug.[16]

The psychopharmacological explanation refers to the pharmacological effects of some drugs that can result in aggressive and/or disinhibited behavior.[15] There is good evidence that some substances such as antidepressants, benzodiazepines, cocaine, and alcohol precipitate behavioral disinhibition,[17] increasing the risk of violence, property crimes, and public disorder crimes. In particular, the disinhibiting effects of alcohol and methamphetamine have been found to increase the chances of perpetrating violence.[16,18,19] There is also emerging evidence of a significant relationship between benzodiazepines and violence,[20] particularly when used in conjunction with alcohol.[21] One Australian study of injecting drug users recently released from prison found that illicit benzodiazepine use significantly increased the risk of committing property crime since release.[22] Approximately 40% of the 1,884 police detainees interviewed as part of the Australian DUMA program in 2009 attributed their offense to being affected by alcohol and/or other drugs at the time.[16] Of 4,237 substance-attributable charges made against these police detainees, the substance attributed to the largest proportion of offenses (29.3%) was alcohol.[16]

Systemic crime is a type of crime that occurs as part of the system of drug distribution and use.[15] This concept is most frequently used to explain violence that is often a deeply embedded characteristic of some drug subcultures, stemming from turf wars in street drug markets, debt collection, and gang affiliation.[4,15] One such example is the systemic violence evident in Mexico, where homicide rates nearly tripled between 2007 and 2012—an estimated 31% to 50% being linked to Mexican drug trafficking organizations.[23]

Expanding on Goldstein's Framework

In recent years Goldstein's work has faced a number of critics,[24-26] suggesting that the drugs-crime relationship is far more nuanced than previously thought, mediated by a number of individual, environmental, cultural, and socio-economic factors. For example, although there is wide-ranging evidence to support the notion that alcohol can have a significant aggressive psychopharmacological effect, there is also an abundance of literature that highlights the role of other factors in alcohol-related violence: individual factors such as masculinity; broader cultural factors such as the acceptability of public drunkenness and aggression; and situational factors embedded in the social and physical drinking environment.[27]

The framework also fails to acknowledge the distinct relationship that exists between certain types of crimes and certain types of drugs.[25] One meta-analysis of the drugs-crime relationship found heroin, crack, and cocaine to be the three drugs most frequently linked with crime, particularly property crime and prostitution.[4] Furthermore, while incarcerated drug users often reoffend soon after release from prison,[28,29] there is evidence that certain types of drugs and patterns of drug use increase the risk of re-incarceration. One Australian study found that risky cannabis, amphetamine, and/or opioid use prior to incarceration significantly increases the risk of re-incarceration after controlling for a number of demographic and criminogenic factors.[30]

Co-occurring drug dependence and mental illness also increase risk of reoffending for those recently released from prison.[31] Among people diagnosed with schizophrenia in particular, substance use disorders are associated with an increased risk of violent behavior[32,33] and conviction for offending.[34] One Australian study found that among regular injecting drug users, psychological distress was associated with an increased risk of criminal behavior.[35]

There are also a number of social mechanisms that contribute to drug use, crime, and the targeting of drug users in law enforcement efforts. For instance, residing in an area of socio-economic deprivation can increase involvement in crime and exposure to a local drug subculture that provides easy access to drugs and opportunities for drug dealing as illegitimate employment.[36,37] Such neighborhoods are also frequently targeted by police.[38]

INTERNATIONAL DRUG POLICY: PUNISH, TREAT, OR TOLERATE?

Historically, international drug treaties have played a significant role in the global prohibition of certain drugs. By the late 20th century, it was evident that global drug prohibition was ineffective in preventing drug use, with most countries (including many developing nations), experiencing extensive drug-related harms.[39] Most noteworthy was the discovery of HIV/AIDS in the early 1980s. This international health epidemic was considered the "greatest threat to global public health since the Black Plague."[39] The immediate focus on reducing the spread of HIV among injecting drug users led to the introduction of harm reduction principles in international drug policy.

Harm reduction refers to measures designed to reduce the harms related to drug use without necessarily reducing drug use itself.[40] Examples include needle exchange programs, drug consumption rooms, and peer administration of naloxone (in the case of overdose). Harm reduction responses can be effective in reducing the possibility of (or effectively responding to) overdose and the spread of infectious disease[41] and are generally aimed at those drug users "not (yet) willing or capable of stopping drug use."[42] Harm reduction philosophy presents an inherent friction with many countries' punitive responses to drug use, which aim to reduce (and ideally stop) drug supply and demand.

Table 1.1 presents incarceration rates, and adoption of harm reduction policy and practice, for 33 countries. These are countries with a population of greater than 4 million and ones for which sufficient information is publicly available to complete the table. Table 1.1 suggests that many countries now make reference to harm reduction strategies in their national drug policy documentation. However, harm reduction drug policy does not always translate into the implementation of harm reduction practices at scale commensurate with demand, particularly in prison settings. Among the reasons for this are a lack of government and international donor funding, and/or perceived conflict between harm reduction and criminal justice goals in many countries.[43]

Nevertheless, there is a high demand for harm reduction practices in prisons, with a substantial number of injecting drug users continuing to inject when incarcerated[44,45] or initiating injecting drug use in prison,[46-48] increasing the risk of infectious disease transmission (eg, hepatitis C) through the sharing of needles. The risky behaviors that many incarcerated drug users engage in highlight the need for appropriate, evidence-informed policy responses and practices that address the urgent treatment requirements of this population.

The data in Table 1.1 suggest that there is a greater focus on harm reduction and rehabilitation (including in prison) in countries with lower imprisonment rates, particularly in Western Europe. This may be related to drug diversion and treatment options that are provided in place of incarceration, or alternatively, these services may prevent re-incarceration. The following examples from four countries provide a more detailed exploration of this relationship and the development of drug policies and related criminal justice consequences.

United States

In the United States, public opinion, moral panic, and the need for political popularity played a significant role in Richard Nixon's response to the "illicit drug problem." As part of his 1971 presidential election campaign, Nixon offered a "heavy-handed law enforcement and incarceration" approach in a war on drugs.[52] Since that time, prison numbers in the United States have increased six fold, with little corresponding decrease in crime or drug use.[53] American drug policy has remained largely unchanged over this time, and a number of other countries have adopted a similar policy, despite persuasive evidence that the approach has been ineffective.[39,54]

The so-called war on drugs has had a devastating impact on those already living in hardship in the United States, particularly for people of color, with a significant

Table 1.1. IMPRISONMENT RATES OF SELECTED COUNTRIES AND HARM REDUCTION POLICIES AND PRACTICES IN THE COMMUNITY AND PRISONS

Rank[a]	Country	Prison pop rate/ 100,000[i]	Supportive national harm reduction policies[ii]	Operating needle exchange programs[ii]	Operating opioid substitution programs[ii]	Drug consumption rooms[ii]	Annual prevalence of drug use among prisoners (%)[iii]	Harm reduction practices in prisons[ii,iv]
1	United States	716	✓	✓	✓	✓	—	Very limited
10	Russian Federation	475	x	✓	x	x	14.80	No
21	Thailand	398	✓	✓	✓	x	—	No
31	Ukraine	305	✓	✓	✓	x	—	No
36	South Africa	294	x	✓	✓	x	—	Very limited
40	Iran	284	✓	✓	✓	x	—	High
47	Brazil	274	✓	✓	x	x	—	No
63	Israel	223	✓	✓	✓	x	51.80	No
67	Mexico	210	✓	✓	✓	x	—	No
74	New Zealand	192	✓	✓	✓	x	5.50	Moderate
80	Hungary	186	✓	✓	✓	x	8.40	Very limited
82	Kyrgyzstan	181	✓	✓	✓	x	15.00	High
83	Turkey	179	✓	x	✓	x	—	Very limited
91	Romania	155	✓	✓	✓	x	2.00	Very limited
102	England and Wales	148	✓	✓	✓	x	—	Moderate
103	Argentina	147	✓	✓	x	x	64.40	No
106	Spain	147	✓	✓	✓	✓	—	High
107	Vietnam	145	✓	✓	✓	x	—	Very limited
116	Malaysia	132	✓	✓	✓	x	39.00	Limited

(continued)

Table 1.1. CONTINUED

Rank[a]	Country	Prison pop rate/ 100,000[i]	Supportive national harm reduction policies[ii]	Operating needle exchange programs[ii]	Operating opioid substitution programs[ii]	Drug consumption rooms[ii]	Annual prevalence of drug use among prisoners (%)[iii]	Harm reduction practices in prisons[ii,iv]
119	Australia	130	✓	✓	✓	✓	70.00	Moderate
128	China	121	✓	✓	✓	x	25.60	Very limited
133	Canada	118	✓	✓	✓	✓	56.70	Moderate
139	Greece	111	✓	✓	✓	x	—	Very limited
146	Italy	106	✓	✓	✓	x	23.80	Limited
152	France	98	✓	✓	✓	x	—	Limited
162=	Switzerland	82	✓	✓	✓	✓	—	High
162=	Netherlands	82	✓	✓	✓	✓	57.00	Limited
165	Egypt	80	✓	✓	x	x	—	Very limited
168	Germany	79	✓	✓	✓	✓	33.00	Moderate
174	Denmark	73	✓	✓	✓	✓	8.00	Moderate
180	Sweden	67	✓	✓	✓	x	42.00	Limited
188	Indonesia	59	✓	✓	✓	x	17.00	Limited
214	India	30	✓	✓	✓	x	—	Very limited

[a] Global incarceration rate ranking; [i] 49; [ii] 43; [iii] 50; [iv] 51.

increase in imprisonment rates, familial poverty, health problems, and unemployment on release from prison.[55-57] US drug policy has also resulted in an increase in the proportion of prisoners who are drug dependent. Between 1996 and 2006, the percentage of "substance-involved" persons in federal, state, and local prisons rose from 78.6% to 84.8%, and in 2006, 65% of prisoners were considered drug dependent based on criteria from the fourth edition of the *Diagnostic and Statistical Manual of Mental Disorders (DSM-IV)*. These individuals had either committed a crime while under the influence, committed acquisitive crime to buy drugs, or violated alcohol or other drug laws.[5]

In addition to punitive drug laws, the United States has the highest rate of imprisonment in the world (see Table 1.1), with 70% of all persons convicted of offenses in the United States in 2010 receiving prison sentences.[58] High imprisonment rates come at a significant economic cost. The National Drug Intelligence Center (NDIC) estimates that drug-related crime alone imposes $113 billion a year in costs to the criminal justice system and victims in the United States. By comparison, treatment costs are estimated at only $14.6 billion.[59] However, with rehabilitation being a secondary sentencing goal to incapacitation and retribution,[58] only a small proportion of eligible offenders benefit from such opportunities in the community, and only 11% of substance-involved prisoners receive any type of addiction treatment, most of which is not evidence based.[5] Furthermore, only 16.6% of correctional facilities in the United States provide specialized, evidence-based treatment.[5]

The United States' policy approach to addressing drug use and related crime has focused on curbing the sale, distribution, and use of illicit drugs, with insufficient emphasis on treatment and harm reduction. This heavy focus on supply and demand reduction has reduced neither drug use nor drug-related crime. The US model highlights that mass incarceration is one of the least cost-effective responses to drug-related crime, diverting funding away from more cost-effective options such as drug treatment.[37] Despite the potential for substantial savings and evidence for the effectiveness of treatment and diversion strategies, rehabilitation of offenders remains a secondary sentencing goal in the United States, with the primary response of incarceration playing a role in rising prison populations.

Australia

Australia's stance on drugs has seen little change since 1985 and has shaped government responses to illicit drug production, distribution, and use. The 2010–2015 National Drug Strategy "encompasses the three equally important pillars of demand reduction, supply reduction and harm reduction being applied together in a balanced way."[60] However, drug policy spending in 2009–2010 clearly demonstrates that the three pillars are not considered equal, with only 2% of funds being dedicated to harm reduction measures, and almost two thirds of funding being dedicated to law enforcement. Remaining funds were split between prevention (10%), treatment (22%), and other (1%), with no significant change in the funding structure since 2002–2003.[61]

At present Australia faces a number of drug-related challenges. A 2014 report by the Australian Crime Commission stated that crystal methamphetamine is "emerging as a pandemic akin to the issue of 'crack' cocaine in the United States."[62] The increased use of this particular drug in Australia and its strong relationship with property and violent crime are reflected in the 2013–2014 DUMA report, which showed the highest recorded rate of amphetamine use among adults detained by police since the DUMA project started in 1999, with 37% of detainees testing positive for amphetamines—a 13% increase since 2011–2012.[8] These findings are supported by data collected in 2014 from a national sample of 898 injecting drug users as part of the Illicit Drug Reporting System (IDRS).[63] The IDRS data suggest a significant increase in methamphetamine use among people who inject drugs (PWID) since 2010, when 60% of the sample reported using in the 6 months prior to being surveyed, compared with 70% of the 2014 sample.[63]

Given the rapid increase in methamphetamine use in Australia, and the drug's ability to suppress the immune system and increase the risk of hepatitis C,[64] it is perhaps not surprising that the prevalence of hepatitis C among injecting drug users in Australia doubled between 2009 and 2013.[65] In response, the number of needle exchange sites in the Australian community almost doubled between 2012 and 2014.[43] Despite prisoners being considered a priority population for infectious disease intervention, needle exchange programs and some other harm reduction strategies used in the Australian community have failed to transfer to prisons.[66] As at 2015, there is still one Australian jurisdiction that does not offer opioid substitution treatment (OST; ie, methadone or buprenorphine) to male prisoners, despite a significant increase in the use of OST in the community since 2012,[43] and despite compelling evidence that OST is associated with a reduction in prison drug injecting and syringe sharing.[67–69]

One cost-benefit analysis of treating Australian Indigenous offenders for problematic drug and alcohol use in community residential rehabilitation services found that diversion from prison would result in significant savings per offender of $96,446, lower recidivism rates, and improved health outcomes.[70] However, this and other evidence of better outcomes for this high-risk and high-needs group, through diversion to treatment, has failed to translate to policy and practice at scale, and imprisonment is still the primary response to drug-related crime in Australia.

Similar to the United States, the prioritization of law enforcement in responding to drugs in Australia has played a role in the significant and continual growth of the prison population since 2000, from a rate of 114 prisoners per 100,000 population to 151 per 100,000 estimated population in 2015.[71] This considerable increase has resulted in over-crowding in prisons, with prisons in 2015 at 104.4% of capacity.[72]

Great Britain

In Great Britain, the national drug strategy "Tackling Drugs Together" was introduced in 1995 by the Conservative government and inherited by the Labour government 2 years later.[73] This strategy represented a significant (and detrimental) shift away from harm minimization following the HIV epidemic, toward law enforcement and punishment.[74] More recently, a shift in drug policy has focused on recovery and abstinence, with "the repositioning of treatment to serve crime reduction and public protection goals."[73] Justice-involved drug users are offered treatment across all sections of the criminal justice system, including arrest referral and coerced treatment for probationers through drug treatment and testing orders.

While imprisonment rates in Great Britain and Wales increased significantly between 2000 and 2010, from 124 prisoners per 100,000 population to 153 per 100,000 population, more recent figures show a slight decline to a rate of 148 per 100,000 population in 2014.[75] These figures are consistent with the view that the recent shift toward treatment for justice-involved drug users may be playing a role in preventing or delaying incarceration. Despite this decline, prisons in Great Britain are still over-crowded, with an occupancy rate of 110.6%.[75] Similar to the United States and Australia, Great Britain prioritizes law enforcement as a key response to drug use. However, a recent shift in its national drug strategy and the expansion of treatment options for offenders may be helping to curb incarceration rates.

The Netherlands

Few countries have achieved a harmonious balance between law enforcement and public health responses to problematic drug use. The Dutch model is arguably one of the more successful examples to date. The 1970s saw the Netherlands face a heroin epidemic that left the country in a state of crisis. A revision of the Opium Act in 1976 distinguished between "hard" drugs as those that present significant risks to the user's health such as heroin, and "soft" drugs such as cannabis.[76] The revision also outlined a stronger law enforcement approach to hard drug offenses compared to soft drug offenses, resulting in a more liberal drug policy approach overall.[77]

By 1986, however, 30% of injecting drug users in Amsterdam were infected with HIV. In response, most cities established needle exchange programs by the late 1980s, and OST became the leading response to heroin addiction.[78] While this approach was reasonably effective, an increase in organized crime and drug-related crime by hard drug users in the mid-1990s led to a number of adjustments to the Dutch drug policy goals.[76] While the protection of public health continued to be a primary focus, the control of drug-related crime became a strong secondary focus. Attempts to balance these two goals in recent years have resulted in some unintended consequences, such as the development of thriving professional cultivation and export industries for "skunk". However, there have also been a number of positive outcomes, including a reduction or stabilization of drug use in youth, a decrease in the number of coffee shops selling marijuana (and promoting drug tourism), and a decrease in the number of hard drug users and related crime.[76] Furthermore, the Netherlands currently has the lowest HIV incidence in Europe.[78]

These positive outcomes also correspond to a significant drop in the prison population rate since 2006, from 125 prisoners per 100,000 population to 69 prisoners per 100,000 population in 2014.[79] As shown in Table 1.1, the Netherlands has one of the lowest imprisonment rates in the world and a healthy prison occupancy rate of 77% in 2013.[79] These reductions in imprisonment rates not only are related to reductions in hard drug use and related crime, but also reflect sentencing practices that embrace harm reduction and rehabilitation practices. Only 10% of convicted offenders in the Netherlands are sentenced to prison, with most offenders receiving community-based orders, fines, suspended sentences, and diversion.[58] Furthermore, 91% of sentences are for 1 year or less.[58]

The Dutch model provides good evidence that prioritizing harm reduction in the community and criminal justice system leads to far more successful outcomes than incarceration focused on retribution. Dedication to harm reduction strategies over the past five decades has led to lower incarceration rates, lower HIV prevalence, and a reduction in injecting drug use and drug-related crime. Although policy responses must be tailored to the local context, the Dutch model provides some important lessons and has a number of policy implications for other countries, particularly the United States.[58] First, prison should be used as a sanction of last resort (reserved for serious offenders) and for minimal time. This may require an increase in the use of prosecutors' discretion and the scenarios in which they can apply it. Second, opportunities for appropriate community-based sanctions and quality treatment should be expanded. Third, to increase the chances of rehabilitation and successful transition back to the community, "normalization" should be an underlying principle to prisoner management, with prison life resembling life in the community as much as possible.[58]

CONCLUSION

There has been a distinct shift in recent decades in the way some Western countries such as the United States and Australia manage and treat drug users, with law enforcement being the favored response. The prioritization of imprisonment as a response has led to growing prison populations with no impact on drug use or drug-related crime rates in the community. At the same time, some Western European countries have embraced harm reduction strategies in the community and in prison, reaping benefits such as lower imprisonment rates and lower rates of infectious diseases. Globally, however, treatment and harm reduction programs have failed to penetrate most prison settings, even when such programs exist in the community.

Literature reviewed in this chapter highlights the need for dynamic, innovative, and evidence-informed policies that address the complexities of responding to drug users and their needs, both in the community and in the criminal justice system. In many countries, there is increasing interest in reconsidering how governments respond to and manage at-risk, vulnerable populations, such as drug users—from methods founded on punitive principles to those founded on the principles of public health. Current and emerging drug policies need to achieve a delicate balance between primary prevention, treatment, harm reduction, and law enforcement.[80]

REFERENCES

1. Stevenson B. *Drug Policy, Criminal Justice and Mass Imprisonment*. Geneva, Switzerland: Global Commission on Drug Policies; 2011.
2. Goldstein A. *Addiction: From Biology to Drug Policy*. New York, NY: Oxford University Press; 2001.
3. Department of Health. *3.1 Classifying Drugs by Their Effect on the Central Nervous System*. Canberra, Australia: Australian Government; 2004.
4. Bennett T, Holloway K, Farrington D. The statistical association between drug misuse and crime: a meta-analysis. *Aggress Violent Beh*. 2008;13(2):107–118.
5. The National Center on Addiction and Substance Abuse at Columbia University (CASA). *Behind Bars II: Substance Abuse and America's Prison Population*. New York, NY: CASA; 2010.
6. Makkai T, Payne J. Key Findings from the Drug Use Careers of Offenders (DUCO) Study. *Trends Issues Crime Crim Just*. 2003;(267):1–8.
7. Office of National Drug Control Policy. *2013 Annual Report, Arrestee Drug Abuse Monitoring Program II*. Washington, DC: Executive Office of the President; 2014.
8. Coghlan S, Gannoni A, Goldsmid S, Patterson E, Willis M. *Drug Use Monitoring in Australia: 2013–14 Report Drug Use Among Police Detainees*. Canberra, Australia: Australian Institute of Criminology; 2015.
9. Bennett T, Holloway K. *Drug Use and Offending: Summary Results of the First Two Years of the NEW-ADAM Programme*. Findings 179. Home Office Research, Development and Statistics Directorate. London, England: Home Office; 2004.
10. D'Amico EJ, Edelen MO, Miles JNV, Morral AR. The longitudinal association between substance use and delinquency in high-risk youth. *Drug Alcohol Depen*. 2008;93(1):85–92.
11. Hales J, Nevill C, Pudney S, Tipping S. *Longitudinal Analysis of the Offending, Crime and Justice Survey 2003–06*. Research Report 19. London, England: Home Office; 2009.
12. Baltieri DA. Order of onset of drug use and criminal activities in a sample of drug-abusing women convicted of violent crimes. *Drug Alcohol Rev*. 2014;33(2):202–210.
13. Swan AC, Goodman-Delahunty J. The Relationship between drug use and crime among police detainees: does gender matter? *Int J Forensic Ment Health*. 2013;12(2):107.
14. Quinn JF, Sneed Z. Drugs and crime: an empirically based, interdisciplinary model. *J Teach Addict*. 2008;7(1):16–30.
15. Goldstein P. The drugs/violence nexus: a tripartite conceptual framework. *J Drug Issues*. 1985;15(4):493–506.
16. Payne J, Gaffney A. How much crime is drug or alcohol related? self-reported attributions of police detainees. *Trends Issues Crime Crim Just*. 2012;(439):1–6.
17. Gillet C, Polard E, Mauduit N, Allain H. Acting out and psychoactive substances: alcohol, drugs, illicit substances. *Encephale*. 2001;27(4):351–359.
18. Boyum DA, Caulkins JP, Kleiman MAR. Drugs, crime and public policy. In: Wilson JQ, Petersilia J, eds. *Crime and Public Policy*. New York, NY: Oxford University Press; 2010:368–410.
19. Duke AA, Giancola PR, Morris DH, Holt JCD, Gunn RL. Alcohol dose and aggression: another reason why drinking more is a bad idea. *J Stud Alcohol Drugs*. 2011;72(1):34–43.
20. Lundholm L, Haggård U, Möller J, Hallqvist J, Thiblin I, Rättsmedicin. The triggering effect of alcohol and illicit drugs on violent crime in a remand prison population: a case crossover study. *Drug Alcohol Depen*. 2013;129(1–2):110–115.
21. Forsyth AJM, Khan F, McKinlay B. Diazepam, alcohol use and violence among male young offenders: "The devil's mixture." *Drugs-Educ Prev Polic*. 2011;18(6):468–476.
22. Kirwan A, Quinn B, Winter R, Kinner SA, Dietze P, Stoové M. Correlates of property crime in a cohort of recently released prisoners with a history of injecting drug use. *Harm Reduct J*. 2015;12(23):1–6.

23. Heinle K, Molzahn C, Shirk, DA. *Drug Violence in Mexico: Data and Analysis Through 2014.* San Diego, CA: University of San Diego; 2015.
24. Bennett T, Holloway K. The causal connection between drug misuse and crime. *Brit J Criminol.* 2009;49(4):513–531.
25. MacCoun R, Kilmer B, Reuter P. *Research on Drugs-Crime Linkages: The Next Generation.* Washington, DC: National Institute of Justice; 2003.
26. Parker RN, Auerhahn K. Alcohol, drugs, and violence. *Annu Rev Sociol.* 1998;24(1):291–311.
27. Graham K, Homel R. *Raising the Bar: Preventing Aggression in and Around Bars, Clubs and Pubs.* 2nd ed. London, England: Taylor and Francis; 2011.
28. Deitch D, Koutsenok I, Ruiz A. The relationship between crime and drugs: what we have learned in recent decades. *J Psychoactive Drugs.* 2000;32(4):391–397.
29. Kinner S. *The post-release experience of prisoners in Queensland.* Trends & issues in crime and criminal justice no. 325. Canberra, Australia: Australian Institute of Criminology; 2006.
30. Thomas EG, Spittal MJ, Taxman FS, Kinner SA. Health-related factors predict return to custody in a large cohort of ex-prisoners: new approaches to predicting re-incarceration. *Health Justice.* 2015;3(1):1–13.
31. Smith N, Trimboli L. Comorbid substance and non-substance mental health disorders and re-offending among NSW prisoners. *Crim Just Bulletin.* 2010;(140):1–16.
32. Fazel S, Långström N, Hjern A, Grann M, Lichtenstein P. Schizophrenia, substance abuse, and violent crime. *JAMA.* 2009; 301(19):2016–2023.
33. Swanson JW, Swartz MS, Van Dorn RA, et al. A national study of violent behavior in persons with schizophrenia. *Arch Gen Psychiatry.* 2006;63(5):490–499.
34. Wallace C, Mullen PE, Burgess P. Criminal offending in schizophrenia over a 25-year period marked by deinstitutionalization and increasing prevalence of comorbid substance use disorders. *Am J Psychiatry.* 2004;161(4):716–727.
35. Kinner SA, George J, Campbell G, Degenhardt L. Crime, drugs and distress: patterns of drug use and harm among criminally involved injecting drug users in Australia. *Aust N Z J Public Health.* 2009;33(3):223–227.
36. Dunlap E, Johnson BD, Kotarba JA, Fackler JL. Macro-level social forces and micro-level consequences: poverty, alternate occupations, and drug dealing. *J Ethnicity Subst Abuse.* 2010;9(2):115–127.
37. Stevens A, Trace M, Bewley-Taylor D. *Reducing Drug Related Crime: An Overview of the Global Evidence.* The Beckley Foundation Drug Policy Programme Report 5. 2005.
38. Stevens A. *Drugs, Crime and Public Health: The Political Economy of Drug Policy.* New York, NY: Routledge; 2011.
39. Wodak A. Ethics and drug policy. *Psychiatry.* 2007;6(2):59–62.
40. Weatherburn D. Dilemmas in harm minimization. *Addiction.* 2009;104(3):335–339.
41. Korf DJ, Bunning EC. Coffee shops, low-threshold methadone and needle exchange: controlling illicit drug use in the Netherlands. In: Inciardi JA, Harrison LD, eds. *Harm Reduction: National and International Perspectives.* London, England: Sage Publications; 1999:125–133.
42. Bunning E, van Brussel GHA. The effects of harm reduction in Amsterdam. *Eur Addict Res.* 1995;1(3):92–98.
43. Stone K. *The Global State of Harm Reduction 2014.* London, England: Harm Reduction International; 2014.
44. Carpentier C, Royuela L, Noor A, Hedrich D. Ten years of monitoring illicit drug use in prison populations in Europe: issues and challenges. *How J Crim Just.* 2012;51(1):37–66.
45. Kinner SA, Jenkinson R, Gouillou M, Milloy MJ. High-risk drug-use practices among a large sample of Australian prisoners. *Drug Alcohol Depen.* 2012;126(1–2):156–160.

46. Allwright S, Bradley F, Long J, Barry J, Thornton L, Parry JV. Prevalence of antibodies to hepatitis B, hepatitis C, and HIV and risk factors in Irish prisoners: results of a national cross sectional survey. *BMJ*. 2000;321(7253):78–82.
47. Boys A, Farrell M, Bebbington P, et al. Drug use and initiation in prison: results from a national prison survey in England and Wales. *Addiction*. 2002;97(12):1551–1560.
48. Gore SM, Bird AG, Ross AJ. Prison Rites: Starting to inject inside. *BMJ*. 1995;311(7013):1135–1136.
49. Walmsley R. *World Prison Population List*. 10th ed. London, England: International Centre for Prison Studies; 2013.
50. United Nations Office on Drugs and Crime. *World Drug Report 2014*. Geneva, Switzerland: UNODC; 2014.
51. Jurgens R. Out of sight, out of mind: harm reduction in prisons and other places of detention. In: Cook C, ed. *The Global State of Harm Reduction 2010: Key Issues for Broadening the Response*. London, England: International Harm Reduction Association; 2010:105–112.
52. Mauer M. Two-tiered justice: race, class and crime policy. In: Hartman C, Squires GD, eds. *The Integration Debate: Competing Futures for American Cities*. New York, NY: Routledge; 2010:169–183.
53. Sabol WJ, Couture H. Prison inmates at mid-year 2007. *Bureau of Justice Statistics Bulletin*. Washington, DC, Department of Justice; 2008.
54. Reuter P. Why has US drug policy changed so little over 30 years? *Crime Justice*. 2013;42(1):75–140.
55. Moore LD, Elkavich A. Who's using and who's doing time. *Am J Public Health*. 2008;98(5):782–786.
56. Nunn KB. Race, crime and the pool of surplus criminality: or why the "war on drugs" was a "war on blacks." *J Gender Race Just*. 2002;6(2):381–445.
57. Western B, Kleykamp M, Rosenfeld J. *Crime, Punishment, and American Inequality*. Princeton, NJ: Russell Sage Foundation; 2003.
58. Subramanian R, Shames A. *Sentencing and Prison Practices in Germany and the Netherlands: Implications for the United States*. New York, NY: Vera Institute of Justice; 2013.
59. National Drug Intelligence Center. *The Economic Impact of Illicit Drug Use on American Society*. Washington, DC: Department of Justice; 2011.
60. Commonwealth of Australia. *National Drug Strategy 2010–2015: A Framework for Action on Alcohol, Tobacco and Other Drugs*. Canberra, Australia: Commonwealth of Australia; 2011.
61. Ritter A, McLeod R, Shanahan M. *Government Drug Policy Expenditure in Australia— 2009/10*. DPMP Monograph 24. Sydney, Australia: National Drug and Alcohol Research Centre; 2013.
62. Australian Crime Commission (ACC). *2012–13 Illicit Drug Data Report*. Canberra, Australia: ACC; 2014.
63. Stafford J, Burns L. *Australian Drug Trends 2014: Findings from the Illicit Drug Reporting System (IDRS)*. Australian Drug Trend Series No. 127. Sydney, Australia: National Drug and Alcohol Research Centre; 2015.
64. Ye L, Peng JS, Wang X, Wang YJ, Luo GX, Ho WZ. Methamphetamine enhances hepatitis C virus replication in human hepatocytes. *J Viral Hepatitis*. 2008;15:261–270.
65. Torresi J. *Inquiry Into Hepatitis C in Australia*. Victoria, Australia: Australasian Society for Infectious Diseases; 2015.
66. Moore M. *Report for the ACT Government Into Implementation of a Needle and Syringe Program at the Alexander Maconochie Centre*. Canberra, Australia: Public Health Association of Australia; 2011.
67. Kinner SA, Moore E, Spittal MJ, Indig D. Opiate substitution treatment to reduce in-prison drug injection: a natural experiment. *Int J Drug Policy*. 2013;24:460–463.

68. Larney S. Does opioid substitution treatment in prisons reduce injecting-related HIV risk behaviours? a systematic review. *Addiction*. 2010;105:216–223.
69. Stallwitz A, Stöver H. The impact of substitution treatment in prisons—a literature review. *Int J Drug Policy*. 2007;18:464–474.
70. Australian National Council on Drugs. *An Economic Analysis for Aboriginal and Torres Strait Islander Offenders: Prison vs Residential Treatment*. Canberra, Australia: Australian National Council on Drugs; 2013.
71. Institute for Criminal Policy Research. *World Prison Brief—Australia 2015*. London, England: ICPR; 2015.
72. Steering Committee for the Review of Government Service Provision PC. *Report on Government Services 2015*. Canberra, Australia: Productivity Commission; 2015.
73. Duke K. From crime to recovery: the reframing of British drugs policy? *J Drug Issues*. 2013;43(1):39–55.
74. Duke K. Out of crime and into treatment? the criminalization of contemporary drug policy since Tackling Drugs Together. *Drugs-Educ Prev Polic*. 2006;13(5):409–415.
75. Institute for Criminal Policy Research. *World Prison Brief—United Kingdom: England and Wales 2015*. London, England: ICPR; 2015.
76. van Ooyen-Houben M, Kleemans E. Drug policy: the "Dutch Model." *Crime Justice*. 2015;44:165–226.
77. Lyman MD. *Drugs in Society: Causes, Concepts, and Control*. Cincinnati, OH: Anderson Publishing; 2014.
78. Grund J, Breeksema J. *Coffee Shops and Compromise: Separated Illicit Drug Markets in the Netherlands*. New York, NY: Open Society Foundations; 2013.
79. Institute for Criminal Policy Research. *World Prison Brief—Netherlands 2015*. London, England: ICPR; 2015.
80. Ritter A, McDonald D. Illicit drug policy: scoping the interventions and taxonomies. *Drugs-Educ Prev Polic*. 2008;15:15–35.

CHAPTER 2

The Global Epidemiology of Drug Use in Prison

CHLOÉ CARPENTIER, MA, MSc, LUIS ROYUELA, MSc,
LINDA MONTANARI, MA, AND PHILIP DAVIS, PhD

On any given day at least 11 million people are estimated to be held in prison (remanded or convicted) at the global level.[1] In Europe more than 1.7 million inmates were held in penal institutions on September 1, 2012, 16% of whom were pre-trial detainees. About 17% of the inmates given a final sentence for criminal offenses were convicted of drug offenses, with this proportion varying from 4% to 39% between countries. Twenty-one of the 36 countries for which information is available report proportions over 15%, indicating that drug-related crime is an important category of custodial offense in many European countries.[2]

In most countries, experience of illicit drug use is more widespread in the prison population than in the general community. For example, in Europe, depending on the country, 0.7% to 35.6% of the general adult population have ever used cannabis and 0.3% to 9.6% have used it in the last year, while the proportion who have ever used cocaine varies between 0.3% and 6.8% and for heroin remains below 1% in all European countries.[3,4] In comparison, the levels of drug use among prisoners are much higher: depending on the studies, 15% to 79% of prisoners report illicit drug use at any time outside prison and 11% to 75% in the year before prison. For specific drugs the proportions are 14% to 70% (at any time outside prison) and 6% to 54% (in the year before prison) for cannabis, 8% to 57% and 2% to 43% for cocaine, and 4% to 37% and 2% to 52% for heroin (note that data are not consistent across studies, which explains why the upper range in the prevalence of heroin in the year before prison is higher than its use at any time outside prison). More recent use of cannabis, measured by consumption in the month prior to incarceration, is reported by 1% to 73% of surveyed inmates in Europe, which is much higher than the range of 0.1% to 4.6% found in the general population of adults.[3,5]

Illicit drugs are more difficult to obtain in prison than they are outside, and for many drug users, incarceration results in their stopping drug use or using less frequently. However, a number of inmates continue to use once inside, while some switch to other substances (sometimes more harmful) and others take up more efficient (and also more harmful) modes of administration such as injecting. Intravenous drug use is reported in many prisons around the globe, and risk behaviors, including sharing of injection equipment, combined with high prevalence of blood-borne viruses (eg, HIV, hepatitis C), "make prisons a high-risk environment"[6] for the transmission of infectious diseases. Because there are frequent contacts with the local community, these particularly risky patterns of drug use represent a potential health risk for the general population as well.

For many individuals, a stay in prison may represent an opportunity for addressing some of their often complex health and social problems. These may include substance use disorders, psychiatric comorbidity, and diverse problems of a psychological, social, and/or economic nature that may affect the many inmates suffering from some form of social exclusion. The prison setting therefore presents an opportunity for detecting, intervening, and referring prisoners with substance use problems to treatment. Assessing the needs of those who are incarcerated is essential; this is a prerequisite for planning the most appropriate interventions and ensuring the best assistance to drug users in prison.[7]

A number of reviews of drug use and prison have been carried out at both regional and global levels, but none has focused on drug use *within* prison. A recent European analysis of 53 studies of illicit drug use in prison populations between the years 2000 and 2008[8] reviewed data on drug use *prior* to imprisonment and drug use *in* prison. While highlighting the heterogeneity of the samples and the diversity of the data collection methodologies used, it showed that illicit drug use *in* prison is not unusual but tends to be lower than reported drug use before incarceration; most studies reported prevalence rates between 20% and 40% for illicit drug use *in* prison and around 50% before incarceration. An international systematic review of 13 studies using standardized diagnostic criteria[9] estimated the prevalence of illicit drug abuse and dependence to be between 10% and 48% in male prisoners and 30% and 60% in female prisoners, and the prevalence for alcohol abuse and dependence, respectively, to be between 18% and 30% in males and 10% and 24% in females. These data may be compared with an estimated 5.5% of the European population suffering from alcohol use disorders in the last year.[10] Baybutt and colleagues,[11] in their recent review of tobacco use in prison settings, stressed that tobacco consumption *in* prison remains two to four times higher than in the community, with prevalence rates ranging from 64% to more than 90%, and rates in female prisoners at best comparable, if not higher.

This chapter compiles the results of a comprehensive search for studies dealing with drug use within prisons. A review of methodological details and issues surrounding these studies is presented, as well as an examination of the extent of use of various drugs within the prison setting.

METHODS

Two methods were used to identify studies on drug use in prison. First, we used the reporting instrument implemented by the European Monitoring Centre for Drugs and Drug Addictions (EMCDDA) since 1999 across the European Union (EU) member states, Norway, and Turkey. It is a flexible instrument that allows European countries to report, on an annual basis, aggregated data on the prevalence of illicit drug use in any prison population. Data are reported by substance or by the generic category of "any illicit drug." In addition to lifetime, past year, and past month prevalence measures, it is possible to report—provided an exact definition is specified— regular drug use, injecting drug use, or any other pattern of drug use. A distinction is made between drug use *prior* to imprisonment and drug use *in* prison.

Second, we searched the available literature to uncover data on drug use in prison from studies falling outside the EMCDDA routine reporting system, in particular in non-EU Europe and in the other global regions. We searched the Psychology & Behavioral Sciences Collection, which provides access to nearly 540 full-text journals, as well as PubMed, Google Scholar, and the websites of some South American university journals. The search was conducted between December 2013 and March 2014, using keywords from seven languages (English, French, German, Italian, Portuguese, Spanish, Swedish). More than 500 documents were reviewed, including papers from peer-reviewed journals, policy reports, scientific reports, and other gray literature.

The present review is limited to studies carried out from 2004 to 2013. However, we exceptionally included studies from 2000–2003 in countries where more recent data were not available. While the focus of this review is mainly on the use of illicit drugs in prison, the consumption of alcohol and tobacco in prison is also addressed whenever possible. The term *prison* was defined in a broad sense, covering all closed institutions such as youth detention centers and establishments where remanded and convicted adults are detained, but excluding such institutions as compulsory drug detention and treatment centers or asylum seeker detention centers because these would not be representative of the general prison populations. A prerequisite for inclusion in this analysis was the availability of data on the prevalence of drug use *in* prison as a percentage of the general prison population; we therefore excluded studies based on samples of drug users or of persons undergoing drug treatment because this would introduce a bias and likely overestimate drug use *in* prison. Different patterns of drug use were reviewed, including injecting, with a distinction made between substances where possible.

RESULTS
Review of Methodologies

Europe is by far the global region where most assessments of drug use in prison have been carried out in the last decade; two-thirds (40) of the studies included in the present review come from 19 European countries. These represent more than half of the total number of countries (31) for which data are available. In the Americas, data from 11 studies referring to 7 countries were uncovered, while the remaining three world regions account for 8 studies (5 countries) in total. In some instances assessments were conducted in only 1 country in an entire region (Oceania, Africa; Table 2.1). The wide range of methodologies used in the 59 studies that met the

Table 2.1. GENERAL CHARACTERISTICS OF STUDIES REVIEWED

Country	Reference	Year of data collection	Coverage and sampling	Definition of (drug use) *in prison*	Measurement and indicators	Substances	Population covered
			Europe				
Belgium	Van Malderen, 2011[27]	2010	National survey in all the 32 Belgian prisons. Representative sample of 10% of all prisoners in each prison, representative sample for gender, penal status, and age (n = 1,251).	Current imprisonment	DU: LT, LY, LM, RG IDU: LM	Illicit drugs, alcohol	On remand, convicted, and mentally disordered. Males and females.
Belgium	Todts et al., 2009[26]	2008	National survey in all the 32 Belgian prisons. Representative sample of 10% of all prisoners in each prison (n = 1,078).	Current imprisonment	DU: LT	Illicit drugs	On remand and convicted, including mentally disordered.
Belgium	Todts et al., 2007[62]	2006	National survey in all the 32 Belgian prisons. Representative sample of 10% of all prisoners in each prison (n = 902).	Current imprisonment	DU: LT IDU: LT	Illicit drugs	On remand and convicted, including mentally disordered.
Bosnia and Herzegovina	Vidic et al., 2011[51]	2011	National survey in 10 prisons. Random sample (n = 620).	Current imprisonment	DU: LT IDU: RG	Illicit drugs	Sentenced to more than 2 months.
Czech Republic	National Monitoring Centre for Drugs and Drug Addiction, the Czech Prison Service, 2013[22]	2012	National survey in all 36 prisons. Random sample (n = 1,641).	Any imprisonment	DU: LT, IDU: LT	Illicit drugs	Males and females.

Country	Reference	Sample	Time reference	Codes	Substance	Population
France	Sannier et al., 2009[33]	Survey in 1 prison. Self-selected sample (n = 205).	Current imprisonment	DU: CU	Tobacco	Prisoners consulting the primary care unit.
France	Lukasiewicz et al., 2007[29]	National survey in 23 (out of 188) prisons. Random sample (n = 998).	Current imprisonment	DU: LY	Illicit drugs, alcohol	All adults.
Germany	Radun et al., 2007[46]	Survey in 6 prisons in 3 out of 16 federal states. Quota sample (n = 1,457).	n.a. ("in prison")	IDU: LT	Illicit drugs	On remand and convicted.
Greece	Sunora, 2001[63]	Survey in 1 prison. Random sample (n =136).	n.a. ("in prison")	DU: LT	Illicit drugs	On remand and convicted.
Greece	Papadodima et al., 2010[64]	Survey in 1 prison (Chalkida). All prisoners self-administered questionnaire (n =162).	Current imprisonment	DU: CU (To)	Tobacco	On remand and convicted.
Hungary	Paksi, 2009[43]	National survey in 22 prisons from all regions. Random sample (n = 503).	Current imprisonment	DU: LT, LY, LM IDU: LT, LY	Illicit drugs	Convicted (final decision). Adults. Hungarian nationality.
Hungary	Elekes and Paksi, 2004[42]	National survey in 11 prisons. Random sample (n = 609).	Current imprisonment	DU: LT, LY, LM IDU: LT	Illicit drugs	Convicted. Males. Adults. Hungarian nationality.
Ireland	Drummond et al., 2014[32]	National survey in all prisons. Random sample (n = 824).	n.a. ("in prison")	DU: LY, LM, CU (To)	Illicit drugs, tobacco	On remand and convicted. Males and females.
Italy	Nobile et al., 2011[65]	Survey in 4 prisons in 1 region (Calabria) among all prisoners (n = 605).	n.a. ("inside prison")	DU: LT, CU (To)	Illicit drugs, tobacco	Males.
Latvia	Snikere, 2011[48]	National survey in 11 (out of 15) prisons. Self-selected sample (n = 1,965).	Current imprisonment	DU: LT, LY, LM	Illicit drugs	Convicted.

(continued)

Table 2.1. CONTINUED

Country	Reference	Year of data collection	Coverage and sampling	Definition of (drug use) *in prison*	Measurement and indicators	Substances	Population covered
Latvia	Snikere et al., 2003[66]	2003	National survey in 11 (out of 15) prisons. Self-selected sample (n = 2,867).	Current imprisonment	DU: LT, LY, LM IDU: LT	Illicit drugs	Convicted.
Lithuania	Lithuanian Reitox National Focal Point, 2011[67]	2011	Survey in 1 prison. Random sample (n = 329).	Current imprisonment	DU: LT	Illicit drugs	Convicted. Males.
Lithuania	Narkauskaite et al., 2010[21]	2009	Survey in 1 prison for women. Self-selected sample (n = 71).	Current imprisonment	DU: LT, CU (To) IDU: LT	Illicit drugs, tobacco	Convicted. Females. 20–60 years.
Luxembourg	Origer and Removille, 2007[47]	2005	National survey in 2 state prisons (n = 246).	Current imprisonment	DU: LT IDU: LT	Illicit drugs	All prisoners.
Norway	Friestad and Kjelsberg, 2009[55]	2003	National study in Norwegian prisons. Random sample (n = 225).	Current imprisonment	DU: LM	Alcohol	Males.
Poland	Sieroslawski, 2007[24]	2007	National survey in 41 prisons. Random sample (n = 1,240).	Current imprisonment	DU: LT	Illicit drugs	On remand and convicted. Males. Adults.
Poland	Sieminska et al., 2006[38]	2006	Survey in 3 prisons. Random sample (n = 907).	Current imprisonment	DU: LT, OTH	Illicit drugs, alcohol	On remand and convicted. Males. Adults.
Poland	Sieroslawski, 2001[68]	2001	National survey in 38 prisons. Random sample (n = 1,189).	Current imprisonment	DU: LT IDU: LT	Illicit drugs	On remand and convicted. Males. Adults.

Country	Study	Year	Sample	Imprisonment	Use	Drug	Population
Portugal	Torres et al., 2008[25]	2007	National survey in 44 prisons. Random sample (n = 1,986).	Current imprisonment	DU: LT, LY, LM, RG; IDU: LT	Illicit drugs	On remand and convicted.
Portugal	Torres and Gomes, 2002[37]	2001	National survey in 47 prisons. Random sample (n = 2,057).	Current imprisonment	DU: LT, LY, LM, RG; IDU: LT	Illicit drugs	On remand and convicted.
Romania	RMCDD, 2012[23]	2011	National survey in 27 prisons (maximum security/close/remand, semi-open, and open, minors and youths, reform centers and hospitals). Probabilistic, stratified, and multistage sampling (n = 2,064).	Current imprisonment	DU: LT, LY, LM	Illicit drugs	On remand and convicted. Males and females. Minors (<=17 years), young offenders (18–21 years) and adults (22–64 years).
Romania	RMCDD, 2007[69]	2006	National survey in 27 prisons (maximum security/close/remand, semi-open, and open, minors and youths, reform centers and hospitals). Probabilistic, stratified, and multistage sampling (n = 3,218).	Current imprisonment	DU: LT, LY, LM	Illicit drugs	All prisoners.
Russian Federation	Dolan et al., 2004[70]	2000–2001	Survey in 3 prisons (Siberia). Convenience sample (n = 153 in 2000; n = 124 in 2001).	Current imprisonment	IDU: LT, LM	Illicit drugs	Males, females and juvenile males.
Russian Federation	Frost and Tchertkov, 2002[50]	2001	Survey in 10 prisons. Representative sample resulting from different methods depending on the prison center: convenience, random, cluster, proportional (n = 1,044).	Current imprisonment	IDU: LT, LM	Illicit drugs	Juveniles. Males. 17–30 years.

(continued)

Table 2.1. CONTINUED

Country	Reference	Year of data collection	Coverage and sampling	Definition of (drug use) in prison	Measurement and indicators	Substances	Population covered
Spain	DGPNSD, 2013[36]	2011	National survey in 72 prisons. Random sample (*n* = 4,980) (women overrepresented).	Current imprisonment	DU: LT, LY, LM, RG IDU: LM	Illicit drugs, alcohol, tobacco	All prisoners.
Spain	Caravaca et al., 2013[57]	2012	Survey in 1 prison (region of Murcia). Random sample (*n* = 21).	Current imprisonment	DU: LM	Illicit drugs, tobacco	Females.
Spain	Solbes, 2008[71]	2008	Regional survey in 4 prisons of 1 region (Andalucía). Self-selected sample (*n* = 206).	Current imprisonment	DU: LM	Illicit drugs	Juveniles (< 21 years). Males (*n* = 196) and females (*n* = 10).
Spain	DGPNSD, 2006[19]	2006	National survey in 66 prisons. Random sample (*n* = 4,934) (women overrepresented).	Current imprisonment	DU: LT, LY, LM, RG IDU: LM	Illicit drugs, alcohol, tobacco	All prisoners.
Spain	Vicens et al., 2011[31]	2007–2008	National survey in 5 (regions of Aragón, Catalonia, and Madrid) prisons. Random sample (*n* = 707).	Current imprisonment	DU: LM	Illicit drugs, alcohol	Convicted males (Spanish and foreigners) 18–75 years.
Spain	López-Barrachina et al., 2007[72]	2005	Survey in 2 prisons (region of Aragón). Self-selected sample (*n* = 236).	Current imprisonment	DU: LT	Illicit drugs, alcohol	Males (75% of sample) and females (25%).
United Kingdom (England and Wales)	Singleton et al., 2005[34]	2001–2002	National survey in 49 prisons. Representative random sample (*n* =1457).	Current imprisonment	DU: LT, LM, OTH IDU: OTH	Illicit drugs	On remand and convicted. Males and females.

Country	Study	Year	Sample	Reference period	Measure	Substance	Population
United Kingdom (England)	Plugge et al., 2009[13]	2004–2005	Survey in 2 remand prisons. All admissions during certain predefined periods (n = 505).	Previous imprisonments	IDU: LT	Illicit drugs	On remand. Females.
United Kingdom (England)	Borrill et al., 2003[44]	2001	National survey in 10 prisons. Random sample (n =301).	n.a. ("in prison")	DU: LT IDU: LT	Illicit drugs	On remand and convicted. Females.
United Kingdom (Northern Ireland)	O'Mahony et al., 2005[73]	2005	Survey in 31 prisons. Random sample (n = 200).	Current imprisonment	DU: LM	Illicit drugs	On remand and convicted. Males (n = 180) and females (n = 20). Young offenders.
United Kingdom (Scotland)	Scottish Prison Service, 2008[28]	2008	National survey in all prisons (n = 4,198).	Current imprisonment	DU: LM IDU: LT, LM	Illicit drugs	All prisoners. Young offenders and adults. 16–79 years.
Americas							
Canada	Guyon et al., 2010[74]	n.a.	Survey in 3 prisons in 1 state (Quebec). Self-selected sample (n = 113).	Current imprisonment	DU: CU (To)	Tobacco	Both prisoners on remand and convicted to a max. sentence of 2 years. Males (n = 73) and females (n = 40).
Canada	Martin et al., 2005[45]	2001	Survey in 1 prison (Burnaby Correctional Centre for Women) in 1 state (British Columbia). Self-selected sample (n = 126).	Current prison	DU: LT IDU: LT	Illicit drugs, alcohol	Females.

(continued)

Table 2.1. CONTINUED

Country	Reference	Year of data collection	Coverage and sampling	Definition of (drug use) in prison	Measurement and indicators	Substances	Population covered
Chile	León-Mayer and Cortés, 2014[53]	2009	Survey in 1 prison among all prisoners (n = 209).	Current imprisonment	DU: LT, OTH (Alc)	Illicit drugs, alcohol	Males.
Chile	Mundt et al., 2013[30]	2012	Nationwide survey in 7 closed correctional facilities. Random sample of prisoners (n = 1008).	Current imprisonment	DU: LY	Illicit drugs, alcohol, tobacco	On remand and convicted. Males (n = 855) and females (n = 153). 1564 years.
Grenada	Crawford-Daniel and Alexis, 2010[35]	2010	Survey in 1 prison. Multistage sampling combination of a simple random sample for males and census for females (enumeration) (n = 104).	n.a. ("in prison")	DU: LY, LM, RG	Illicit drugs, alcohol, tobacco	On remand and convicted. Males and females.
Mexico	Azaola and Bergman, 2009[18]	2009	Survey in 16 prisons (9 federal and 7 in one state). Multistage systematic sampling (women overrepresented) (n = 1,312).	Current imprisonment	DU: LM	Illicit drugs, alcohol	Convicted. Males (n = 1,090) and females (n = 222).
Panama	Peren de Rios, 2001[41]	2000	Survey in 1 prison among all inmates (n = 305).	Current imprisonment	DU: CU	Illicit drugs	On remand and convicted. Males. 18–70 years.
Uruguay	Macri Troya and Berthier Vila, 2010[52]	2005	Survey in 1 prison (50% of national prison population). Random sample (n = 291).	n.a. ("in prison")	IDU: LT	Illicit drugs	Males. 18–74 years.
USA	Seal et al., 2004[16]	n.a.	Survey in 5 prisons in 4 states (California, Mississippi, Rhode Island, Wisconsin). Convenience sample (n = 80).	Any imprisonment since adults (+ 18 y.o.)	DU: LT	Illicit drugs, alcohol	Dischargees (to be released within 30 to 60 days). Males. 18–29 years.

USA	Simpler and Langhimrichsen-Rohling, 2005[49]	n.a.	Survey in 2 prisons (state-level). Self-selected sample (n = 103).	Current imprisonment	DU: LT	Illicit drugs, alcohol	Males.
USA	Kauffman et al., 2011[12]	2008	Survey in 2 low to medium security prisons in Ohio. All admissions in 14 weeks (n = 200).	n.a. ("during incarceration")	DU: LT, CU, RG	Tobacco	Males.
Oceania							
Australia	AIHW, 2013[14]	2012	Survey in 74 public and private prisons in all states and territories except Western Australia. All dischargees (n = 387).	n.a. ("while in prison")	DU: LT, CU (To) IDU: LT	Illicit drugs, alcohol, tobacco	Convicted. Dischargees (to be released within 4 weeks). Adults (18 and over).
Australia	Indig et al., 2010[20]	2008–2009	Survey in 30 prisons of New South Wales (26 for males and 4 for females). Stratified random sample (n = 996) (oversampling of women and Aboriginal people).	n.a. ("in prison")	DU: LT, CU (To), RG (To) IDU: LT	Illicit drugs, alcohol, tobacco	On remand and convicted. Males and females. Adults (18 and over).
Australia	Kinner et al., 2012[15]	2008–2010	Survey in 7 prisons of Queensland. All dischargees (n = 1,322) (oversampling of women).	Both "all imprisonments" and "current imprisonment"	DU: CU (To) IDU: LT	Illicit drugs, tobacco	Convicted. Dischargees (to be released within 6 weeks). Adults.
Africa							
Nigeria	Ebiti and Taiwo, 2008[39]	2005	Survey in 1 medium security prison in the South of Nigeria. Random sample (n = 249).	Current imprisonment	DU: LT, CU	Illicit drugs, alcohol, tobacco	On remand and convicted. Males (n = 235) and females (n=14).

(continued)

Table 2.1. CONTINUED

Country	Reference	Year of data collection	Coverage and sampling	Definition of (drug use) in prison	Measurement and indicators	Substances	Population covered
Nigeria	Amdzaranda et al., 2009[56]	2006	Survey in 1 medium security prison among all inmates ($n = 303$).	Current imprisonment	DU: LM	Illicit drugs, alcohol, tobacco	On remand and convicted. Males ($n = 292$) and females ($n = 11$). 15–70 years.
Asia							
Afghanistan	UNODC, 2010[40]	2010	Survey in 1 prison. Stratified random sample ($n = 92$).	Current imprisonment	DU: CU	Illicit drugs	n.a.
Dubai	Almarri et al., 2009[54]	2006	Survey in 1 prison. Convenience sample ($n = 107$).	Current imprisonment	DU: CU (To)	Tobacco	Males. 19–62 years.
Thailand	Thaisri et al., 2003[17]	2001–2002	Survey in 1 prison (largest in the country). Self-selected sample ($n = 689$).	Current imprisonment	IDU: LT	Illicit drugs	Convicted (with 5 years still to serve). Males. 20–50 years.

DU: drug use; **IDU**: injecting drug user; **LT**: lifetime prevalence; **LY**: last-year prevalence; **LM**: last-month prevalence; **RG**: regular drug use; **CU**: current drug use; **OTH**: other drug use; **To**: tobacco; **Alc**: alcohol; **n.a.**: not available.

inclusion criteria prevents any simple synthesis of results. Research in prison settings is affected by a number of issues, including the non-representativeness of the respondents with respect to the national prison populations and the bias introduced by the self-selection of survey respondents in some studies. However, illicit behaviors such as drug use in prison are likely to be under-reported given that disclosure may lead to further sanctions or penalties.

Most data pertain to individuals in prison on a specific date or during a short period of time. All studies reviewed are cross-sectional surveys, except 2 that were conducted among prison entrants at admission[12,13]; 3 that were conducted among dischargees either before release[14,15] or after release[16]; and 1 estimate that was based on a month follow-up cohort study within prison.[17] Eleven studies were repeated once or twice.[18-25] Of these, 2 in Belgium[26,27] and 1 in Scotland are currently carried out on an annual basis.[28]

Coverage and sampling strategies vary considerably between studies. Although some purport to be "national," this often refers to the intended geographical coverage and does not guarantee that the sample is representative of the national prison population, which would depend on the sampling procedure adopted. Variations in the approach to sampling include surveying the entire prison population of all prisons in a country, reported in one instance[28]; sampling from all prisons; surveying the entire population of selected prisons; and applying a two-stage sampling strategy whereby prisons are selected first and the population to be sampled is then chosen. Random sampling is reported in half of the studies, while 10 studies were based on self-selected samples, and 9 included all prisoners meeting the inclusion criteria. For some studies there is no information available on the sampling strategy adopted. The size of the prison population sampled is not available for most of the studies listed in Table 2.1, and sample sizes—which vary from less than 50 to nearly 5,000—reflect different proportions of the prison population in different countries.

Representativeness of samples is also an issue. The penal establishments sampled are sometimes not representative of the prison system as a whole. In addition, although most of the reported studies refer to both remanded and convicted detainees, a few refer only to convicted prisoners, and 1 covers only remanded prisoners.[13] Inclusion may also be limited by age, with studies carried out in prisons for adults or for young offenders. Both genders are included in most of the studies, but the reported data rarely distinguish between males and females. When only one gender is included, males are more often targeted (16 studies) than are females (4 studies; see Table 2.1). This is perhaps explained by the fact that in many countries males represent the majority of the prison population.

In nearly all studies, drug use is measured by self-report, using either a questionnaire or a clinical interview, and in some instances, standard diagnostic instruments (*DSM-IV* and/or ICD-9) are used to qualify it.[29-31] Oral fluid testing was used in one study together with self-report,[32] and in another instance, tobacco consumption was assessed by screening airflow imitation via a spirometer.[33]

Although all the studies included in this review report on drug use *in* prison, this is operationalized in different ways, leading to potentially large differences in terms of what is measured. Data from a large majority of studies refer to drug use in the *current imprisonment* or in the *current prison*, while 10 studies do not define "*in* prison," 3 refer to drug use *at any time in prison*, and 1 refers to *previous imprisonment episodes* only. This is likely to have a major influence on the results and affect comparability between drug use prevalence estimates. For example, in an Australian study carried out in 2008–2010, 23% of dischargees reported injecting drug use at any time in prison, and 13% reported doing so during the current incarceration episode.[15]

Drug use is reported in a number of ways. The most common measure in the studies reviewed here is any illicit drug use ever *in* prison (lifetime prevalence), followed by illicit drug use in the past month. Other less frequent measures include use in the past year, use multiple times in the past month or week,[27] use in the past week,[34] and use in the past day.[35] Regular consumption is defined variously as daily use (in particular for tobacco), use every day in the past month,[19,25,36,37] and on-going or current use. In rare cases, measures of drug abuse or dependence including consumption *in* prison are reported.[29,31,38] Injecting drug use is addressed in nearly half of the identified studies, mostly by reporting those who have ever injected *in* prison, and in a few cases drug injectors in the past month (see Table 2.1).

Data on Drug Use Prevalence

Data from the 59 studies listed in Table 2.1 show that drug use continues at some level within the prison setting, with large variations in the prevalence of drug use between samples. The proportion of inmates having ever used an illicit drug *in* prison lies between 20% and 45% in most studies. Seven studies in five countries (Czech Republic, Hungary, Romania, Bosnia and Herzegovina, Australia) report levels below 15%, while 5 studies in four countries (Spain, Luxembourg, Chile, United States, Nigeria) report prevalence estimates above 50% (Table 2.2). As in the community, cannabis remains the illicit drug most frequently reported, with lifetime/ever use *in* prison varying from below 1% in Romania to 63% in Spain. Lifetime use of cocaine *in* prison was reported for <1% to 57% of inmates, that of heroin for <1% to 31%, and that of amphetamines for 1% to 23%. Prison inmates reporting having used an illicit drug during the past year *in* prison represent 2% to 67% of the surveyed prison population, with the highest prevalence levels reported in studies from Ireland and Grenada. Recent use of illicit drugs, defined as drug use *in* the past month in prison, ranges from 0.7% in Romania to 43% (cannabis only) in Ireland and 65% in Spain (see Table 2.2). Illicit drug use in the past week was reported by 25% of prisoners in 1 study in England and Wales,[34] and cannabis use in the past day by 30% in another study in Grenada.[35]

The proportion of inmates reporting regular illicit drug use (daily) *in* prison remains around 10% in the few European studies measuring the frequency of use *in* prison.[25,27,36,37] The prevalence of "current" illicit drug use *in* prison was assessed in 3 studies: it varied from 16% in Nigeria[39] to 34% in Afghanistan[40] and 48% in Panama.[41]

Given the potential for transmission of blood-borne viral infections, injecting drug use is a particularly significant issue in the prison environment. In most studies

Table 2.2. ILLICIT DRUG USE IN PRISON: LIFETIME, LAST-YEAR, AND LAST-MONTH PREVALENCE AMONG ALL PRISONERS

Country	Reference	Year of data collection	Ever use in prison (%)						Past 12 months use in prison (%)						Past 30 days use in prison (%)					
			ANY	CAN	HER	COC	AMP	XTC	ANY	CAN	HER	COC	AMP	XTC	ANY	CAN	HER	COC	AMP	XTC
Europe																				
Belgium	Van Malderen, 2011[27]	2010	32.9	31.3	13.3	9	8.2	4	14.7						11.8					
Belgium	Todts et al., 2009[26]	2008	34.9	31.9	11.6	8.6	5.4	3.6												
Belgium	Todts et al., 2007[62]	2006	29	27.3	12	8.8	7.1	5												
Bosnia and Herzegovina	Vidic et al., 2011[51]	2011	11																	
Czech Republic	National Monitoring Centre for Drugs and Drug Addiction, the Czech Prison Service, 2013[22]	2012	14.4	10.9	2.9	1.4	10.3	1.7												
France	Lukasiewicz et al., 2007[29]	2003–2004							27.9	26.7										
Greece	Sunora, 2001[63]	2000	46																	
Hungary	Paksi, 2009[43]	2008	14.3	12.3	0.5	1.4	3.7	4.5	8.4	6.4	0.4	0.6	1.8	2.1	3.2	2.5	0.2	0.2	0.9	0.4
Hungary	Elekes and Paksi, 2004[42]	2004	7.9	6.3	0.7	0.7	0.9	2.8	4.7	3.4	0.2	0.4	0.4	1.3	3	1.2		0.2		0.3
Italy	Nobile et al., 2011[65]	2005	52.9	23.5		41.2		8.8												
Ireland	Drummond et al., 2014[32]	2011							66.7	28.8	20.3				43.2	10.9	4.8			
Latvia	Snikere, 2011[48]	2010	31.8	24.2	10.1	2.9	19	7.6	17.8	11.7	5.9	1	10.3	2.9	8.5	5.9	1.7	0.6	3	1.4
Latvia	Snikere et al., 2003[66]	2003	28	12	4		12	7	15	5	2		8	4	6	2	1		2	1

(continued)

Table 2.2. CONTINUED

Country	Reference	Year of data collection	Ever use in prison (%)						Past 12 months use in prison (%)						Past 30 days use in prison (%)					
			ANY	CAN	HER	COC	AMP	XTC	ANY	CAN	HER	COC	AMP	XTC	ANY	CAN	HER	COC	AMP	XTC
Lithuania	Lithuanian Reitox National Focal Point, 2011[67]	2011	29.8																	
Luxembourg	Origer and Removille, 2007[47]	2005	56																	
Poland	Sieroslawski, 2007[24]	2007	20.3	18.3	2.4	2.9	14.8	7.3												
Poland	Sieminska et al., 2006[38]	2006	22																	
Poland	Sieroslawski, 2001[68]	2001	22.5	21.3	2.5	5	15.4	4.7												
Portugal	Torres et al., 2008[25]	2007	35.7	29.8	13.5	9.9	2.3	2.7	33.5	29	11.5	7.6	2.1	2.1	27.4	23.3	7.3	3.8	0.7	0.8
Portugal	Torres and Gomes, 2002[37]	2001							52	44	33	26	10	10	30	24	15.5	7	1.5	1
Romania	RMCDD, 2012[23]	2011	4.5	1.3	2.2	0.4		1.1	2	0.5	1	0.1		1.1	0.7	0.1	0.4	0.1		
Romania	RMCDD, 2007[69]	2006	2	0.6	1	0.2		0.2	2	0.4	0.8	0.4			0.7	0.1	0.5	0.1		
Spain	DGPNSD, 2013[36]	2011	63.2		31.4	57.4	22.7	24.7							21.3	21.3	2.4	1.3	0.2	0.2
Spain	Caravaca et al., 2013[57]	2012													65.1	33.3	9	19	19	2
Spain	Solbes, 2008[71]	2008													60					
Spain	DGPNSD, 2006[19]	2006													27.7	27.7	4.8	2.9	0.3	0.3
Spain	Vicens et al., 2011[31]	2007–2008													17	14.4	3.4	15		
United Kingdom (England and Wales)	Singleton et al., 2005[34]	2001–2002	39	32	21	1	1	3												

Country	Reference	Year														
United Kingdom (England)	Borrill et al., 2003[44]	2001	21	27	2	1	45	1			40	38	4			15
United Kingdom (Northern Ireland)	O'Mahony et al., 2005[73]	2005														
United Kingdom (Scotland)	Scottish Prison Service, 2008[28]	2008									21	13	15	3	9	2
Americas																
Canada	Martin et al., 2005[45]	2001					36									
Chile	León-Mayer and Cortés, 2014[53]	2009					76.1									
Chile	Mundt et al., 2013[30]	2012							12.2							
Grenada	Crawford-Daniel and Alexis, 2010[35]	2010							67	41		11				
Mexico	Azaola and Bergman, 2009[18]	2009									11.9	9.3	1.8			
USA	Seal et al., 2004[16]	n.a.					50.6									
USA	Simpler and Langhinrichsen-Rohling, 2005[49]	n.a.	37.9	4.9	5.8	7.8	51.5									
Oceania																
Australia	AIHW, 2013[14]	2012					13									
Australia	Indig et al., 2010[20]	2008–2009	31.4	15.4	5.9	9.6	42.5	3.7								

(continued)

Table 2.2. CONTINUED

Country	Reference	Year of data collection	Ever use in prison (%)						Past 12 months use in prison (%)						Past 30 days use in prison (%)					
			ANY	CAN	HER	COC	AMP	XTC	ANY	CAN	HER	COC	AMP	XTC	ANY	CAN	HER	COC	AMP	XTC
Africa																				
Nigeria	Amdzaranda et al., 2009[56]	2006														7	1.3	2.3		
Nigeria	Ebiti and Taiwo, 2008[39]	2005	60	37.3	4	9.2	3.6								16	12				
Asia																				
Afghanistan	UNODC, 2010[40]	2010													28.3					

ANY: illicit drug; **CAN**: cannabis; **HER**: heroin; **COC**: cocaine; **AMP**: amphetamines; **XTC**: ecstasy.

reporting such data, drug users who report injecting *in* prison represent around 10% or less of the prison population. The lowest proportions—below 3%—are reported in Belgium[27] (last month), Hungary[42,43] (lifetime, last year), Portugal[25] (lifetime), Spain[36] (last month), and the United Kingdom[13,34,44] (injecting in prison, in current prison). In a few studies, however, these proportions reach much higher levels: at just above 20% in Canada[45] (lifetime), Germany[46] (last month), and Australia[15] (lifetime), and over 30% in Luxembourg[47] (lifetime) and Thailand[17] (lifetime). In all the studies that distinguish between different substances, heroin is the drug most often injected *in* prison, followed by amphetamines, except in Latvia, where amphetamines (lifetime) prevail.[48]

The majority of those who report illicit drug use or injecting *in* prison commenced use in the community and continue during incarceration. However, a few studies show that some inmates started using illicit drugs within prison: 0.5% (1 person) in the United States,[49] 3% in Australia,[20] 4% in Lithuania,[21] 5% (cannabis) and 7% (heroin) in Belgium,[27] and 10% in Grenada, where another 20% reinitiated (or relapsed to) drug use *in* prison.[35] In a Russian study, 1% of inmates started injecting drugs *in* prison,[50] which compares with nearly 4% in Bosnia and Herzegovina[51] and close to 12% (heroin) in Thailand.[17]

In addition to illicit drugs, many prisoners use other psychoactive substances such as alcohol and tobacco. The proportion of inmates reporting having used alcohol *in* prison is extremely variable in the studies reviewed here: low prevalences—under 10%—are reported in studies in Australia,[14,20] Belgium,[27] Chile,[30] Mexico,[18] Spain,[36] and Uruguay[52]; while high prevalences—above 55%—are reported in other studies in Chile,[53] Dubai,[54] Nigeria,[39] and Norway.[55]

Tobacco is the psychoactive substance most widely consumed *in* prison,[11] with up to 90% of inmates[33] reporting current smoking, and most of the other studies reviewed here suggesting prevalence rates for current smoking above 60%. However, comparatively low proportions of tobacco smokers in the prison population are reported in three studies—4% in Chile[30] and around 14% in Nigeria[56] and Spain.[57]

DISCUSSION

Our systematic review of drug use in prison has highlighted the scarceness of data on use of psychoactive substances within the prison setting. While there are many studies reporting on drug use prior to incarceration or drug use in prisoners without further specification (and thus covering both outside and *in*-prison use), studies that measure the prevalence of drug consumption *in* prison are relatively rare. The geographical distribution of the studies reporting on drug use *in* prison is also striking—most of them were carried out in Europe, but even there the picture is patchy and very heterogeneous, preventing sound comparative analysis. In many large Western countries including Canada and the United States, there were only two or three assessments in the last 15 years, none of which were at a national level.

The data reviewed in this chapter reveal substantial heterogeneity, both between and within countries, in the methodologies used to assess drug use *in* prison. As in the European review of 2012,[8] comparability between surveys remains a major challenge. Whether by intention or as a result of the sampling strategies used, the studies analyzed here refer to very different populations. Data may be generated from reception, cross-sectional, or release surveys; they may be ad hoc or repeated; local or national; from a selection of penal institutions that may or may not be representative of the national prison population; and using a documented sampling method or not. Drug use may refer to the current incarceration, previous episodes of incarceration, or all the incarcerations during an individual's life. The populations sampled differ in terms of legal status (on remand, convicted), length of incarceration, main offense, and socio-economic and demographic characteristics.

The data analyzed reveal very wide prevalence ranges, with 20-fold differences in some cases between studies. It is likely that, at least partially, these differences reflect the broad range of methodologies used to sample prisoners and assess the prevalence and patterns of substance use in prison. In the absence of a standard methodology, the scope for comparative analysis is extremely limited. Both the scarcity of the available data and their large variation prevent the emergence of a clear picture of drug use in prison at a global level. In addition, the difficulty in distinguishing between the effect of methodologies and true differences between populations and countries makes interpretation a major challenge.

Understanding the cultural, social, and political context of each country or penal institution is essential to interpreting the data emerging from that context. Drug use in prison needs to be compared to drug use in the general community; it is essential to understand whether, for example, the studies with the highest prevalence of drug use in prison were conducted in the countries where the prevalence of drug use in the general population is also comparatively high. Sanctions against drug use in prison is another area that needs to be reviewed as it may lead to selective underreporting where fear of disclosure is high, which may differentially affect prisons and countries. As far as alcohol is concerned, consumption is certainly not socially accepted everywhere, in particular where religion forbids its use, which may both reduce use in the general community and further discourage users from disclosing their consumption, either in the community or in prison. In a context in which tobacco has become part of the prison environment in many countries, with cigarettes often being used as currency in prison, and the drug being widely consumed to combat boredom and manage stressful situations, countries with a low prevalence of in-prison tobacco use are the exception. These patterns may change markedly in the coming years, with increasing implementation of tobacco control policies (total or partial smoking bans) in prison settings.[11,58,59]

Despite the methodological caveats discussed here, our analysis shows that levels of drug consumption are sometimes very high in prison settings. This raises a number of issues both for society at large and for the prison system itself, including issues of control (smuggling of illicit drugs and alcohol), safety and order (violent and risky behaviors under the influence), public health (spread of infectious diseases, exposure to tobacco smoking), and treatment provision (equivalence and continuity of care with the community). Understanding the size and nature of the problem is a prerequisite for taking the appropriate measures.

CONCLUSION

Available data on drug use *in* prison are scarce and patchy, with large variations in methodology. This diversity hampers comparison and may in part account for the wide range of prevalence estimates observed in the literature. While assessing the extent of and trends in drug use *in* prison is key to assessing needs and planning appropriate responses, there is a lack of consensus on how this should be done. Common measures on drug use and its consequences in prison populations are needed, possibly through the development of internationally agreed upon data collection instruments. Given the current climate of economic crisis in many countries, funding for large multi-centric international studies using a unique methodology is unlikely to be obtained. The next best option is therefore to develop a standard instrument or parameters for comparable measures that could be used in any prison survey or routine data collection, with a view to generating standardized data and enhancing the potential for carrying out comparative analysis across countries.[8]

The EMCDDA has recently reviewed the data collection instruments used in a number of studies to assess drug use in prison populations in Europe and beyond.[60] Based on this review the center, together with a group of international experts, developed the European Common Questionnaire on Drug Use Among Prisoners.[61] The model questionnaire targets both licit and illicit psychoactive substances and covers a number of issues, including consumption outside and within prison, drug injecting and other risk behaviors, health status, and use of health and drug treatment services, including harm reduction services. An annex to the questionnaire provides a discussion of good principles and methodological recommendations for conducting drug assessments in prison. The questionnaire can be used on its own or as part of a survey covering broader issues in prison. Although it was developed within a European perspective, experiences from other world regions were taken into account, making it a good candidate for dissemination across the world. The implementation of such a tool would facilitate international comparisons and provide the sound information needed for the development and implementation of drug interventions in various prison settings across the globe.

ACKNOWLEDGMENTS

The authors wish to thank the Reitox network of national focal points for its invaluable contribution to the EMCDDA monitoring of drug use in the prison population in Europe.

REFERENCES

1. Walmsley R. *World Prison Population List.* 4th ed. London, England: International Centre for Prison Studies; 2013.
2. Aebi M, Delgrande N. *SPACE I—Council of Europe Annual Penal Statistics: Prison Populations.* Strasbourg, France: Council of Europe; 2014.

3. European Monitoring Centre for Drugs and Drug Addiction. *Statistical Bulletin 2014*. Luxembourg City, Luxembourg: Publications Office of the European Union; 2014.

4. Montanari L, Royuela L, Pasinetti M, Giraudon I, Wiessing L, Vicente J. Drug use and related consequences among prison populations in European countries. In: Enggist S, Moller L, Galea G, Udesen C, eds. *Prisons and Health*. Copenhagen, Denmark: WHO Regional Office for Europe; 2014:107–112.

5. European Monitoring Centre for Drugs and Drug Addiction. *European Drug Report: Trends and Developments 2014*. Luxembourg City, Luxembourg: Publications Office of the European Union; 2014.

6. Jürgens R, Ball A, Verster A. Interventions to reduce HIV transmission related to injecting drug use in prison. *Lancet Infect Dis*. 2009;9(1):57–66.

7. Moller L, Stover H, Jurgens R, Gatherer A, Nikogosian H. *Health in Prisons: A WHO Guide to the Essentials in Prison Health*. Copenhagen, Denmark: WHO Regional Office for Europe; 2007.

8. Carpentier C, Royuela L, Noor A, Hedrich D. Ten years of monitoring illicit drug use in prison populations in Europe: issues and challenges. *Howard J*. 2011;51(1):37–66.

9. Fazel S, Bains P, Doll H. Substance abuse and dependence in prisoners: a systematic review. *Addiction*. 2006;101(2):181–191.

10. Graham L, Parkes T, McAuley A, Doi L. *Alcohol Problems in the Criminal Justice System: An Opportunity for Intervention*. Copenhagen, Denmark: WHO Regional Office for Europe; 2012.

11. Baybutt M, Ritter C, Stover H. Tobacco use in prison settings: a need for policy implementation. In: Enggist S, Moller L, Galea G, Udesen C, eds. *Prisons and Health*. Copenhagen, Denmark: WHO Regional Office for Europe; 2014:138–147.

12. Kauffman RM, Ferketich AK, Murray DM, Bellair PE, Wewers ME. Tobacco use by male prisoners under an indoor smoking ban. *Nicotine Tob Res*. 2011;13(6):449–456.

13. Plugge E, Yudkin P, Douglas N. Changes in women's use of illicit drugs following imprisonment. *Addiction*. 2009;104(2):215–222.

14. Australian Institute for Health and Welfare. *The Health of Australia's Prisoners 2012*. Cat. no. PHE 170. Canberra, Australia: AIHW; 2013.

15. Kinner SA, Jenkinson R, Gouillou M, Milloy MJ. High-risk drug-use practices among a large sample of Australian prisoners. *Drug Alcohol Depend*. 2012;126(1–2):156–160.

16. Seal DW, Belcher L, Morrow K, et al. A qualitative study of substance use and sexual behavior among 18- to 29-year-old men while incarcerated in the United States. *Health Educ Behav*. 2004;31(6):775–789.

17. Thaisri H, Lerwitworapong J, Vongsheree S, et al. HIV infection and risk factors among Bangkok prisoners, Thailand: a prospective cohort study. *BMC Infect Dis*. 2003;3(25):1–8.

18. Azaola E, Bergman M. *Delincuencia, marginalidad y desempeño institucional: Resultados de la tercera encuesta a población en reclusión en el Distrito Federal y el Estado de México*. Mexico City, Mexico: Centro de Investigación y Docencia Económicas; 2009.

19. Delegación del Gobierno para el Plan Nacional sobre Drogas (DGPNSD). *Encuesta sobre salud y consumo de drogas a los internados en instituciones penitenciarias (ESDIP) 2006 [Survey on Health and Drugs Among Prison Inmates 2006]*. Madrid, Spain: Spanish Government, Ministry of Health and Consumption, Ministry of the Interior; 2006.

20. Indig D, Topp L, Ross B, et al. *2009 NSW Inmate Health Survey: Key findings report*. Sydney, Australia: Justice Health NSW; 2010.

21. Narkauskaite L, Juozulynas A, Mackiewicz Z, Venalis A, Utkuviene J. Prevalence of psychoactive substances use in a Lithuanian women's prison revisited after 5 years. *Med. Sci. Monit*. 2010;16(11):Ph91–96.

22. National Monitoring Centre for Drugs and Drug Addiction, The Czech Prison Service. *Report to the EMCDDA by the Reitox National Focal Point Czech Republic: Drug Situation 2013*. Prague: National Focal Point Czech Republic; 2013.

23. Romanian Monitoring Centre for Drugs and Drug Addiction (RMCDD). *National Report on Drug Situation in Prisons*. Bucharest, Romania: National Anti-Drug Agency; 2012.
24. Sieroslawski J. *Problem narkotykow i narkomanii w zakladach karnych i aresztach sledczych [Drugs and Drug Addiction Problems in Prisons and Detention Centres]*. Warsaw, Poland: Institute of Psychiatry and Neurology; 2007.
25. Torres A, Maciel D, Sousa I, Cruz R. *Drogas e prisoes: Portugal 2001.2007 [Drugs and Prisons: Portugal 2001.2007]*. Lisbon, Portugal: Portuguese Institute for Drugs and Drug Addictions; 2008.
26. Todts S, Gilbert P, Malderen VS, Huyck VC, Saliez V, Hogge M. *Usage de drogues dans les prisons belges: monitoring des risques sanitaires—2008 [Drug Use in Belgian Prisons: Monitoring Health Risks]*. Brussels, Belgium: Federal Public Service Justice; 2009.
27. Van Malderen S. *Monitoring Drug Use and Related Problems in Belgian Prisons as a Tool for Policy Making: Difficulties and Challenges*. Brussels, Belgium: Federal Public Service Justice; 2011.
28. Scottish Prison Service. *11th Prisoner Survey 2008: Executive Summary*. Edinburgh, Scotland: Scottish Prison Service; 2008.
29. Lukasiewicz M, Falissard B, Michel L, Neveu X, Reynaud M, Gasquet I. Prevalence and factors associated with alcohol and drug-related disorders in prison: a French national study. *Subst Abuse Treat Prev Policy*. 2007;2(1):1–10.
30. Mundt AP, Alvarado R, Fritsch R, et al. Prevalence rates of mental disorders in Chilean prisons. *PLoS ONE*. 2013;8(7):e69109.
31. Vicens E, Tort V, Dueñas RM, et al. The prevalence of mental disorders in Spanish prisons. *Crim Behav Ment Health*. 2011;21(5):321–332.
32. Drummond A, Codd M, Donnelly N, et al. *Study on the Prevalence of Drug Use, including Intravenous Drug Use, and Blood Borne Viruses Among the Irish Prisoner Population*. Dublin, Ireland: National Advisory Committee on Drug and Alcohol; 2014.
33. Sannier O, Gignon M, Defouilloy C, Hermant A, Manaouil C, Jardé O. Obstructive lung diseases in a French prison: results of systematic screening. *Rev Pneumol Clin*. 2009;65(1):1–8.
34. Singleton N, Pendry E, Simpson T, et al. *The Impact of Mandatory Drug Testing in Prisons*. London, England: Home Office; 2005.
35. Crawford-Daniel W, Alexis J. *Review and Evaluation of the Drug Use Survey Used to Develop Protocols by the OAS/CICAD: Pilot Study at Her Majesty's Prison Richmond Hill*. St George's, Grenada: St George's University; 2010.
36. Delegación del Gobierno para el Plan Nacional sobre Drogas (DGPNSD). *Encuesta sobre salud y consumo de drogas en internados en instituciones penitenciarias ESDIP 2011 [Survey on Health and Drugs Among Prison Inmates 2011]*. Madrid, Spain: Spanish Government, Ministry of Health and Consumption, Ministry of the Interior; 2013.
37. Torres A, Gomes M. *Drogas e prisoes em Portugal [Drugs and Prisons in Portugal]*. Lisbon, Portugal: Portuguese Institute for Drugs and Drug Addictions (IPDT); 2002.
38. Sieminska A, Jassem E, Konopa K. Prisoners' attitudes towards cigarette smoking and smoking cessation: a questionnaire study in Poland. *BMC Public Health*. 2006;6(181):1–9.
39. Ebiti N, Taiwo A. *Psychoactive Substance Use Among Inmates in a Nigerian Prison Population*. Lagos, Nigeria: Federal Neuropsychiatric Hospital; 2008.
40. United Nations Office on Drugs and Crime (UNODC). *Drug Use Survey 2010. Sarpoza Prison, Kandahar, Afghanistan. Assessment of Drug Use Levels and Associated High-Risk Behaviours Amongst the Prison Population of Sarpoza, Kanfahar*. Vienna, Austria: UNODC; 2010.
41. Peren de Rios D. *Análisis de las condiciones laborales en la evolución de la situación de salud de la población penitenciaria de David, provincia de Chiriquí, años: 1995 a 1991*. David, Panama: Vicerrectoria de investigacion y postgrado/Medicina; 2001.

42. Elekes Z, Paksi B. *Jogerosen ehtelt fogvatartottak kábitószer-és egyéb szenvedélyszer használata.* Budapest, Hungary: Research Library for Penalty Authorities; 2004.
43. Paksi B. *A jogerosen ehteltt fogvatartottak kabitoszer-és egyeb szenvedélyszer használata Magyarországon 2008-ban [Drug Use Among Convicted Detainees in Hungary in 2008.* Budapest, Hungary: Corvinus University Institute of Behavioural Science and Communication Theory, Centre of Behavioural Research; 2009.
44. Borrill J, Maden A, Martin A, et al. *Differential Substance Misuse Treatment Needs of Women, Ethnic Minorities and Young Offenders in Prison: Prevalence of Substance Misuse and Treatment Needs.* London, England: Home Office; 2003.
45. Martin RE, Gold F, Murphy W, Remple V, Berkowitz J, Money D. Drug use and risk of bloodborne infections: a survey of female prisoners in British Columbia. *Can J Public Health.* 2005;96(2):97–101.
46. Radun D, Weilandt C, Eckert J, Schuettler C, Weid F. *Cross-Sectional Study on Seroprevalence Regarding Hepatitis B, Hepatitis C, and HIV, Risk Behaviour, Knowledge and Attitudes About Bloodborne Infections Among Adult Prisoners in Germany.* Stockholm, Sweden: European Scientific Conference on Applied Infectious Disease Epidemiology—Preliminary Results; 2007.
47. Origer A, Romeville R. *Prévalence et propagation des hépatites A, B, C et du HIV au sein de la population des Usagers Problématiques de Drogues d'acquisition illicite au Luxembourg [Prevalence and Diffusion of Hepatitis A, B, C and of HIV Among Problem Drug Users in Luxembourg].* Luxembourg: PF/CES/CPR-Santé; 2007.
48. Snikere R. *Narkotiku lietošanas izplatiba ieslodzijuma vietas Latvija. [Drug Use Prevalence in Latvia's Prisons].* Riga, Latvia: Veselibas ekonomikas centrs, Sociologisko petijumu instituts; 2011.
49. Simpler AH, Langhinrichsen-Rohling J. Substance use in prison: how much occurs and is it associated with psychopathology? *Addiction Res Theory.* 2005;13(5):503–511.
50. Frost L, Tchertkov V. Prisoner risk taking in the Russian Federation. *AIDS Educ Prev.* 2002;14(5 Suppl B):7–23.
51. Vidic V, Ler Z, Ravlija J. *Research on Risk Behavior of Prison Inmates in Relation to HIV/SPI Bosnia and Herzegovina, 2011.* Mostar, Bosnia and Herzegovina: Institute for Public Health Federation B&H; 2011.
52. Macri Troya M, Berthier Vila R. HIV infection and associated risk behaviours in a prison in Montevideo, Uruguay. *Rev Esp Sanid Penit* 2010;12(1):21–28.
53. León-Mayer E, Cortés MSFJ. Descripción multidimensional de la población carcelaria chilena. *Psicoperspectivas.* 2014;13(1):68–81.
54. Almarri TSK, Oei TPS, Amir T. Validation of the alcohol use identification test in a prison sample living in the Arabian Gulf region. *Subst Use Misuse.* 2009;44(14):2001–2013.
55. Friestad C, Kjelsberg E. Drug use and mental health problems among prison inmates—results from a nation-wide prison population study. *Nord J Psychiatry.* 2009;63(3):237–245.
56. Amdzaranda PA, Fatoye FO, Oyebanji AO, Ogunro AS, Fatoye GK. Factors associated with psychoactive substance use among a sample of prison inmates in Ilesa, Nigeria. *Nigerian Postgrad Med J.* 2009;16(2):109–114.
57. Caravaca F, Sánchez F, Luna A. La situación de las mujeres en las prisiones de Murcia ¿más vulnerables que los hombres? *Boletín Criminológico* 2013;146(6).
58. Butler T, Yap L. Smoking bans in prison: time for a breather? *MJA.* 2015;203(8):313.
59. de Andrade D, Kinner SA. Systematic review of health and behavioural outcomes of smoking cessation interventions in prisons. *Tob Control.* 2016;0:1–7.
60. Royuela L, Montanari L, Miriam R, Vicente J. *Drug Use in Prison: Assessment Report.* Lisbon, Portugal: EMCDDA; 2014.
61. Montanari L, Royuela L, Miriam R, Vicente J. *European Questionnaire on Drug Use Among Prisoners (EQDP).* Lisbon, Portugal: EMCDDA; 2014.

62. Todts S, Hariga F, Pozza M, Leclercq D, Glibert P, Micalessi M. *Use in Belgian Prisons: Monitoring Health Risks 2006: Final Report*. Brussels, Belgium: Modus Vivendi; 2007.

63. Sunora G. *Katagrafi apotelesmaton diereunisis kai protasi programmatos sti Dikastiki Fulaki Koridallou [Recording of the Results of Research and Submission of a Programme to the Criminal Prison of Koridallos]*. Athens, Greece: Médecins Sans Frontières; 2001.

64. Papadodima SA, Sakelliadis EI, Sergentanis TN, Giotakos O, Sergentanis IN, Spiliopoulou CA. Smoking in prison: a hierarchical approach at the crossroad of personality and childhood events. *Eur J Pub Health*. 2010;20(4):470–474.

65. Nobile CGA, Flotta D, Nicotera G, Pileggi C, Angelillo IF. Self-reported health status and access to health services in a sample of prisoners in Italy. *BMC Public Health*. 2011;11(529):1–8.

66. Snikere R, Trapencieris M, Vanaga S. *Survey of prison inmates: drug abuse prevalence' in: Latvia Population Survey Report 2003*. Riga: Institute of Philosophy and Sociology, University of Latvia; 2003.

67. Lithuanian Reitox National Focal Point. *2011 National Report to the EMCDDA*. Vilnius: Government of the Republic of Lithuania; 2011.

68. Sieroslawski J. *Projekt badan nad problemem narkomanii w zakladach karnych i aresztach sledczych: Raport za rok 2001 [Research Project on Drug Addition in Prisons and Detention Centres: Report for the Year 2001]*. Warsaw, Poland: Institute of Psychiatry and Neurology; 2001.

69. Romanian Monitoring Centre for Drugs and Drug Addiction (RMCDD). *2007 National Report on Drug Situation*. Bucharest, Romania: National Anti-Drug Agency; 2007.

70. Dolan KA, Bijl M, White B. HIV education in a Siberian prison colony for drug dependent males. *Int J Equity Health*. 2004;3(7):1–6.

71. Solbes V. Estudio socioeducativo de los jóvenes internados en las prisiones andaluzas. *Revista Española de Investigación Criminológica*. 2008;3(6):1–25.

72. López-Barrachina R, Lafuente O, Garcia-Latas J. From the myth of Narcissus to personality disorders in Aragonese prisons: an introductory profile of personality disorders amongst people deprived of their liberty. *Rev Esp Sanid Penit*. 2007;9(2):53–63.

73. O'Mahoney D, Fox C, Chapman T. *Report of the Fifth Survey of the Male Inmate Population in Hydebank Wood Centre*. Belfast, Ireland: Hydebank Wood Centre; 2005.

74. Guyon L, Brochu S, Royer A, Cantinotti C, Chayer L, Lasnier B. *L'interdiction de fumer en établissement de détention québécois*. Quebec, Canada: Institut National de Santé Publique du Québec; 2010.

CHAPTER 3

Injecting While Incarcerated

M-J MILLOY, PhD

INTRODUCTION

Just before Christmas in the winter of 1982, a team of scientists, research nurses, and interviewers from the United States Centers for Disease Control, Vanderbilt School of Medicine, and the Tennessee state government began a trek to each of the prisons scattered throughout the southern US state.[1] Public health officials had recommended that the state begin immunizing prisoners against the hepatitis B virus (HBV), which previous reports had found to be endemic among incarcerated populations.[2,3] While a vaccine had recently been developed, it was expensive, and officials lacked the data on risk factors and transmission patterns needed for a cost-effective targeted immunization program. Between December 1982 and February 1983 the team, led by Michael D. Decker, a physician at Vanderbilt's medical school, visited the state's 10 prisons for men. At each facility they obtained a census of all men currently held and, using simple random sampling, constructed a representative sample of the prisoners. Prison health and administrative records were obtained for each participant, and a private interview elicited information on sensitive behaviors—especially "homosexual activity" and "intravenous drug abuse"—both prior to and during the current sentence. Serum specimens were gathered for testing for HBV surface antigen. By the spring of 1983, the completed survey contained information on 6,503 men held in the Tennessee prison system. According to the interview data, 37% reported engaging in injection drug use prior to incarceration, and 28% while incarcerated. Plotting the frequency of in-prison injection drug use against the prevalence of HBV seropositivity revealed a clear dose-dependent relationship.

Previous serosurveys of prisoners had hinted at the contribution of injection drug use in prison as a risk factor.[2,4] In 1970 an investigation into HBV at an unnamed prison for men in California noted that "illicit use of drugs by inmates of this institution has been occasionally detected."[2] However, the study by Decker et al. was the first to systematically assess the use of injection drugs while incarcerated.[1] In a pattern soon to be repeated dozens of times in investigations of HIV, these researchers found that a substantial proportion of inmates arrived at prison gates with a history of injection drug use. Although many of these individuals did not continue injection drug use once incarcerated, those who did faced highly elevated risks of infection with blood-borne pathogens owing to the lack of sterile injection equipment. In another similarity to future investigations of HIV, Decker et al.'s survey did not lead to any public health intervention—they recommended against a mass vaccination for Tennessee's prisoners, arguing that their statistical model determined the prisoners' infection risk was not related to imprisonment.[1]

In the more than 30 years since Decker et al.'s report, in excess of 80 studies, most assessing risk factors for HIV infection among people held in closed settings and people who inject drugs (PWID), have investigated using injection drugs while incarcerated.[1,5-87] For PWID, a wealth of evidence has confirmed that arrest and incarceration are nearly inevitable given the emphasis placed on criminal justice–led approaches to psychoactive drug use in nearly all global settings.[88-91] Incarceration, despite the best efforts of prison-based healthcare providers, has been consistently identified as an amplifier for experiencing injection drug–associated harms, including infection with hepatitis C virus (HCV) and HIV[19,92-94]; discontinuation of opioid substitution therapy and antiretroviral treatment for those living with HIV/AIDS[95-98]; and both non-fatal[99,100] and fatal overdose.[101,102] Despite the central role played by injection while incarcerated (IWI) in producing these drug-related harms and the development of effective public health–based responses to IWI, there has yet to be effective scale-up. In this chapter I will review the scientific literature on incarceration among PWID, focusing on empirical analyses of the phenomenon of IWI.

IWI: PREVALENCE, RISKS, INTERVENTIONS

Around the world, in all countries with substantial numbers of PWID, injection drug use not only is a contributor to substantial and significant amounts of morbidity and mortality,[103,104] but also is primarily classified by government authorities as a crime and is the focus of a diverse array of official responses by various government sectors, including criminal justice. Although executions of people who use injection drugs have been reported,[105] in resource-rich settings, from which the vast majority of the investigations into IWI are produced, the typical state response is incarceration. Beginning in the 1950s, a succession of moral panics about some psychoactive drugs, including heroin, cannabis, crack cocaine, and crystal methamphetamine, resulted in official responses based on prohibition, backed by arrest and incarceration. The public order approach to some psychoactive drugs is best exemplified by the so-called war on drugs spawned by US president Richard Nixon in the early 1970s, which, along with mandatory minimum sentences for crack cocaine use imposed by Ronald Reagan in the early 1980s, has resulted in drastic increases in the number of individuals exposed to correctional facilities.[88] At the end of 2014 in the United States, for example, more than 1.5 million people were held in state or federal facilities, an increase of more than 1,000% since 1980.[106] Many millions more were under the supervision of the criminal justice system in community settings. In total, more than half of the prisoners in the United States were serving sentences for drug crimes.[106]

Among PWID, exposure to the many facets of the criminal justice system, including police, short-term holding cells, long-term jails, prisons, and penitentiaries, is the rule.[6,21,107,108] The prohibition of injection drug use creates criminals in two ways: directly, by defining drug use as a crime; and indirectly, as prohibition inflates drug prices in the illicit market,[109] forcing many PWID to turn to prohibited forms of income generation, such as sex work, drug dealing, and theft and fraud.[110-113] Thus, typical is the experience of PWID participating in a multicenter study conducted in five European cities in the mid-1990s, in which 60% to 90% of PWID reported being held in custody at some point since beginning to inject.[114] In New York City, in a sample of 365 men drawn from a methadone clinic, almost all poor and many of African heritage, almost all had been exposed to the criminal justice system: 94% had ever been arrested, and almost three-quarters had a history of incarceration.[115] In Australia, where the incarceration rate is less than one-quarter of that in the United States,[116] 51% of a national sample of 909 community-recruited PWID reported a history of incarceration, and 43% reported engaging in (primarily low-level, acquisitive) crime in the past month.[117] Similar levels of incarceration have been reported in surveys of PWID recruited from community settings in Tijuana, Mexico[62]; Vancouver, Canada[118]; Glasgow, Scotland[22]; three cities in Afghanistan[58]; Amsterdam[80]; Bangkok, Thailand[79]; Helsinki, Finland[119]; and Tehran, Iran.[86] As might be expected from the high rates of imprisonment faced by PWID, surveys of prisoners have consistently found that many report a history of injection drug use.[8,9,11,20,30,35,47,48,79,82] In one of the largest representative studies of men held in closed settings ever conducted, Weild et al. reported in 2000 that nearly one-quarter of prisoners in 8 of 135 facilities in England and Wales had ever injected drugs.[82] In the central Canadian provinces of Ontario and Quebec, three large cross-sectional studies of prisoners found that more than 30% reported a history of injection drug use.[17,120,121]

Despite the substantial burdens of injection drug use among prisoners, as well as histories of incarceration experienced by PWID, the characteristics of the correctional experience for injectors has never been well described. There is evidence to suggest that the typical sentence is short and that PWID typically experience many incarceration episodes over the course of their injection careers.[11,18,22,26,55,56] For example, among 50 PWID with a history of incarceration recruited from drug treatment settings in London, the mean number of incarceration events was 2.4, and the average total time spent in custody was 20.6 months, with the average length of a single custodial sentence 8.6 months.[18] Most charges were related to drug use, both directly and indirectly, for example, acquisitive crimes such as shoplifting, burglary, and small-scale fraud.[18] In Ireland, a representative sample of imprisoned men found that 85% were imprisoned on drug charges.[56] As in Ireland, injectors represent a substantial fraction of prisoners in many countries. Prison populations are primarily male[106,122,123]; drawn disproportionately from racial, ethnic and sexual minorities[124-126]; and are exposed to an array of political, social, and economic inequities, including poverty and lack of social support, as well as physical and mental comorbidities[127-129];

and survive in environments often marked by overcrowding, violence, and in some instances torture.[128,130-133]

While prisons are officially illicit drug-free, alcohol-free and, increasingly, tobacco-free environments, studies of general correctional populations, imprisoned PWID, and retrospective surveys of once-incarcerated drug users in community settings have identified that a substantial proportion of individuals report injection drug use while incarcerated.[1,6,8–10,18,21,22,26,29,33,35,39,43,47,49,56,58,59,62,67,70,71,73,79,84,85] In fact, I am unaware of any published investigation of IWI that has failed to detect it. In studies of PWID drawn from community or treatment settings in many locales, IWI is common. For example, among 642 PWID recruited from street settings in Los Angeles County in the United States, approximately 15% released from detention in the previous 12 months reported IWI.[49] Among 50 PWID in London recruited from drug treatment clinics, 94% reported that they had ever taken an illicit drug while imprisoned, including 33 (70%) intravenously.[18] Similarly, in a study among PWID in Glasgow, more than half reported being held in custody in the previous 6 months; of those, 16% had injected while imprisoned.[22] The same prevalence was reported in a study in 2003 of 1,865 PWID in northern Thailand recruited from drug treatment clinics.[6] More recently, among 623 PWID recruited from three cities in Afghanistan, 63% had ever been imprisoned; among those, more than one-quarter reported IWI.[58] Even studies conducted among imprisoned PWID, who have an obvious incentive to not report drug use within prison walls, have reported IWI. Of 3,176 adults held in one of eight prisons in England and Wales in 1997 and 1998, 24% reported ever injecting drugs; of those, 30% reported injecting in prison.[82] Substantial levels of IWI have been reported from surveys of imprisoned PWID in other settings, including Scotland (43%)[10]; Greece (60%)[47]; Australia (85% and 50%)[33,84]; and Denmark (60%).[20] Although many of these individuals were established injectors, a fraction of individuals reporting IWI in many surveys in fact initiated injection while incarcerated.[5,9,12,35,36,54,56] In a representative sample of 1,205 prisoners in Ireland, approximately 20% of PWID reported that their first injection occurred within a correctional facility.[56] A large cross-sectional study of 3,142 prisoners in England and Wales found that initiating drug use while incarcerated was common; and 6% of cannabis users, 26% of heroin users, and 4% of injectors reported initiating inside prison walls.[12]

This phenomenon of injecting while incarcerated is transformed into a risk factor for blood-borne pathogens by the lack of sterile injection equipment. In 1994, surveying HIV infection among people held in Austrian prisons, Pont et al. noted that any strategy to prevent further cases would need to face the "tabooed facts of everyday prison life," namely, that "in the circumstances prevailing in prisons and penitentiaries, intravenous drug use . . . cannot altogether be eradicated."[63] Unfortunately, efforts to interdict drugs flowing into prisons were having the effect of reducing the availability of sterile injection equipment.[63] Because the vast majority of prisons prohibit distribution of sterile injection equipment,[134,135] borrowing and lending used syringes is commonplace among imprisoned PWID.[5,18,22,26,29,30,39,43,49,70,79,82] For example, among PWID reporting IWI in a survey of male inmates in Thailand, 95% reported using shared injection equipment.[79] Surveys comparing incarcerated and non-incarcerated PWID have generally concluded that incarceration heightens levels of unsafe injections.[26,31,40,43,63,64,85] For example, among 1,745 HIV-negative injection drug users recruited from community settings and followed prospectively in Vancouver, Canada, periods of incarceration were associated with a 26% increase in the likelihood of syringe sharing.[85] In the 4 weeks prior to their current sentence, less than half (46%) of incarcerated PWID in Sydney reported sharing injection equipment, while 75% reported sharing in prison.[26] This dynamic was echoed in a later analysis of 234 imprisoned male drug users in Scotland in the early 1990s.[71] Of those, one-third reported injecting prior to imprisonment; 11% reported IWI. However, 24% of PWID reported sharing in the community versus 76% of individuals reporting IWI. "In general terms," Shewan et al. concluded, "drug users appear less likely to inject in prison than in the community, but those who do are more likely to share equipment."[71] A decade later, Hellard et al. studied HCV transmission in Australian prisons and restated the same dynamic: "Prisoners who injected drugs outside of prison continue to inject in prison, but in a less safe manner."[40]

Elevated use of contaminated injection equipment while incarcerated has translated into strong associations between incarceration and positive HIV serostatus.[11,15,24,26,29,44,59,63,66,72–74,79,81,86,87] For example, in a survey of 611 community-based PWID attending drug treatment clinics in Iran, reporting a history of sharing injection equipment while incarcerated was associated with a 12-fold crude increase in the risk of HIV infection, leading the authors to call for harm reduction services available in the community to be extended to correctional settings.[87] In a similar study conducted among 741 PWID recruited from drug treatment settings in Berlin, 35% of those reporting IWI were HIV-positive versus 22% who had not injected in prison settings.[74] In a follow-up prospective study of community-recruited PWID in Berlin, sharing injection equipment in prison was associated with a 10 times greater likelihood of HIV seroconversion.[72] More recently, a number of studies have described similar dynamics governing HCV seroconversion among PWID.[5,13,20,37,50,52,60,72,75,77,82] For example, in a survey of 1,131 PWID in 10 European cities conducted in 2006, IWI was a significant independent risk factor for being HCV antibody–positive.[52] This was further detailed in a molecular analysis of four in-custody transmission events in Australia, in which three were associated with drug injection and equipment sharing among prisoners.[13]

Despite the clear importance of in-prison injecting among PWID, the micro risk environment of IWI has never been fully described. For example, very few studies have examined in detail the use of psychoactive substances by imprisoned individuals, including motivations for drug use, preferences, and changes in drug use patterns associated with incarceration. In their study of imprisoned Scottish drug users, Shewan et al. found that the likelihood of injecting while incarcerated was positively linked to a range of factors, including greater number of substances used in prison and being discontinued from methadone upon incarceration.[71] The two most detailed analyses of IWI were conducted using surveys of prisoners held in Australia and Thailand.[14,45] In 2003, Buavirat et al. used a case-control study to determine that being tattooed in prison and sharing needles in holding cells prior to incarceration strongly predicted HIV infection.[14] This finding was supported the following year in a study that fit a four-level injection risk scale (ie, < daily, ≥ daily, ≥ daily with syringe sharing; IWI) to data gathered during a prospective study involving community-recruited Thai PWID and found that HIV incidence doubled at each step.[19] In 2012, in a study involving 1,322 Australian prisoners, IWI was independently associated with male gender, being unemployed prior to incarceration, a history of needle/syringe sharing, being HCV-antibody-positive, using ≥ three illicit drugs prior to incarceration, and in-prison tattooing.[45] Notably, the association between IWI and in-prison tattooing illuminates a pathway for blood-borne pathogens to spread beyond people who use injection drugs.

In non-correctional settings, a variety of interventions have been developed for PWID that have been shown to reduce the frequency and intensity of injection drug use (most notably pharmacotherapies such as methadone for opioid-dependent individuals)[136] and curb the incidence of harms associated with injecting, including sterile syringe provision.[137] Unfortunately, with only a few notable exceptions, many of these strategies have yet to be scaled up within correctional systems, limited by logistical, financial, or ideological constraints.[138,139] For example, studies evaluating in-prison opioid substitution therapy found significant reductions in in-prison opioid use.[27,28,46] In a controlled trial in 2003, all eligible prisoners were randomly assigned to either in-prison methadone or treatment-as-usual and followed for 4 months.[27] Among those on methadone, rates of heroin use, as ascertained by self-report and hair analysis, were significantly lower, along with declines in IWI and syringe sharing. This benefit was replicated in an analysis of a natural experiment involving more than 2000 prisoners in Australia, in which individuals incarcerated in a jurisdiction that allowed in-prison opioid substitution therapy reported lower levels of lifetime IWI than individuals incarcerated in a jurisdiction that prohibited in-prison opioid substitution therapy.[46] Unfortunately, although in-prison methadone has also been associated with a number of important benefits, including lower post-release risk behaviors for HIV transmission,[140] and has long been designated an essential medication by the World Health Organization,[138] it remains either unavailable or sub-optimally delivered in many settings. For example, standard practice in US correctional facilities is forced withdrawal from methadone upon incarceration.[141]

As with opioid substitution therapy, provision of strategies to mitigate the risks of blood-borne virus transmission, in particular sterile syringe distribution, remain unutilized in almost all settings, even in jurisdictions where community-based distribution networks are widespread.[134,139] In 2006, a global review found that only 11 countries, almost all in central Asia or Western Europe, had established prison-based needle exchange programs.[134] In most cases, evaluations of prison-based needle exchange programs have identified reductions in syringe sharing secondary to IWI.[142-145] For example, in Berlin, self-reported levels of contaminated syringe sharing dropped from 71% at baseline to 0% at the 12-month follow-up period.[145]

Faced with persistent levels of in-prison illicit drug use, IWI, syringe sharing, and outbreaks of blood-borne pathogens, many correctional systems have avoided controversial if effective harm reduction–based interventions and chosen instead largely unproven efforts to reduce levels of in-prison drug use and viral transmission. Most common is the provision of bleach and other disinfectants to imprisoned PWID.[134] Unfortunately, evidence supporting the use of bleach to prevent viral transmission was judged by the WHO to be weak, undercut by poor access and inadequate use by

PWID.[135] As in non-correctional settings, substantial efforts have gone toward stemming the supply of illicit drugs, including heightened security measures and improved surveillance measures to detect drugs and drug use. Unfortunately, no evidence exists to suggest that these efforts have reduced levels of illicit drug use among prisoners.[139]

CONCLUSION

Her Majesty's Prison Glenochil sits in the Scottish lowlands, approximately halfway between Glasgow and Edinburgh, and currently houses nearly 700 men on short- and long-term sentences. In the spring and summer of 1993, it was the site of the first documented outbreak of HIV driven by in-prison injecting.[36,76] Between April and June, eight symptomatic cases of acute hepatitis B infection were followed by two HIV seroconversions in the midst of reports of IWI and syringe sharing received by the prison doctor.[76] The well-documented epidemiological investigation and public health response echo many of the dynamics identified in this review of the prevalence of and risks associated with IWI. In the wake of the first case of HIV, 162 prisoners received testing for HIV; 76 had ever injected drugs, including 33 within the walls of the prison. Of those, 14 were newly diagnosed with HIV; based on testing dates and prison records, 6 of 14 incident infections were thought to have definitely occurred in Glenochil, and another 2 probably in another prison prior to transfer.[76] (A molecular analysis conducted in 1997 found that all but one of the individuals were infected with closely related viral isolates.[146]) Among 76 PWID, 7 began injecting during their current sentence, including 2 who were among the seroconverters. Of the 69 who injected outside Glenochil, only 26 continued to do so, but almost all reported sharing their syringes with an unknown number of other prisoners. Of the newly infected, almost all came from Glasgow, where the prompt implementation of an extensive sterile needle distribution system in 1988 was thought to have prevented the rapid spread of HIV among PWID seen in Edinburgh in the late 1980s. After the introduction of a "public health response" among the men held at Glenochil prison, including bleach tablets to clean injecting equipment—but not methadone maintenance or sterile syringes—follow-up testing revealed no further HIV infections.[34] "[PWID] spend large parts of their lives in prison," concluded Taylor et al., who investigated the outbreak. "The effort and imagination that has already been expended on preventing HIV transmission among injectors outside the prison setting should be afforded to the prevention of the spread of infection inside."

REFERENCES

1. Decker MD, Vaughn WK, Brodie JS, Hutcheson RH, Schaffner W. Seroepidemiology of hepatitis B in Tennessee prisoners. *J Infect Dis*. 1984;150(3):450–459.
2. Hok KA, Nieman R, Lackey JO, Cabasso VJ. Australia antigen in a closed adult population monitored for serum glutamic oxalacetic transaminase. *Appl Microbiol*. 1970;20(1):6–10.
3. Nelson M, Cooke B. The incidence of Australia antigen in blood donors and in certain high-risk patient populations. *Med J Aust*. 1971;1(18):950–954.

4. Koplan JP, Walker JA, Bryan JA, Berquist KR. Prevalence of hepatitis B surface antigen and antibody at a state prison in Kansas. *J Infect Dis*. 1978;137(4):505–506.

5. Allwright S, Bradley F, Long J, Barry J, Thornton L, Parry JV. Prevalence of antibodies to hepatitis B, hepatitis C, and HIV and risk factors in Irish prisoners: results of a national cross sectional survey. *BMJ*. 2000;321(7253):78–82.

6. Beyrer C, Jittiwutikarn J, Teokul W, et al. Drug use, increasing incarceration rates, and prison-associated HIV risks in Thailand. *AIDS Behav*. 2003;7(2):153–161.

7. Birchard K. Inmates in Irish prisons face drug abuse and disease. *Lancet*. 1999;354(9180):753.

8. Bird AG, Gore SM, Burns SM, Duggie JG. Study of infection with HIV and related risk factors in young offenders' institution. *BMJ*. 1993;307(6898):228–231.

9. Bird AG, Gore SM, Cameron S, Ross AJ, Goldberg DJ. Anonymous HIV surveillance with risk factor elicitation at Scotland's largest prison, Barlinnie. *AIDS*. 1995;9(7):801–808.

10. Bird AG, Gore SM, Hutchinson SJ, Lewis SC, Cameron S, Burns S. Harm reduction measures and injecting inside prison versus mandatory drugs testing: Results of a cross sectional anonymous questionnaire survey. *BMJ*. 1997;315(7099):21–24.

11. Bird AG, Gore SM, Jolliffe DW, Burns SM. Anonymous HIV surveillance in Saughton Prison, Edinburgh. *AIDS*. 1992;6(7):725–733.

12. Boys A, Farrell M, Bebbington P, et al. Drug use and initiation in prison: results from a national prison survey in England and Wales. *Addiction*. 2002;97(12):1551–1560.

13. Bretaña NA, Boelen L, Bull R, et al. Transmission of hepatitis C virus among prisoners, Australia, 2005–2012. *Emerg Infect Dis*. 2015;21(5):765–774.

14. Buavirat A, Page-Shafer K, van Griensven GJP, et al. Risk of prevalent HIV infection associated with incarceration among injecting drug users in Bangkok, Thailand: case-control study. *BMJ*. 2003;326(7384):1–5.

15. Burattini M, Massad E, Rozman M, Azevedo R, Carvalho H. Correlation between HIV and HCV in Brazilian prisoners: evidence for parenteral transmission inside prison. *Rev Saude Publica*. 2000;34(5):431–436.

16. Butler T, Spencer J, Cui J, Vickery K, Zou J, Kaldor J. Seroprevalence of markers for hepatitis B, C and G in male and female prisoners—NSW, 1996. *Aust N Z J Public Health*. 1999;23(4):377–384.

17. Calzavara LM, Burchell AN, Schlossberg J, et al. Prior opiate injection and incarceration history predict injection drug use among inmates. *Addiction*. 2003;98(9):1257–1265.

18. Carvell AL, Hart GJ. Risk behaviours for HIV infection among drug users in prison. *BMJ*. 1990;300(6736):1383–1384.

19. Choopanya K, Des Jarlais DC, Vanichseni S, et al. Incarceration and risk for HIV infection among injection drug users in Bangkok. *J Acquir Immune Defic Syndr*. 2002;29(1):86–94.

20. Christensen PB, Krarup HB, Niesters HG, Norder H, Georgsen J. Prevalence and incidence of bloodborne viral infections among Danish prisoners. *Eur J Epidemiol*. 2000;16(11):1043–1049.

21. Clarke JG, Stein MD, Hanna L, Sobota M, Rich JD. Active and former injection drug users report of HIV risk behaviors during periods of incarceration. *Subst Abuse*. 2001;22(4):209–216.

22. Covell RG, Frischer M, Taylor A, et al. Prison experience of injecting drug users in Glasgow. *Drug Alcohol Depend*. 1993;32(1):9–14.

23. Darke S, Kaye S, Finlay-Jones R. Drug use and injection risk-taking among prison methadone maintenance patients. *Addiction*. 1998;93(8):1169–1175.

24. Davies AG, Dominy NJ, Peters A, Bath GE, Burns SM, Richardson AM. HIV in injecting drug users in Edinburgh: prevalence and correlates. *J Acquir Immune Defic Syndr*. 1995;8(4):399–405.

25. Dolan KA, Teutsch S, Scheuer N, et al. Incidence and risk for acute hepatitis C infection during imprisonment in Australia. *Eur J Epidemiol*. 2010;25(2):143–148.

26. Dolan KA, Donoghoe M, Stimson GV. Drug injecting and syringe sharing in custody and in the community: an exploratory survey of HIV risk behaviour. *How J Crim Just*. 1990;29(3):177–187.

27. Dolan KA, Shearer J, MacDonald M, Mattick RP, Hall W, Wodak AD. A randomised controlled trial of methadone maintenance treatment versus wait list control in an Australian prison system. *Drug Alcohol Depend*. 2003;72(1):59–65.

28. Dolan KA, Wodak AD, Hall WD. Methadone maintenance treatment reduces heroin injection in New South Wales prisons. *Drug Alcohol Depend*. 1998;17(2):153–158.

29. Dufour A, Alary M, Poulin C, et al. Prevalence and risk behaviours for HIV infection among inmates of a provincial prison in Quebec City. *AIDS*. 1996;10(9):1009–1015.

30. Edwards A, Curtis S, Sherrard J. Survey of risk behaviour and HIV prevalence in an English prison. *Int J STD AIDS*. 1999;10(7):464–466.

31. Ford PM, Pearson M, Sankar-Mistry P, Stevenson T, Bell D, Austin J. HIV, hepatitis C and risk behaviour in a Canadian medium-security federal penitentiary. Queen's University HIV Prison Study Group. *QJM*. 2000;93(2):113–119.

32. Frost L, Tchertkov V. Prisoner risk taking in the Russian Federation. *AIDS Educ Prev*. 2002;14(5)(suppl B):7–23.

33. Gaughwin MD, Douglas RM, Liew C, et al. HIV prevalence and risk behaviours for HIV transmission in South Australian prisons. *AIDS*. 1991;5(7):845–851.

34. Goldberg D, Taylor A, McGregor J, Davis B, Wrench J, Gruer L. A lasting public health response to an outbreak of HIV infection in a Scottish prison? *Int J STD AIDS*. 1998;9(1):25–30.

35. Gore SM, Bird AG, Burns S, Ross AJ, Goldberg D. Anonymous HIV surveillance with risk-factor elicitation: at Perth (for men) and Cornton Vale (for women) prisons in Scotland. *Int J STD AIDS*. 1997;8(3):166–175.

36. Gore SM, Bird AG, Burns SM, Goldberg DJ, Ross AJ, Macgregor J. Drug injection and HIV prevalence in inmates of Glenochil prison. *BMJ*. 1995;310(6975):293–296.

37. Gore SM, Bird AG, Cameron SO, Hutchinson SJ, Burns SM, Goldberg DJ. Prevalence of hepatitis C in prisons: WASH-C surveillance linked to self-reported risk behaviours. *QJM*. 1999;92(1):25–32.

38. Gore SM, Bird AG, Ross AJ. Prison rites: starting to inject inside. *BMJ*. 1995;311(7013):1135–1136.

39. Hart GJ, Sonnex C, Petherick A, Johnson AM, Feinmann C, Adler MW. Risk behaviours for HIV infection among injecting drug users attending a drug dependency clinic. *BMJ*. 1989;298(6680):1081–1083.

40. Hellard ME, Hocking JS, Crofts N. The prevalence and the risk behaviours associated with the transmission of hepatitis C virus in Australian correctional facilities. *Epidemiol Infect*. 2004;132(3):409–415.

41. Hutchinson SJ, Goldberg DJ, Gore SM, et al. Hepatitis B outbreak at Glenochil prison during January to June 1993. *Epidemiol Infect*. 1998;121(1):185–191.

42. Kang S-Y, Deren S, Andia J, Colón HM, Robles R, Oliver-Velez D. HIV transmission behaviors in jail/prison among Puerto Rican drug injectors in New York and Puerto Rico. *AIDS Behav*. 2005;9(3):377–386.

43. Kennedy DH, Nair G, Elliott L, Ditton J. Drug misuse and sharing of needles in Scottish prisons. *BMJ*. 1991;302(6791):1507.

44. Kheirandish P, Seyedalinaghi SA, Hosseini M, et al. Prevalence and correlates of HIV infection among male injection drug users in detention in Tehran, Iran. *J Acquir Immune Defic Syndr*. 2010;53(2):273–275.

45. Kinner SA, Jenkinson R, Gouillou M, Milloy M-J. High-risk drug-use practices among a large sample of Australian prisoners. *Drug Alcohol Depend*. 2012;126(1–2):156–160.

46. Kinner S, Moore E, Spittal MJ, Indig D. Opiate substitution treatment to reduce in-prison drug injection: a natural experiment. *Int J Drug Policy*. 2013;24(5):460–463.

47. Koulierakis G, Gnardellis C, Agrafiotis D, Power KG. HIV risk behaviour correlates among injecting drug users in Greek prisons. *Addiction*. 2000;95(8):1207–1216.

48. Long J, Allwright S, Barry J, et al. Prevalence of antibodies to hepatitis B, hepatitis C, and HIV and risk factors in entrants to Irish prisons: a national cross sectional survey. *BMJ*. 2001;323(7323):1209–1213.

49. Lopez-Zetina J, Kerndt P, Ford W, Woerhle T, Weber M. Prevalence of HIV and hepatitis B and self-reported injection risk behavior during detention among street-recruited injection drug users in Los Angeles County, 1994–1996. *Addiction*. 2001;96(4):589–595.

50. Luciani F, Bretaña NA, Teutsch S, et al. A prospective study of hepatitis C incidence in Australian prisoners. *Addiction*. 2014;109(10):1695–1706.

51. Malliori M, Sypsa V, Psichogiou M, et al. A survey of bloodborne viruses and associated risk behaviours in Greek prisons. *Addiction*. 1998;93(2):243–251.

52. March JC, Oviedo-Joekes E, Romero M. Factors associated with reported hepatitis C and HIV among injecting drug users in ten European cities. *Enferm Infecc Microbiol Clin*. 2007;25(2):91–97.

53. Martin RE, Gold F, Murphy W, Remple V, Berkowitz J, Money D. Drug use and risk of bloodborne infections: a survey of female prisoners in British Columbia. *Can J Public Health*. 2005;96(2):97–101.

54. Miller ER, Bi P, Ryan P. Hepatitis C virus infection in South Australian prisoners: seroprevalence, seroconversion, and risk factors. *Int J Infect Dis*. 2009;13(2):201–208.

55. Milloy M-J, Kerr T, Salters K, et al. Incarceration is associated with used syringe lending among active injection drug users with detectable plasma HIV-1 RNA: a longitudinal analysis. *BMC Infect Dis*. 2013;13(1):1–10.

56. Murphy M, Gaffney K, Carey O, Dooley E, Mulcahy F. The impact of HIV disease on an Irish prison population. *Int J STD AIDS*. 1992;3(6):426–429.

57. Narkauskaitė L, Juozulynas A, Mackiewicz Z, Venalis A, Utkuvienė J. Prevalence of psychoactive substances use in a Lithuanian women's prison revisited after 5 years. *Med Sci Mon*. 2010;16(11):PH91–96.

58. Nasir A, Todd CS, Stanekzai MR, et al. Prevalence of HIV, hepatitis B and hepatitis C and associated risk behaviours amongst injecting drug users in three Afghan cities. *Int J Drug Policy*. 2011;22(2):145–152.

59. Navadeh S, Mirzazadeh A, Gouya MM, Farnia M, Alasvand R, Haghdoost A-A. HIV prevalence and related risk behaviours among prisoners in Iran: results of the national biobehavioural survey, 2009. *Sex Transm Infect*. 2013;89(suppl 3):iii33–36.

60. O'Sullivan BG, Levy MH, Dolan KA, et al. Hepatitis C transmission and HIV post-exposure prophylaxis after needle- and syringe-sharing in Australian prisons. *Med J Aust*. 2003;178(11):546–549.

61. Plourde C, Brochu S. Drugs in prison: a break in the pathway. *Subst Abuse Misuse*. 2002;37(1):47–63.

62. Pollini RA, Alvelais J, Gallardo M, et al. The harm inside: injection during incarceration among male injection drug users in Tijuana, Mexico. *Drug Alcohol Depend*. 2009;103(1–2):52–58.

63. Pont J, Strutz H, Kahl W, Salzner G. HIV epidemiology and risk behavior promoting HIV transmission in Austrian prisons. *Eur J Epidemiol*. 1994;10(3):285–289.

64. Power KG, Markova I, Rowlands A, McKee KJ, Anslow PJ, Kilfedder C. Intravenous drug use and HIV transmission amongst inmates in Scottish prisons. *Brit J Addict*. 1992;87(1):35–45.

65. Rahman MZ, Ditton J, Forsyth AJ. Variations in needle sharing practices among intravenous drug users in Possil (Glasgow). *Brit J Addict*. 1989;84(8):923–927.

66. Robles RR, Colón HM, Diaz N, et al. Behavioural risk factors and HIV infection of injection drug users at detoxification clinics in Puerto Rico. *Int J Epidemiol*. 1994;23(3):595–601.

67. Rotily M, Weilandt C, Bird SM, et al. Surveillance of HIV infection and related risk behaviour in European prisons: a multicentre pilot study. *Eur J Epidemiol*. 2001;11(3):243–250.

68. Rowell TL, Wu E, Hart CL, Haile R, El-Bassel N. Predictors of drug use in prison among incarcerated black men. *Am J Drug Alcohol Abuse*. 2012;38(6):593–597.
69. Sarang A, Rhodes T, Platt L, et al. Drug injecting and syringe use in the HIV risk environment of Russian penitentiary institutions: qualitative study. *Addiction*. 2006;101(12):1787–1796.
70. Shewan D, Gemmell M, Davies JB. Behavioural change amongst drug injectors in Scottish prisons. *Soc Sci Med*. 1994;39(11):1585–1586.
71. Shewan D, Macpherson A, Reid MM, Davies JB. Patterns of injecting and sharing in a Scottish prison. *Drug Alcohol Depend*. 1995;39(3):237–243.
72. Stark K, Bienzle U, Vonk R, Guggenmoos-Holzmann I. History of syringe sharing in prison and risk of hepatitis B virus, hepatitis C virus, and human immunodeficiency virus infection among injecting drug users in Berlin. *Int J Epidemiol*. 1997;26(6):1359–1366.
73. Stark K, Müller R, Guggenmoos-Holzmann I, Deininger S, Meyer E, Bienzle U. HIV infection in intravenous drug abusers in Berlin: risk factors and time trends. *Wien Klin Wochenschr*. 1990;68(8):415–420.
74. Stark K, Müller R, Wirth D, Bienzle U, Pauli G, Guggenmoos-Holzmann I. Determinants of HIV infection and recent risk behaviour among injecting drug users in Berlin by site of recruitment. *Addiction*. 1995;90(10):1367–1375.
75. Sutton AJ, McDonald SA, Palmateer N, Taylor A, Hutchinson SJ. Estimating the variability in the risk of infection for hepatitis C in the Glasgow injecting drug user population. *Epidemiol Infect*. 2012;140(12):2190–2198.
76. Taylor A, Goldberg D, Emslie J, et al. Outbreak of HIV infection in a Scottish prison. *BMJ*. 1995;310(6975):289–292.
77. Taylor A, Munro A, Allen E, et al. Low incidence of hepatitis C virus among prisoners in Scotland. *Addiction*. 2013;108(7):1296–1304.
78. Teutsch S, Luciani F, Scheuer N, et al. Incidence of primary hepatitis C infection and risk factors for transmission in an Australian prisoner cohort. *BMC Public Health*. 2010;10(1):1–9.
79. Thaisri H, Lerwitworapong J, Vongsheree S, et al. HIV infection and risk factors among Bangkok prisoners, Thailand: a prospective cohort study. *BMC Infect Dis*. 2003;3(25):1–8.
80. Van Haastrecht HJ, Bax JS, van den Hoek AA. High rates of drug use, but low rates of HIV risk behaviours among injecting drug users during incarceration in Dutch prisons. *Addiction*. 1998;93(9):1417–1425.
81. Vanichseni S, Kitayaporn D, Mastro TD, et al. Continued high HIV-1 incidence in a vaccine trial preparatory cohort of injection drug users in Bangkok, Thailand. *AIDS*. 2001;15(3):397–405.
82. Weild AR, Gill ON, Bennett D, Livingstone SJ, Parry JV, Curran L. Prevalence of HIV, hepatitis B, and hepatitis C antibodies in prisoners in England and Wales: a national survey. *Commun Dis Public Health*. 2000;3(2):121–126.
83. Wohl AR, Johnson D, Jordan W, et al. High-risk behaviors during incarceration in African-American men treated for HIV at three Los Angeles public medical centers. *J Acquir Immune Defic Syndr*. 2000;24(4):386–392.
84. Wolk J, Wodak A, Morlet A, Guinan JJ, Gold J. HIV-related risk-taking behaviour, knowledge and serostatus of intravenous drug users in Sydney. *Med J Aust*. 1990;152(9):453–458.
85. Wood E, Li K, Small W, Montaner JS, Schechter MT, Kerr T. Recent incarceration independently associated with syringe sharing by injection drug users. *Public Health Rep*. 2005;120(2):150–156.
86. Zamani S, Kihara M, Gouya MM, et al. High prevalence of HIV infection associated with incarceration among community-based injecting drug users in Tehran, Iran. *J Acquir Immune Defic Syndr*. 2006;42(3):342–346.
87. Zamani S, Kihara M, Gouya MM, et al. Prevalence of and factors associated with HIV-1 infection among drug users visiting treatment centers in Tehran, Iran. *AIDS*. 2005;19(7):709–716.

88. Drucker E. Drug prohibition and public health: 25 years of evidence. *Public Health Rep.* 1999;114(1):14–29.
89. Mauer M, King R. *A 25-Year Quagmire: The War on Drugs and Its Impact on American Society.* Washington, DC: The Sentencing Project; 2007.
90. Reuter P. What drug policies cost: estimating government drug policy expenditures. *Addiction.* 2006;101(3):315–322.
91. Stevenson B. *Drug Policy, Criminal Justice and Mass Imprisonment.* Geneva, Switzerland: Global Commission on Drug Policy; 2011.
92. Bruneau J, Roy E, Arruda N, Zang G, Jutras-Aswad D. The rising prevalence of prescription opioid injection and its association with hepatitis C incidence among street-drug users. *Addiction.* 2012;107(7):1318–1327.
93. Hagan H. The relevance of attributable risk measures to HIV prevention planning. *AIDS.* 2003;17(6):911–913.
94. Tyndall MW, Currie S, Spittal P, et al. Intensive injection cocaine use as the primary risk factor in the Vancouver HIV-1 epidemic. *AIDS.* 2003;17(6):887–893.
95. Baillargeon J, Giordano TP, Rich JD, et al. Accessing antiretroviral therapy following release from prison. *JAMA.* 2009;301(8):848–857.
96. Fu JJ, Zaller ND, Yokell MA, Bazazi AR, Rich JD. Forced withdrawal from methadone maintenance therapy in criminal justice settings: a critical treatment barrier in the United States. *J Subst Abuse Treat.* 2013;44(5):502–505.
97. Milloy M-J, Kerr T, Buxton J, et al. Dose-response effect of incarceration events on nonadherence to HIV antiretroviral therapy among injection drug users. *J Infect Dis.* 2011;203(9):1215–1221.
98. Polonsky M, Azbel L, Wickersham JA, et al. Challenges to implementing opioid substitution therapy in Ukrainian prisons: personnel attitudes toward addiction, treatment, and people with HIV/AIDS. *Drug Alcohol Depend.* 2015;148:47–55. https://www.ncbi.nlm.nih.gov/pubmed/25620732
99. Kinner SA, Milloy MJ, Wood E, Qi J, Zhang R, Kerr T. Incidence and risk factors for non-fatal overdose among a cohort of recently incarcerated illicit drug users. *Addict Behav.* 2012;37(6):691–696.
100. Winter RJ, Stoove M, Degenhardt L, et al. Incidence and predictors of non-fatal drug overdose after release from prison among people who inject drugs in Queensland, Australia. *Drug Alcohol Depend.* 2015;153:43–49. https://www.ncbi.nlm.nih.gov/pubmed/26105708
101. Binswanger IA, Stern MF, Deyo RA, et al. Release from prison—a high risk of death for former inmates. *N Engl J Med.* 2007;356(2):157–165.
102. Binswanger IA, Blatchford PJ, Mueller SR, Stern MF. Mortality after prison release: opioid overdose and other causes of death, risk factors, and time trends from 1999 to 2009. *Ann Intern Med.* 2013;159(9):592–600.
103. Mathers BM, Degenhardt L, Phillips B, et al. Global epidemiology of injecting drug use and HIV among people who inject drugs: a systematic review. *Lancet.* 2008;372(9651):1733–1745.
104. Mathers BM, Degenhardt L, Bucello C, Lemon J, Wiessing L, Hickman M. Mortality among people who inject drugs: a systematic review and meta-analysis. *Bull World Health Organ.* 2013;91(2):102–123.
105. Gallahue P. *The Death Penalty for Drug Offences: Global Overview 2011.* London, England: Harm Reduction International; 2011.
106. Carson E. *Prisoners in 2014.* Washington, DC: US Department of Justice; 2015.
107. Pallas JR, Farinas-Alvarez C, Prieto D, Delgado-Rodriguez M. Coinfections by HIV, hepatitis B and hepatitis C in imprisoned injecting drug users. *Eur J Epidemiol.* 1999;15(8):699–704.
108. Genberg BL, Astemborski J, Vlahov D, Kirk GD, Mehta SH. Incarceration and injection drug use in Baltimore, Maryland. *Addiction.* 2015;110(7):1152–1159.
109. Miron J. *The Effect of Drug Prohibition on Drug Prices: Evidence From the Markets for Heroin and Cocaine.* Washington, DC: National Bureau of Economic Research; 2003.

110. Bretteville-Jensen AL, Sutton M. The income-generating behaviour of injecting drug-users in Oslo. *Addiction*. 1996;91(1):63–79.

111. Sherman SG, Latkin CA. Drug users' involvement in the drug economy: implications for harm reduction and HIV prevention programs. *J Urban Health*. 2002;79(2):266–277.

112. DeBeck K, Shannon K, Wood E, Li K, Montaner J, Kerr T. Income generating activities of people who inject drugs. *Drug Alcohol Depend*. 2007;91(1):50–56.

113. Ompad DC, Nandi V, Cerda M, Crawford N, Galea S, Vlahov D. Beyond income: material resources among drug users in economically-disadvantaged New York City neighborhoods. *Drug Alcohol Depend*. 2012;120(1–3):127–134.

114. Ball A. *Multi-Centre Study on Drug Injecting and Risk of HIV Infection*. Geneva, Switzerland: World Health Organization; 1995.

115. Epperson M, El-Bassel N, Gilbert L, Orellana ER, Chang M. Increased HIV risk associated with criminal justice involvement among men on methadone. *AIDS Behav*. 2008;12(1):51–57.

116. Walmsley R. *World Prison Population List*. 11th ed. London, England: Institute for Criminal Policy Research; 2015.

117. Kinner SA, George J, Campbell G, Degenhardt L. Crime, drugs and distress: patterns of drug use and harm among criminally involved injecting drug users in Australia. *Aust N Z J Public Health*. 2009;33(3):223–227.

118. Koehn JD, Bach P, Hayashi K, et al. Impact of incarceration on rates of methadone use in a community recruited cohort of injection drug users. *Addict Behav*. 2015;46:1–4. https://www.ncbi.nlm.nih.gov/pubmed/25746159

119. Kivela P, Krol A, Simola S, et al. HIV outbreak among injecting drug users in the Helsinki region: social and geographical pockets. *Eur J Public Health*. 2007;17(4):381–386.

120. Calzavara L, Ramuscak N, Burchell AN, et al. Prevalence of HIV and hepatitis C virus infections among inmates of Ontario remand facilities. *CMAJ*. 2007;177(3):257–261.

121. Poulin C, Alary M, Lambert G, et al. Prevalence of HIV and hepatitis C virus infections among inmates of Quebec provincial prisons. *CMAJ*. 2007;177(3):252–256.

122. Boe R, Nafekh M, Vuong B. *The Changing Profile of the Federal Inmate Population*. Ottawa: Government of Canada; 2003.

123. Australian Bureau of Statistics. *Prisoners in Australia (4517.0)*. Canberra: Government of Australia;2015.

124. Hogg RS, Druyts EF, Burris S, Drucker E, Strathdee SA. Years of life lost to prison: racial and gender gradients in the United States of America. *Harm Reduct J*. 2008;5(4):1–5.

125. Wacquant L. The new "peculiar institution": on the prison as a surrogate ghetto. *Theor Criminol*. 2000;4(3):377–389.

126. Weatherburn DJ. The role of drug and alcohol policy in reducing Indigenous over-representation in prison. *Drug Alcohol Rev*. 2008;27(1):91–94.

127. Albertie A, Bourey C, Stephenson R, Bautista-Arredondo S. Connectivity, prison environment and mental health among first-time male inmates in Mexico City. *Glob Public Health*. 2017;12(2):170–184.

128. de Viggiani N. Unhealthy prisons: exploring structural determinants of prison health. *Sociol Health Illn*. 2007;29(1):115–135.

129. Duhamel A, Renard JM, Nuttens MC, Devos P, Beuscart R, Archer E. Social and health status of arrivals in a French prison: a consecutive case study from 1989 to 1995. *Rev Epidemiol Sante Publique*. 2001;49(3):229–238.

130. Cashmore AW, Indig D, Hampton SE, Hegney DG, Jalaludin BB. Workplace violence in a large correctional health service in New South Wales, Australia: a retrospective review of incident management records. *BMC Health Serv Res*. 2012;12(245):1–10.

131. Rabe K. Prison structure, inmate mortality and suicide risk in Europe. *Int J Law Psychiatry*. 2012;35(3):222–230.

132. McCarthy M. US prison directors' group calls for reduced use of solitary confinement. *BMJ*. 2015;351(h4765):1–2.
133. Way BB, Sawyer DA, Barboza S, Nash R. Inmate suicide and time spent in special disciplinary housing in New York State prison. *Psychiatr Serv*. 2007;58(4):558–560.
134. Lines R, Jurgens R, Betteridge G. *Prison Needle Exchange: Lessons From a Comprehensive Review of the Evidence*. Montreal, Canada: Canadian HIV/AIDS Legal Network; 2006.
135. Jurgens R. *Effectiveness of Interventions to Address HIV in Prisons*. Geneva, Switzerland: World Health Organization; 2007.
136. Sees KL, Delucchi KL, Masson C, et al. Methadone maintenance vs 180-day psychosocially enriched detoxification for treatment of opioid dependence: a randomized controlled trial. *JAMA*. 2000;283(10):1303–1310.
137. Des Jarlais DC, Marmor M, Paone D, et al. HIV incidence among injecting drug users in New York City syringe-exchange programmes. *Lancet*. 1996;348(9033):987–991.
138. Jurgens R, Ball A, Verster A. Interventions to reduce HIV transmission related to injecting drug use in prison. *Lancet Infect Dis*. 2009;9(1):57–66.
139. Jurgens R, Betteridge G. Prisoners who inject drugs: public health and human rights imperatives. *Health Hum Rights*. 2005;8(2):46–74.
140. Wilson ME, Kinlock TW, Gordon MS, O'Grady KE, Schwartz RP. Postprison release HIV-risk behaviors in a randomized trial of methadone treatment for prisoners. *Am J Addict*. 2012;21(5):476–487.
141. Rich JD, McKenzie M, Larney S, et al. Methadone continuation versus forced withdrawal on incarceration in a combined US prison and jail: a randomised, open-label trial. *Lancet*. 2015;386(9991):350–359.
142. Dolan KA, Rutter S, Wodak AD. Prison-based syringe exchange programmes: a review of international research and development. *Addiction*. 2003;98(2):153–158.
143. Menoyo C, Zulaica D, Parras F. Needle exchange programs in prisons in Spain. *Can HIV AIDS Policy Law Rev*. 2000;5(4):20–21.
144. Nelles J, Fuhrer A, Hirsbrunner H. How does syringe distribution in prison affect consumption of illegal drugs by prisoners? *Drug Alcohol Depend*. 1999;18:133–139.
145. Stark K, Herrmann U, Ehrhardt S, Bienzle U. A syringe exchange programme in prison as prevention strategy against HIV infection and hepatitis B and C in Berlin, Germany. *Epidemiol Infect*. 2006;134(4):814–819.
146. Yirrell DL, Robertson P, Goldberg DJ, McMenamin J, Cameron S, Leigh Brown AJ. Molecular investigation into outbreak of HIV in a Scottish prison. *BMJ*. 1997;314(7092):1446–1450.

CHAPTER 4

Alcohol Use Among Incarcerated Individuals

DAVID WYATT SEAL, PhD, SARAH YANCEY, MPH, MPS,
MANASA REDDY, MPH, AND STUART A. KINNER, PhD

INTRODUCTION

Much of the global population consumes alcohol and does so safely.[1] However, alcohol can increase the risk of cardiac, neurological, and digestive problems (eg, gastritis, pancreatitis), diabetic complications, many cancers, sexual function or menstruation problems, and motor vehicle accidents.[2,3] Worldwide, excessive alcohol consumption contributes to nearly 3.3 million deaths, or 5.9% of all deaths, each year.[4]

While alcohol misuse and dependence affect all segments of society, globally higher rates of alcohol use are observed in justice-involved populations than in the general community. Although measures of alcohol misuse and dependence vary, 18% to 30% of men and 10% to 24% of women entering prisons in the United States, the United Kingdom, and New Zealand are believed to meet criteria for alcohol misuse or dependence, and many more are likely at risk of alcohol-related harm.[5] In countries with displaced Indigenous populations, including Canada, New Zealand, and Australia, the prevalence of alcohol misuse is considerably higher among Indigenous than non-Indigenous prison entrants, suggesting that alcohol may play an important role in the over-representation of these communities in the criminal justice system.[6,7]

Most incarcerated individuals ultimately return to the community, but many individuals in the community with alcohol use disorders do not seek or receive treatment.[8] Correctional facilities, where alcohol is almost universally banned, have a unique opportunity to identify and treat people at high risk for alcohol misuse or dependence. Furthermore, every dollar invested in alcohol misuse or dependence treatment can yield significantly larger savings to the justice system and the community through averted loss of productivity, damage to social structures, and diversion of resources to alcohol rather than social capital.[9-11] Finally, efforts targeting the prevention of relapse after release from prison reduce the burden on the community and the public health sector, especially in the realm of social services.

ALCOHOL AND CRIME

Statistics abound on the association between alcohol use and crime, particularly violent crime. For example, 15% of a national sample of adults with alcohol use disorder in the United States reported criminal involvement in the past year.[6] Another study indicated that 19% to 33% of incarcerated individuals in the United States reported being under the influence of alcohol at the time of their offense.[12] Similarly, an Australian study estimated that alcohol was causally implicated in the offenses of almost 1 in 10 prisoners nationally.[13] Findings such as these have led some to posit a link between alcohol misuse and "impulsive crimes" (eg, assault, domestic violence, and vandalism).[14] Certainly, alcohol consumption impairs judgment and accounts for a large proportion of accidental injury-related morbidity and mortality.[15] However, drawing a definitive causal link between alcohol misuse and crime has been more difficult due to the many other confounding factors that lead to involvement in criminal activity.

Other researchers have argued that it is more useful to consider the broader context in which people who are disproportionately incarcerated engage in risky behaviors, as well as the motivating factors behind their offending behavior. Examining socio-economic, demographic, environmental, and cultural factors can provide a more encompassing contextual framework to identify links between violent crime and alcohol use, and physical or sexual abuse. For example, a growing body of literature in the United States and Australia has shown that community-level alcohol outlet density is associated with violent crime such as robbery, assault, and sexual offenses.[16–22]

EPIDEMIOLOGY OF ALCOHOL USE, MISUSE, AND DEPENDENCE
Alcohol Use, Misuse, and Dependence in the General Population

There is considerable variation across contexts and studies in the terms and measures used to describe harmful alcohol consumption. The Alcohol Use Disorders Identification Test (AUDIT) is a commonly used measure of alcohol-related risk that has been validated across gender, age, and cultural contexts.[23,24] The test assesses quantitative and qualitative dimensions of alcohol consumption to classify drinking behaviors into non-hazardous drinking, hazardous drinking, harmful use, and alcohol dependence. The AUDIT has been used in several large studies of prisoners in Australia.[25,26] In contrast, the US Bureau of Justice Statistics typically reports alcohol misuse and dependence according to the *Diagnostic and Statistical Manual of Mental Disorders (DSM)*,[12] which identifies those at greatest risk of alcohol-related harm but fails to capture harmful patterns of alcohol consumption that fall short of a clinical diagnosis.

Drinking alcohol may function as a way of coping with stress or pain, as social currency, or simply as a form of recreation. As with many kinds of drug misuse and dependence, a number of interconnected and overlapping risk factors, including many of those overrepresented in corrections, can contribute to alcohol misuse and dependence. Some of these include social and environmental factors, such as having a social network in which alcohol misuse is normative, genetic predisposition to dependence, and/or other psychiatric illnesses such as depression or post-traumatic stress disorder. In general, men drink at greater rates and in greater quantity than women, but the number of women who drink at risky levels has been increasing in recent years in some population-level samples.[1,4] Childhood physical abuse and sexual abuse have been found to be strong predictors of early drinking initiation and substance use dependence among both men and women.[27-32] Similarly, living in communities where alcohol misuse and dependence are common and/or growing up in households with family members who have problematic drinking patterns are also risk factors for future adult alcohol misuse and dependence.[27,28,33,34] There is also evidence that paternal arrest and incarceration increase the risk of early initiation to alcohol use in boys.[25]

Across Western countries, the relationship between socio-economic status (SES) and alcohol use is mixed. Evidence suggests that binge drinking is more common in people with lower SES, but frequency and total consumption of alcohol are greater among people of higher SES.[35-37] Nonetheless, the adverse effects of alcohol are disproportionately borne by the poor, even when quantity of alcohol consumption is controlled for.[1,4,38] On an individual level, those marginalized from the rest of society may have less social capital or support to buffer the social stigma and diminished productivity that can bring about or be compounded by heavy drinking. For instance, displaced Indigenous populations typically consume alcohol at rates higher than observed in the same nation's non-Indigenous populations.[7,25,39] At a societal level, although high-income countries may have more non-abstainers who drink more often, and low-income countries have more abstainers, low-income countries experience a higher burden of alcohol-related disease, injury incidence, and mortality. Among areas of low economic development, this disproportionate burden may be accounted for in part by other factors that exacerbate alcohol-related harm, such as poor nutrition due to limited access to affordable food and water, and poor availability or accessibility of health care.[40]

Alcohol Use, Misuse, and Dependence Among Incarcerated Populations

Most studies of alcohol use in incarcerated populations focus on the period immediately preceding incarceration. Further, most studies do not distinguish between alcohol use and alcohol misuse or dependence. Nonetheless, research suggests that, in much of the developed world, alcohol use disorders in correctional settings are less prevalent than are other drug use disorders.[5,41] In a 2004 survey in the United States, 32.6% of people incarcerated in state prisons and 18.5% of people incarcerated in federal prisons reported being under the influence of alcohol at the time of their offense. Furthermore, 18.5% of people arrested for drug-related crimes reported being under the influence of alcohol at the time of their arrest.[12] As in community samples, prior alcohol use disorders are more prevalent among incarcerated men than among incarcerated women.[25,41] There is also substantial overlap between substance misuse and mental illness. Studies suggest that 44% to 53% of incarcerated people self-reporting one or more mental problems in the past year concurrently meet criteria for substance misuse or dependence. In contrast, about a third (30% to 36%) of individuals not reporting mental illness have issues with substance misuse or dependence.[25,43–45]

The relationship between age and alcohol use among incarcerated populations is unclear. In the United States, rates of *drug* misuse and dependence tend to be higher among younger people who are incarcerated, while rates of *alcohol* misuse and dependence tend to be higher among incarcerated individuals who are greater than 35 years of age.[33] By contrast, in a national survey of Australian prison entrants in 2012, 46% met criteria for alcohol misuse in the past year according to the AUDIT, with higher rates among those under 35 years of age (48% compared with 40% of older entrants) and among Indigenous people (59% compared with 39% among non-Indigenous entrants).[42] We note, however, that this latter finding may reflect age differences because incarcerated individuals who are Indigenous tend to be younger than incarcerated individuals who are non-Indigenous.[42] In a survey of male entrants to a Scottish prison, 48% of respondents received AUDIT scores consistent with an alcohol use disorder.[46] Younger respondents were more likely to report heavy episodic drinking but were less likely to report behaviors consistent with dependence. A national survey of 998 prisoners in France found that nearly one in five respondents met criteria for an alcohol use disorder.[47]

Because it is a banned substance in the vast majority of correctional facilities, alcohol must be brought in from the outside or manufactured illicitly on the inside. Given its illicit nature, alcohol consumption in correctional settings is particularly risky. There is evidence linking several outbreaks of botulism across US correctional facilities resulting from consumption of "pruno" made behind bars.[48–50] Other studies have documented instances of prisoners using mouthwash or hand sanitizers for alcohol to become intoxicated.[3,4,51] The alcohol content of many of these products, called non-beverage ethanol (NBE), may exceed conventional alcoholic beverages by large margins. For example, several popular brands of mouthwash contain upwards of 30% ethanol content. In contrast, beer ethanol content is typically less 10%, and wine ethanol content is typically 10% to 15%. Indeed, research has shown that drinking many common mouthwashes will result in ethanol intake levels that exceed the acceptable daily limits and can potentially have detrimental health effects, including death.[51]

Despite these risks, two multi-site studies of incarcerated men in the United States found that about one-third of participants reported using alcohol while incarcerated, and most reported drinking on multiple occasions.[52,53] Men reported making their own alcohol while incarcerated or receiving smuggled alcohol from correctional staff.[53] Alcohol use in prison was associated with gang affiliation, violence while incarcerated, experience of sexual abuse in the community, older age, greater number of years incarcerated, and white race.[53]

Regardless of whether they drink during incarceration, many individuals relapse after release, especially in the first few days.[54-56] Poor social support and social environments in which drinking is normative are important risk factors.[56,57] In the community, alcohol-using justice-involved individuals can be hard to reach and often experience unstable living situations (eg, transitory housing, homelessness). Upon returning to the community, these individuals typically face competing priorities and barriers to accessing care[58] such as transportation and securing income, as well as drastically increased availability of alcohol and other drugs, in the context of numerous stressors that may precipitate a return to harmful patterns of use. Correctional facilities can have a positive impact on these outcomes by screening and identifying patients at risk of alcohol-related harm and facilitating linkage to care on the outside prior to release.

ADDRESSING ALCOHOL MISUSE AND DEPENDENCE INSIDE CORRECTIONAL FACILITIES

In US correctional facilities, educational programs are the most widely provided services for addressing alcohol misuse and dependence (in 74% of prisons and 61% of jails), followed by group counseling (in 55% of prisons and 60% of jails).[59] However, Taxman and colleagues suggest that even in facilities where such services are provided, access varies dramatically, and it is estimated that less than a quarter of those incarcerated people have daily access to these services.[59] Relatively few of those with an alcohol use disorder who perceive a need for treatment report receipt of treatment in prison.[6] Another US study reported that only one in six people who met *DSM-IV* criteria for alcohol misuse or dependence participated in treatment after arrest.[33] Uptake of alcohol and/or drug treatment services varies by gender, race, and other factors. In the United States, for example, women and white people are more likely to access treatment services on the inside than are men or people of other races, respectively.[33] Although treatment services vary dramatically across settings, there is growing evidence of inadequate coverage and provision of evidence-based treatments for alcohol misuse and dependence in many correctional settings.

Detoxification and Withdrawal Treatment

Individuals who are alcohol dependent on entry into prison face the difficult transition to immediate sobriety upon incarceration. Alcohol withdrawal can have serious effects on mental and physical health. Acute alcohol withdrawal is a potentially fatal condition that can occur when heavy drinkers abruptly stop drinking. Furthermore, although alcohol intake ceases at the time of arrest, blood alcohol content can continue to increase. Prison intake protocols must therefore ensure that arrested individuals are screened for withdrawal risk and receive prompt treatment if necessary. The Clinical Institute Withdrawal Assessment of Alcohol Scale revised version (CIWA-Ar) is a rapid assessment of alcohol withdrawal risk that can be used at intake. The World Health Organization (WHO) recommends benzodiazepines as a first-line treatment in managing acute alcohol withdrawal (ie, minimizing discomfort as well as preventing seizures or delirium tremens) and oral thiamine.[10] Those suffering severe withdrawal should receive inpatient treatment, to stabilize their health status prior to incarceration. However, data suggest that at least in the United States, possible drug or alcohol dependence is likely to be ignored upon arrest and incarceration.[60,61] In a 1997 survey of US jail administrators, only 28% reported that their facilities had ever offered detoxification services.[61]

Medication-Assisted Treatment (MAT)

Medication-assisted treatments for alcohol dependence include extended-release acamprosate, naltrexone in an oral or injected extended-release form, and disulfiram (Antabuse). Acamprosate and naltrexone are generally used in the management of dependence to reduce cravings. Disulfiram works by creating aversive rather than pleasurable responses to alcohol (ie, nausea). Cochrane reviews of these treatments have confirmed the effectiveness of acamprosate and naltrexone for the treatment of dependence and prevention of relapse.[60,62–64] However, there are few head-to-head comparisons of the efficacy and cost-effectiveness of these treatments. One of the few exceptions was a study conducted in Finland that directly compared these three treatments.[64] In a randomized controlled trial, all three medications resulted in significant reductions in drinking. This study further found that participants randomized to receive acamprosate had the best outcomes during a 12-week supervised medication period but did not differ from participants in the other two groups in a subsequent targeted medication follow-up. Different findings were reported by De Sousa and De Sousa[65,66] in a set of randomized comparison studies in India. These authors found that disulfiram use resulted in better outcomes than acamprosate and naltrexone use across studies.

Despite their effectiveness, there is uncertainty about the extent of MAT use in correctional settings. A multisite survey of criminal justice agencies (eg, jails, prisons, parole/probation, and drug courts) in the United States reported that 78% of jails and 75% of prisons provided MAT for alcohol dependence.[67] However, MAT was primarily administered to pregnant women and individuals experiencing opiate withdrawal in jails or prisons, while those reentering the community from jail or prison were the least likely to receive MAT. Further, MAT for alcohol use was typically limited to individuals experiencing acute withdrawal, but not for longer-term treatment. Factors influencing use of MAT included criminal justice preferences for drug-free treatment, limited knowledge of the benefits of MAT, perceived security concerns, regulations prohibiting use of MAT for certain agencies, and lack of qualified medical staff.

Behavioral Interventions and Counseling

Motivational interviewing is favored for its non-confrontational approach for individuals who may not currently want or be ready to quit their drug or alcohol use.

However, evidence for its effectiveness is mixed. A recent Cochrane review noted significant positive effects immediately post-intervention but diminishing effects over time.[68] Another Cochrane review of motivational interviewing among young adults found no evidence of its effectiveness in reducing substance misuse.[69] In one study of incarcerated adolescents, those who received motivational interviewing had lower rates of drug and alcohol use at follow-up after release compared with individuals who received relaxation training.[70]

A systematic review of 22 randomized controlled trials of brief alcohol interventions for primary care patients not seeking alcohol treatment confirmed a significant reduction compared with controls among male treatment group participants at 1-year follow-up.[71] Although the reviewed studies were conducted in non-correctional settings, brief interventions may be particularly relevant and helpful for those who are only in the system for a short period of time but who screen positive for alcohol misuse at intake. However, one evaluation of a brief intervention conducted among heavy-drinking women leaving jail found no effect compared with a control group.[56] More than 40% relapsed on the day of release. At present, there is little direct evidence for the effectiveness of brief interventions for alcohol use in incarcerated populations.

Social support is consistently recognized as an important factor in whether or not a patient relapses after ceasing drinking. Group approaches can facilitate the building of such support and reinforce positive behaviors. Research indicates that for incarcerated populations, longer programs of group therapy may be the most effective form of treatment to prevent relapse.[72] Such programs are best suited for long-term facilities, and for people upon release from incarceration. Indeed, therapeutic communities have been found to reduce substance use as well as recidivism in the year after release.[73] However, evidence for 12-step programs, such as Alcoholics Anonymous (AA) and other spiritually based interventions, is inconclusive. A Cochrane review concluded that there was no definitive evidence that AA or other types of 12-step programs help patients to initiate and maintain therapy more than other interventions.[74] The review did find that 12-step programs help to reduce alcohol consumption similar to other interventions, but that comparisons to no-treatment control conditions were lacking. The authors concluded that there is no clear evidence to show that AA can help patients to achieve abstinence or reduce alcohol dependence more than other types of interventions.

Combination Approaches

Combination approaches often involve transitional prevention programs that comprehensively address not only specific outcomes (eg, substance misuse and dependence) but also the contextual factors that enable or impede healthy outcomes as individuals reintegrate into the community after release (eg, housing, employment). Transitional programs can assist in the development of individual risk reduction and re-entry plans, provide postrelease case management support, and facilitate referral to community-based organizations capable of meeting individual healthcare, social-psychological, and substance use treatment service needs.[75] An accumulating body of evidence supports the efficacy of comprehensive prevention approaches with individuals being released from prison. Programs that combine prevention and drug treatment in residential work release environments can help men remain drug-free and reduce the likelihood of reincarceration after release from prison.[75-77] However, programs tend to focus on substance use broadly, not alcohol use specifically.

Policy Approaches

In the United States and many other countries, federal, state, and local laws work to shape how the public can access alcohol via regulating the nature of manufacturing and importing of alcohol, setting restrictions on who can drink alcohol, and levying taxes on alcohol. Specific to correctional populations, drug courts have had some success in reducing substance use and criminal behavior during program participation, as well as reducing recidivism. Mandated treatment programs such as California's Proposition 36 (Substance Abuse and Crime Prevention Act) work by channeling all non-violent drug-related offenders into community-based supervision and treatment programs as opposed to formal incarceration. Evaluations of nearly 44,000 Proposition 36 participants have observed lower rates of substance use (including alcohol, marijuana, cocaine, crack, or heroin) and recidivism from baseline to a 12-month follow-up.[72] Research with justice-involved Indigenous people in Australia suggests that compared with incarceration, substance use treatment delivered in the community results in reduced offending, lower mortality, better health-related quality of life, and reduced aggregate costs.[78]

CONCLUSIONS AND RECOMMENDATIONS

In many Western countries, criminal behavior is strongly associated with alcohol use, and a significant percentage of incarcerated individuals have alcohol misuse or dependence issues. However, obtaining a precise estimate of the scope of alcohol-related crime and alcohol misuse in correctional populations is challenging, particularly in resource-poor settings where neither routine surveillance nor epidemiological research is common. As mentioned previously, establishing a direct causal link between alcohol use and crime is complicated by the presence of many other variables influencing involvement with crime, such as other drug use, poor anger management and conflict resolution skills, and mental health issues.[79] Second, many empirical studies do not distinguish between alcohol and other drug use, instead relying on generic reports of substance use, misuse, and/or dependence. More generally, there is wide variability in the measurement of alcohol use, misuse, or dependence across studies and programs, and many evaluations do not use standardized, validated measures. Further, most follow-up assessments are relatively brief and may not capture longer-term patterns of alcohol consumption. Finally, in contrast to the observation that most of the global population consumes alcohol and does so safely,[1] treatment programs for correctional populations are predominantly abstinence-only focused. Such programs may be unrealistic given the widespread use of alcohol in non-incarcerated settings.

Similarly, assessing the effectiveness of alcohol use reduction programs in correctional systems is difficult as many programs prioritize drug use reduction as a primary goal. Further, even within program classifications (eg, behavioral therapy), there are wide differences across correctional settings in the availability of services, the quality of those services, and the fidelity of their delivery.[67,80,81] Relatedly, given the limited treatment resources available in many correctional systems,[82] there is a need to develop effective systems for identifying not only those most in need of treatment but also those who are most likely to respond positively to treatment and avoid relapse to alcohol misuse or dependence after release. If a triage system is used, then screening needs to be conducted using reliable and valid assessment tools with clear and defensible cut-offs for referral to treatment services while incarcerated.

There are unique advantages to treating alcohol misuse and dependence within a correctional system, including mandated attendance at regularly scheduled treatment sessions, restricted alcohol supply, and the relative ease of medical treatment access and follow-up. At the same time, this artificial "alcohol-free" environment cannot offer practice in handling precisely the same triggers that a person will encounter after release into the community. Furthermore, particularly in short-term facilities, treatment disruption or termination is likely if a connection to care on the outside is not facilitated. To realize long-term gains, it is necessary to provide resources in the community for long-term treatment options for sustained follow-up and avoidance of relapse to alcohol misuse and dependence.[57,58] Social workers and community organizations can play an important role in facilitating linkage to care on the outside prior to release, and coordinating wraparound services after release to help address competing needs and priorities (eg, transportation, housing, access to health care).[83,84] Assisting people to maintain sobriety or manage their alcohol consumption following release can help them to avoid recidivism, obtain and maintain employment, and facilitate positive social relationships.[75,77,83,84] Successful reintegration, including continued substance use treatment after release, has been shown to reduce recidivism and reduce societal costs.[33,85]

There are also challenges to alcohol use treatment access for people who have not yet been sentenced, are under community corrections supervision, or are released to transitional treatment programs. Although drug court diversion and other community treatment programs have shown success and can be cost-effective relative to incarceration,[72] they often are met with resistance by criminal justice staff (eg, judges, probation or parole officers, and prosecutors) in many judicial settings. Studies are needed to rigorously evaluate these programs and their cost-effectiveness in relation to incarcerating people whose primary crime is related to drug or alcohol misuse. Even when effective diversion programs are operating, they may be undermined by people's reluctance to enroll in and remain involved in community substance use programs, as well as by social environments that can facilitate continued risky substance use. Finally, little is known about effective treatments for those with co-occurring alcohol use disorders and mental illness, particularly within correctional systems.[86,87]

REFERENCES

1. Rehm J. Alcohol and global health 1—global burden of disease and injury and economic cost attributable to alcohol use and alcohol-use disorders. *Lancet*. 2009;373(9682):2223–2233.
2. Corrao G, Bagnardi V, Zambon A, La Vecchia C. A meta-analysis of alcohol consumptionand the risk of 15 diseases. *Prev Med*. 2004;38(5):613–619.
3. Mohd Hanafiah K, Groeger J, Flaxman AD, Wiersma ST. Global epidemiology of hepatitis C virus infection: new estimates of age-specific antibody to HCV seroprevalence. *Hepatology*. 2013;57(4):1333–1342.
4. World Health Organization. *Global Status Report on Alcohol and Health 2014*. Luxembourg City, Luxembourg: World Health Organization; 2014.
5. Fazel S, Bains P, Doll H. Substance abuse and dependence in prisoners: a systematic review. *Addiction*. 2006;101(2):181–191.
6. Weatherburn, DJ. The role of drug and alcohol policy in reducing Indigenous over-representation in prison. *Drug Alcohol Rev*. 2008;27(1):91–94.
7. Calabria B, Doran C, Vos T, Shakeshaft A, Hall W. Epidemiology of alcohol-related burden of disease among Indigenous Australians. *Aust N Z J Public Health*. 2010;34(suppl 1):s47–s51.
8. Booth BM, Curran GM, Han X, Edlund MJ. Criminal justice and alcohol treatment: results from a national sample. *J Subst Abuse Treat*. 2013;44(3):249–255.
9. Centers for Disease Control and Prevention. *HIV in Correctional Settings CS233254*. Atlanta, GA: Centers for Disease Control and Prevention; 2012.
10. World Health Organization. *Management of Alcohol Withdrawal*. Geneva, Switzerland: World Health Organization; 2012.
11. Australian National Council on Drugs. *Prison vs. Residential Treatment: An Economic Analysis for Aboriginal and Torres Strait Islander Offenders*. Canberra, Australia: ANCD; 2013.
12. Rand MR, Sabol WJ, Sinclair M, Snyder H. *Alcohol and Crime: Data from 2002 to 2008*. Washington, DC: Bureau of Justice Statistics; 2010.
13. Makkai T, Payne J. *Key Findings From the Drug Use Careers of Offenders (DUCO) Study*. Canberra, Australia: Australian Institute of Criminology; 2003.
14. Boden JM, Fergusson DM, Horwood LJ. Alcohol misuse and criminal offending: findings from a 30-year longitudinal study. *Drug Alcohol Depend*. 2013;128(1-2):30–36.
15. Centers for Disease Control and Prevention. Vital signs: drinking and driving among high school students aged >/=16 years—United States, 1991–2011. *MMWR Morb Mortal Wkly Rep*. 2012;61(5):796–800.
16. Franklin FA, Laveist TA, Webster DW, Pan WK. Alcohol outlets and violent crime in Washington DC. *West J Emerg Med*. 2010;11(3):283–290.
17. Gruenewald PE, Freisthler B, Remer L, LaScala EA, Treno A. Ecological models of alcohol outlets and violent assaults: crime potentials and geospatial analysis. *Addiction*. 2006;101(5):666–677.
18. Scribner RA, MacKinnon DP, Dwyer JH. The risk of assaultive violence and alcohol availability in Los Angeles County. *Am J Public Health*. 1995;85(3):335–340.
19. Speer G, LaBouvie G. Spatial dynamics of alcohol availability, neighborhood structure and violent crime. *J Stud Alcohol Drugs*. 2001;62(5):628–636.
20. Livingston M. Alcohol outlet density and assault: a spatial analysis. *Addiction*. 2008;103(4):619–628.

21. Livingston M. A longitudinal analysis of alcohol outlet density and domestic violence. *Addiction*. 2011;106(5):919–925.
22. Livingston M. Alcohol outlet density and harm: comparing the impacts on violence and chronic harms. *Drug Alcohol Rev*. 2011;30(5):515–523.
23. Babor TF, Higgins Biddle JC, Saunders JB, Monteiro MG. *AUDIT: The Alcohol Use Disorders Identification Test: Guidelines for Use in Primary Care*. Geneva, Switzerland: World Health Organization Department of Mental Health and Substance Dependence; 2001.
24. World Health Organization. *Alcohol Problems in the Criminal Justice System- Opportunities for Intervention, Alcohol and Crime*. Geneva, Switzerland: World Health Organization; 2012.
25. Kinner SA, Dietze PM, Gouilloi M, Alati R. Prevalence and correlates of alcohol dependence in adult prisoners vary according to Indigenous status. *Aust N Z J Public Health*. 2012;36(4):329–334.
26. Indig D, Topp L, Ross B, et al. *2009 NSW Inmate Health Survey: Key Findings Report*. Sydney, Australia: Justice Health NSW; 2010.
27. El-Bassel N, Ivanoff A., Schilling RF, Gilbert L, Chen DR. Correlates of problem drinking among drug-using incarcerated women. *Addict Behav*. 1995;20(3):359–369.
28. Mullings JL, Hartley DJ, Marquart JW. Exploring the relationship between alcohol use, childhood maltreatment, and treatment needs among female prisoners. *Subst Use Misuse*. 2004;39(2):277–305.
29. Lown EA, Nayak MB, Korcha RA, Greenfield TK. Child physical and sexual abuse: a comprehensive look at alcohol consumption patterns, consequences, and dependence from the National Alcohol Survey. *Alcohol Clin Exp Res*. 2011;35(2):317–325.
30. Schraufnagel TJ, Davis KC, George WH, Norris J. Childhood sexual abuse in males and subsequent risky sexual behavior: a potential alcohol-use pathway. *Child Abuse Negl*. 2010;34(5):369–378.
31. Sartor CE, Waldron M, Duncan AE, et al. Childhood sexual abuse and early substance use in adolescent girls: the role of familial influences. *Addiction*. 2013;108(5):993–1000.
32. Tripodi SJ, Pettus-Davis C. Histories of childhood victimization and subsequent mental health problems, substance use, and sexual victimization for a sample of incarcerated women in the US. *Int J Law Psychiatry*. 2013;36(1):30–40.
33. Karlberg JC, James DJ. *Substance Dependence, Abuse, and Treatment of Jail Inmates, 2002*. Washington, DC: US Department of Justice; 2005.
34. Shin SH, Edwards EM, Heeren T. Child abuse and neglect: relations to adolescent binge drinking in the National Longitudinal Study of Adolescent Health (AddHealth) Study. *Addict Behav*. 2009;34(3):277–280.
35. Fone DL, Farewell DM, White J, Lyons RA, Dunstan FD. Socioeconomic patterning of excess alcohol consumption and binge drinking: a cross-sectional study of multi level associations with neighborhood deprivation. *BMJ Open*. 2013;3(4):1–9.
36. Giskes K, Turrell G, Bentley R, Kavanagh A. Individual and household-level socioeconomic position is associated with harmful alcholol consumption behaviours among adults. *Aust N Z J Public Health*. 2011;35(3):270–277.
37. Huckle T, You RQ, Casswell S. Socio-economic status predicts drinking patterns but not alcohol related consequences independently. *Addiction*. 2010;105(7):1192–1202.
38. Grittner U, Kuntsche S, Graham K, Bloomfield K. Social inequalities and gender differences in the experience of alcohol-related problems. *Alcohol*. 2012;47(5):597–605.
39. Seale JP, Seale JD, Alvarado M, Vogel RL, Terry NE. Prevalence of problem drinking in a Venezuelan Native American population. *Alcohol Alcoholism*. 2002;37(2):198–204.
40. Room R, Jernigan D, Carlini-Marlatt B, et al. *Alcohol and Developing Societies: A Public Health Approach*. Geneva, Switzerland: World Health Organization and Finnish Foundation for Alcohol Studies; 2002.

41. Binswanger IA, Merrill JO, Krueger PM, White MC, Booth RE, Elmore JG. Gender differences in chronic medical, psychiatric, and substance-dependence disorders among jail inmates. *Am J Public Health*. 2010;100(3):476–482.
42. Australian Institute of Health and Welfare. *The Health of Australia's Prisoners 2012*. Cat. no. PHE 170. Canberra, Australia: AIHW; 2013.
43. Smith N, Trimboli L. Comorbid substance and non-substance mental health disorders and re-offending among NSW prisoners. *Crime Just Bull*. 2010;140:1–16.
44. James DGL. *Mental Health Problems of Prison and Jail Inmates*. NCJ 213600. Washington, DC: US Department of Justice; 2006.
45. Brinded P, Simpson A, Laidlaw T, Fairley N, Malcolm F. Prevalence of psychiatric disorders in New Zealand prisons: a national study. *Aust N Z J Psychiatry*. 2001;35(2):166–173.
46. MacAskill S, Parkes T, Brooks O, et al. Assessment of alcohol problems using AUDIT in a prison setting: more than an "aye or no" question. *BMC Public Health*. 2011;11(865):1–12.
47. Lukasiewicz M, Falissard B, Michel L, et al. Prevalence and factors associated with alcohol and drug-related disorders in prison: a French national study. *Subst Abuse Treat Prev Policy*. 2007;2(1):1–10.
48. Centers for Disease Control and Prevention. Botulism from drinking prison-made illicit alcohol—Utah 2011. *MMWR Morb Mortal Wkly Rep*. 2012;61(39):782–784.
49. Vugia DJ, Mase SR, Cole B, et al. Botulism from drinking pruno. *Emerg Infect Dis*. 2009;15(1):69–71.
50. Centers for Disease Control and Prevention. Notes from the field: botulism from drinking prison-made illicit alcohol—Arizona, 2012. *MMWR Morb Mortal Wkly Rep*. 2013;62(5):88.
51. Lachenmeier DW, Monakhova YB, Markova M, Kuballa T, Rehm J. What happens if people start drinking mouthwash as surrogate alcohol? a quantitative risk assessment. *Food Chem Toxicol*. 2012;51:173–178.
52. Seal DW, Margolis AD, Morrow KM, et al. Substance use and sexual behavior during incarceration among 18- to 29-year old men: prevalence and correlates. *AIDS Behav*. 2008;12(1):27–40.
53. Seal DW, Belcher L, Morrow K, et al. A qualitative study of substance use and sexual behavior among 18- to 29-year-old men while incarcerated in the United States. *Health Educ Behav*. 2004;31(6):775–789.
54. Mallik-Kane K, Visher CA. *Health and Prisoner Reentry—How Physical, Mental, and Substance Abuse Conditions Shape the Process of Reintegration*. Washington, DC: Urban Institute; 2008.
55. Visher C, Kachnowski V, La Vigne N, Travis J. *Baltimore Prisoners' Experiences Returning Home*. Washington, DC: Urban Institute; 2004.
56. Clarke JG, Anderson BJ, Stein MD. Hazardously drinking women leaving jail: time to first drink. *J Correct Health Care*. 2011;17(1):61–68.
57. Binswanger IA, Nowels C, Corsi KF, et al. Return to drug use and overdose after release from prison: a qualitative study of risk and protective factors. *Addict Sci Clin Pract*. 2012;7(3):1–9.
58. Seal DW, Eldrige GD, Kacanek D, Binson D, MacGowan RJ. A longitudinal, qualitative analysis of the context of substance use and sexual behavior among 18-29 year old men after their release from prison. *Soc Sci Med*. 2007;65(11):2394–2406.
59. Taxman FS, Perdoni ML, Harrison, LD. Drug treatment services for adult offenders: the state of the state. *J Subst Abuse Treat*. 2007;32(3):239–254.
60. Rosner S, Leucht S, Lehert P, Soyka M. Acamprosate supports abstinence, naltrexone prevents excessive drinking: evidence from a meta-analysis with unreported outcomes. *J Psychopharmacol*. 2008;22(1):11–23.
61. Fiscella K, Pless N, Meldrum S, Fiscella P. Alcohol and opiate withdrawal in US jails. *Am J Public Health*. 2004;94(9):1522–1524.

62. Rosner S, Hackl-Herrwerth A, Leucht S, et al. Acamprosate for alcohol dependence. *Cochrane Database Syst Rev.* 2010;9:CD004332.
63. Soyka M, Rosner S. Emerging drugs to treat alcoholism. *Expert Opin Emerg Drugs.* 2010;15(4):695–711.
64. Laaksonen E, Koski-Jannes A, Salaspuro M, Ahtinen H, Alho H. A randomized, multicentre, open-label, comparative trial of disulfiram, naltrexone and acamprosate in the treatment of alcohol dependence. *Alcohol Alcohol.* 2007;43(1):53–61.
65. DeSousa A, DeSousa A. A one-year pragmatic trial of naltrexone vs disulfiram in the treatment of alcohol dependence. *Alcohol Alcohol.* 2004;39(6):528–531.
66. DeSousa A, DeSousa A. An open trial comparing disulfiram and acamprosate in the treatment of alcohol dependence. *Alcohol Alcohol.* 2005;40(6):545–548.
67. Friedmann P, Hoskinson R, Gordon M, et al. Medication assisted treatment in criminal justice agencies affiliated with the Criminal Justice–Drug Abuse Treatment Studies (CJ-DATS): availability, barriers, and intentions. *Subst Abuse.* 2012;33(1):9–18.
68. Smedslund G, Berg RC, Hammerstrom KT, et al. Motivational interviewing for substance abuse. *Cochrane Database Syst Rev.* 2011;CD008063.
69. Foxcroft DR, Coombes L, Wood S, Allen D, Almeida Santimano NM. Motivational interviewing for alcohol misuse in young adults. *Cochrane Database Syst Rev.* 2014;8:CD007025.
70. Stein LA, Lebeau R, Colby SM, et al. Motivational interviewing for incarcerated adolescents: effects of depressive symptoms on reducing alcohol and marijuana use after release. *J Stud Alcohol Drugs.* 2011;72(3):497–506.
71. Kaner EF, Dickinson HO, Beyer F, et al. The effectiveness of brief alcohol interventions in primary care settings: a systematic review. *Drug Alcohol Rev.* 2009;28(3):301–323.
72. Belenko S, Hiller M, Hamilton L. Treating substance use disorders in the criminal justice system. *Curr Psychiatry Rep.* 2013;15(11):414.
73. Smith LA, Gates S, Foxcroft D. Therapeutic communities for substance related disorder. *Cochrane Database Syst Rev.* 2006;Cd005338.
74. Ferri M, Amato L, Davoli M. Alcoholics Anonymous and other 12-step programmes for alcohol dependence. *Cochrane Database Syst Rev.* 2006;19:3.
75. Harrison L, Butzin C, Inciardi J, Martin S. Integrating HIV prevention strategies in a therapeutic community work-release program for criminal offenders. *Prison Journal.* 1998;78(3):232–243.
76. Martin S, Butzin C, Inciardi J. Assessment of a multistage therapeutic community for drug involved offenders. *J Psychoactive Drugs.* 1995;27(1):109–116.
77. Ritchie B, Freudenberg N, Page J. Reintegrating women leaving jail into urban communities: a description of a model program. *J Urban Health.* 2001;78(2):290–303
78. Australian National Council on Drugs. *An Economic Analysis for Aboriginal and Torres Strait Islander Offenders: Prison Versus Residential Treatment.* Canberra, Australia: ANCD;2012.
79. Seal DW, Margolis AD, Kacanek D, Binson D. HIV and STD risk behavior among 18-25 year old men released from U.S. prisons: provider perspectives. *AIDS Behav.* 2003;7(2):131–141.
80. Sung HE, Mahoney A, Mellow J. Substance abuse treatment gap among adult parolees: prevalence, correlates and barriers. *Crim Just Rev.* 2011;36(1):40–57.
81. Dixon PS, Flanigan TP, DeBuono BA, et al. Infection with the human immunodeficiency virus in prisoners: meeting the health care challenge. *Am J Med.* 1993;95(6):629–635.
82. McMurran M. What works in substance misuse treatments for offenders? *Crim Behav Ment Health.* 2007;17(4):225–233.
83. Turley A, Thornton T, Johnson C, Azzolino S. Jail drug and alcohol treatment program reduces recidivism in nonviolent offenders: a longitudinal study of Monroe

County, New York's jail treatment drug and alcohol program. *Int J Offender Ther Comp Criminol.* 2004;48(6):721–728.

84. Wexler HK, Magura S, Beardsley MM, Josepher H. ARRIVE: an AIDS education/relapse prevention model for high risk parolees. *Int J Addictions.* 1994;29(3):361–386.

85. McCollister K, Prendergast M, Wexler H, Sacks S. Is in-prison treatment enough? a cost-effectiveness analysis of prison-based treatment and aftercare services for substance-abusing offenders. *Law Policy.* 2003;25(1):63–82.

86. Hunt GE, Siegfried N, Morley K, Sitharthan T, Cleary M. Psychosocial interventions for people with both severe mental illness and substance misuse. *Cochrane Database Syst Rev.* 2013;10:CD001088.

87. Perry AE, Neilson M, Martyn-St James M, et al. Interventions for drug-using offenders with co-occurring mental illness. *Cochrane Database Syst Rev.* 2014;1:CD010901.

CHAPTER 5

Tobacco Use Among Prisoners

JENNIFER CLARKE, MD AND MANASA REDDY, MPH

EPIDEMIOLOGY AND BURDEN OF TOBACCO SMOKING IN CORRECTIONAL POPULATIONS

Tobacco smoking is known to be a major risk factor for a wide range of illnesses: cardiovascular disease, chronic obstructive pulmonary disease, oral disease, and various cancers.[1] It is the leading cause of preventable deaths in the developed world, with 6 million deaths attributable to smoking-related illness globally and 480,000 in the United States each year.[1,2] Nicotine dependence, like most addictions, is a chronically relapsing condition, and most people require multiple quit attempts before they are able to achieve sustained abstinence.[3]

Despite substantial reductions in tobacco smoking rates in many developed countries in recent years, the practice remains highly prevalent, and even normative in the same countries' correctional populations. A recent systematic review found that the prevalence of smoking among detainees in the United States, Australia, and Europe ranged from 64% to 92%, approximately three times as high as in these regions' general populations.[4] In surveys of inmates in the United States in 2005, 38.2% of state and federal inmates reported smoking in the month prior to their arrest.[5] Consequently, tobacco-related illnesses are a significant cause of death among people released from prison.[6]

Given the large proportion of smokers that passes through prisons (one in eight smokers in the United States each year),[7] as well as the high risk and costs of smoking-related illnesses,[8] correctional systems have both the opportunity and an obligation to address this significant public health problem.

Correlates of Smoking

Why are cigarette smokers disproportionately represented in incarcerated populations? In the general population, tobacco smoking is more prevalent in the same disadvantaged groups that are over-represented in corrections: those with mental illness,[9] people who use and inject drugs,[10,11] the poor,[12-14] and individuals with low educational attainment.[13,15,16]

Certain mental illnesses that are disproportionately represented in the prisoner population (eg, post-traumatic stress disorder [PTSD], schizophrenia, and bipolar disorder) are also associated with particularly high rates of smoking. PTSD carries a 30% to 70% lifetime smoking prevalence rate.[17] Among those with schizophrenia, the lifetime prevalence of smoking is 90%.[17] The mechanisms underlying the link between schizophrenia and smoking are unclear, but current research suggests a few possible reasons: nicotine may have a stronger reinforcing effect on patients with schizophrenia, may reduce symptoms of schizophrenia, and, as in the general population, relaxes smokers.[18,19]

Because the same environmental, genetic, and chemical factors are linked to different kinds of addictions, people who smoke often use other drugs as well, ranging from alcohol to injection drugs. For example, smoking rates among those with alcohol use disorders have been estimated at between 78% and 90% in the United States.[20,21] These comorbid addictions place individuals at increased risk for cancers and cardiovascular disease and can cause tobacco addiction treatment to fall by the wayside. Clarke et al. found that among a sample of women in a correctional facility in Rhode Island, those who met criteria for alcohol abuse or dependence in the past 6 months were less likely to be interested in smoking cessation.[22] Indig et al. found that, among male prisoners who participated in a smoking cessation intervention in an Australian prison facility, more than half (56.5%) reported using heroin prior to incarceration.[23] Those who reported heroin use prior to incarceration had poorer smoking cessation outcomes compared with those who did not report heroin use.

Globally, incarcerated individuals are more likely to be poor and to have lower educational attainment. Both of these characteristics are associated with smoking. A 2014 systematic review of the relationship between smoking and poverty by the World Health Organization found a significant association between lower income and smoking (odds ratio [OR] 1.45; 95% confidence interval [95%CI] 1.35–1.55).[24] This effect was stronger in countries with lower mortality (OR 1.48; 95%CI 1.37–1.60) and among women (OR 1.59; 95%CI 1.30–1.93). A 2011 analysis of World Health Survey results from 48 low- and middle-income countries also found higher odds of smoking in men in the lowest-income groups relative to the highest, in both low-income countries (adjusted odds ratio [AOR] 1.67; 95%CI 1.37–2.04) and middle-income countries (AOR 1.36; 95%CI 1.19–1.56), and in women in low-income countries (AOR 2.10; 95%CI 1.30–3.39).[25] People of low socioeconomic status may be more likely to smoke because they may not have health insurance or financial resources to access health care providers who can advise them to stop smoking or provide smoking cessation treatment. Smoking may also serve as a way of coping with the stresses of poverty and may be seen as an acceptable indulgence.

In developed settings such as Australia, Western Europe, and the United States, cigarette smoking is more prevalent in populations with lower educational attainment: in a study of smoking prevalence in nine Western European countries, smoking was twice as common among women at the lowest education level as among those at the highest education level (31.49% vs. 16.61%) and 1.6 times more prevalent among men at the lowest educational level than among men at the highest education level.[26-28] The New England Family Study in the United States found that individuals with less than a high school education smoked a greater number of pack-years (risk ratio [RR] 1.58; 95%CI 1.31–1.91), were less likely to quit smoking (OR 0.34; 95%CI 0.19–0.62), and made fewer quit attempts.[26] However, the authors note that it is unclear whether these relationships are causal. The analysis of World Health Survey results from low- and middle-income countries cited earlier found that respondents were more likely to report smoking if they had little to no education.[25]

Drivers of Smoking in Prison Populations

In addition to mental illness, substance use, poverty, and low educational attainment, triggering factors and pro-smoking social norms are important risk factors for smoking.[29,30]

The stresses of the prison environment can exacerbate the perceived need to smoke: in Sieminska et al.'s survey of nearly 1,000 male inmates in Polish prisons, 75% of respondents reported a greater need to smoke in prison than they did in the community.[31] The most commonly cited factors behind increased smoking in prisons were missing family and friends (66%), lack of freedom (57%), and other factors related to anxiety, boredom due to lack of other drugs or sex, and poor relations with staff and fellow inmates.[31] The desire to save money and the limited availability of cigarettes were cited as motivating factors to quit by 21% to 24% of respondents.[31] Conversely, concern for one's own health has been cited as a factor that encourages smoking cessation among many prisoners. Surveys of prisoners in the United States find that most (70%) report a desire to quit, with 63% reporting an intention to quit in the coming year, and the majority are knowledgeable that smoking increases the risks of cancer and cardiovascular disease.[32] This level of intention to quit is comparable to that in the general population: 69% of smokers in the general US population report wanting to quit.[33]

However, even though most prisoners report a desire to quit, in the absence of smoking bans, few actually do so. This may be due to the psychological roles cigarettes and cigarette smoking play in these settings. First, smokers often use smoking as a strategy to cope with daily stresses both in confinement and in the community, although in fact smoking cessation has been found to reduce stress.[34] Second, smoking provides a way to socialize and build social capital or express solidarity with peer groups, who might otherwise stigmatize an individual, further exacerbating the challenges of incarceration.[35] Cigarettes may be shared as payment or expression of solidarity. Finally, some prisoners see smoking as an expression of independence in confinement.[36]

Smoking Policies and Cessation Services in Prisons

Historically, cigarettes have played a social and economic role in prison culture. In recent years, however, particularly given the threat of litigation due to second-hand smoke exposure (as in *Helling v. McKinney* in 1993), correctional institutions have increasingly adopted smoke-free policies.[37-39] Smoking bans may be total or partial (ie, limited to designated places only, such as outdoor spaces). New Zealand and most Canadian provinces have instituted total bans across all correctional facilities.[40,41] In Australia complete smoking bans have been implemented in prisons in five jurisdictions, with partial bans in the remaining three.[42] In a 2007 survey of US correctional facilities, 60% of all systems reported total bans, and 27% reported indoor bans.[43]

In facilities with total bans, incoming smokers undergo periods of forced abstinence. In some systems the institution of smoke-free policies has been accompanied by the discontinuation of smoking cessation programs. In the same 2007 survey of US correctional facilities cited above, 86% of systems with indoor tobacco bans reported tobacco cessation programs, whereas few with total bans (39%) reported offering sustained programming beyond the initial transitional phase.[43]

Even if individuals spend years in smoke-free facilities, the majority relapse to smoking after release.[44,45] While studies of smoking relapse after release have been relatively limited, studies of people leaving smoke-free correctional facilities have found overwhelmingly high rates of relapse, with rates increasing over time: in Lincoln et al.'s 2009 study of 165 individuals who smoked at the time of incarceration in a tobacco-free facility, nearly 97% reported relapse by follow-up at 6 months after release, compared with 86% at 1 month after release.[7] Enforced tobacco abstinence allows for the completion of the physical withdrawal from nicotine but does not address the behavioral or social motivations or triggers behind the activity of smoking in a way that can sustain abstinence after release. Efforts in facilities with smoking bans should therefore focus on these facets to maintain abstinence after release. Strategies to address these facets are considered later in this chapter. Even with high relapse rates, the benefits of tobacco-free facilities are substantial, by eliminating environmental exposures as well as total lifetime exposure.

In individuals who have undergone forced tobacco abstinence in tobacco-free facilities, half the battle is already won. Given the high risk of relapse after release, emphasis should be placed on addressing the behavioral factors that contribute to relapse independent of chemical dependence. Particularly because justice-involved populations are hard to find and follow in the community, and generally have poorer access to health care than the general population, the correctional setting offers an opportunity to more easily monitor adherence, offer support, and reinforce the importance of smoking cessation. Public health authorities should capitalize on this opportunity to thoroughly and comprehensively address this important issue when the odds of success are considerably increased.

THERAPEUTIC OPTIONS

Although smoking is known to be widespread among correctional populations, relative to the study of other addictions, little research has been published on interventions to address smoking or their effectiveness in this population.

Many public health authorities including the World Health Organization recommend smoke-free environments as well as smoking cessation interventions for inmates.[46] While one study found that among female smokers in Rhode Island, those with multiple incarcerations were less likely to want to quit (odds ratio 0.1; 95% confidence interval 0.01–0.44),[47] high interest in quitting has been documented among prisoners in Australia,[48-50] female prisoners in the southern[51] and northeastern[47] United States, and people who inject drugs.[22] Facilities should capitalize on this time of high interest and offer smoking cessation services. After an overview of the most effective therapies available, we discuss their application in correctional settings.

Approaches

In facilities that permit smoking, and in those that impose enforced abstinence, the approach to smoking cessation should be similar to that in the community. In smoke-free facilities there is no evidence to suggest benefit from the use of pharmacological interventions, and behavioral interventions need to be modified to focus on the prevention of post-release return to smoking.

Pharmacological Approaches to Smoking Cessation. The most commonly used pharmacological aids for smoking cessation available in the community can be grouped into the following categories: (1) nicotine replacement therapy (NRT), for example, the nicotine transdermal patch; (2) antidepressants, such as bupropion and nortriptyline; and (3) partial nicotinic receptor agonists, such as varenicline and cystisine.[52] First-line pharmacotherapies for smoking cessation recommended by the American Agency for Healthcare Research and Quality and the World Health Organization include bupropion sustained release (SR) and NRT (in the form of gum, lozenges, inhalers, nasal spray, or the patch); second-line therapies include clonidine and nortriptyline.[53,54]

In facilities that permit smoking, in addition to patient preference, clinicians should also consider patients' contraindications and previous experience with pharmacotherapies and other conditions including depression. Because depression is highly prevalent in this population, the antidepressants bupropion and nortriptyline may be particularly relevant. Weight gain is also likely an important consideration,[55] particularly given that this population generally displays multiple chronic disease risk factors,[56,57] obesity a key factor among them. Depending on the security level or rules of the facility, patches or gum may not be allowed. Nicotine lozenges may pose the least security risk and the fewest compliance issues.

In a recent review of pharmacological interventions for smoking cessation by the Cochrane Tobacco Addiction Group, both bupropion and NRT yielded superior abstinence rates in the general population compared with placebo.[52] In head-to-head comparisons, bupropion and NRT were found to be equally efficacious. Furthermore, pharmacotherapies for smoking cessation have generally been shown to be cost-effective and cost-saving.[52,58] Typically, varenicline was more effective in supporting abstinence and in other analyses was found more cost-effective than bupropion in the long run.[58] However, the side effects of increased depression, agitation, and anger may make this medication problematic for smokers in correctional facilities. In addition, bupropion has been associated with false positive drug screening tests for amphetamines.[59] Pharmacological interventions are appropriate in settings where tobacco products are allowed or upon entering a facility with a complete tobacco ban. There are no studies on the effectiveness of these products for people being released from a tobacco-free facility.

Behavioral Approaches to Smoking Cessation. Motivational interviewing (MI) and cognitive behavioral therapy (CBT) are the most common and most studied behavioral approaches to smoking cessation, and they can be delivered individually or in groups. In facilities that allow smoking these interventions are very similar to those in the community. Standard community behavioral interventions for smoking cessation may not be appropriate for smoke-free facilities because the focus in the community is usually on stopping smoking.

1. *Motivational interviewing (MI)*—This approach relies on an empathic, non-confrontational style to assess the individual's readiness to change, employing reflective listening, personalized feedback, and exploration of the pros and cons of change to help individuals work through ambivalence. MI emphasizes the individual's choice to change as well as his or her self-efficacy to achieve change. MI is favored for use in individuals who may not be interested in quitting or ready to quit,[60,61] and has been used to positive effect in incarcerated and adolescent populations.[62-64]
2. *Cognitive behavioral therapy*—CBT is based on the idea that behaviors such as smoking and drinking are maladaptive coping mechanisms to restore a sense of balance. CBT trains individuals to recognize environmental events or "triggers" related to their smoking habit and respond by, for example, avoiding or modifying the situation. CBT has been studied extensively and used to positive effect in a range of populations, including incarcerated and adolescent groups.[65-68] However, given that smoke-free settings provide smokers with an artificially smoke-free environment, some strategies to address the habit (eg, delaying time between cigarettes, self-monitoring, or taking a walk) may not be possible to practice before they are needed following release.
3. *Computer and electronic aids*—Such aids have been found to increase the likelihood of cessation compared with offering self-help resources or no intervention at all; however, the effect size is small,[69] and use of these aids may not be feasible in correctional settings.

Combination Approaches. A recent meta-analysis found that people receiving a combination of counseling and medication achieved higher abstinence rates at 6 months than did those receiving either medication or counseling alone (compared with medication alone: OR 1.4; 95%CI 1.2–1.6; compared with counseling alone: OR 1.7; 95%CI 1.3–2.1).[53] However, none of the studies included in this meta-analysis were conducted in correctional settings, and therefore the findings may not be generalizable to correctional settings, particularly those with the condition of forced cessation.

SMOKING CESSATION INTERVENTIONS IN CORRECTIONAL POPULATIONS

Overall, little primary research has been published on the use or efficacy of these approaches in correctional settings. In facilities that do not have smoke-free policies, best practice for addressing addiction will be similar to community standards of medication and behavioral interventions. On a systems level, smoking bans and restrictions, increasing the costs of cigarettes, and media campaigns have all been shown to decrease smoking rates.[70]

To date, few studies of smoking cessation interventions in correctional settings have been published. These have mainly employed a combined pharmaceutical and behavioral approach and randomized controlled designs. All tailored interventions to their target populations and incorporated peer input into the design of accompanying materials. Two studies assessed whether smoking cessation interventions can have a sustained impact on people during incarceration, and one assessed relapse rates after release from a smoke free facility. A brief summary of each of these studies follows:

1. *Cropsey et al., 2008*—Between 2004 and 2006, Cropsey and colleagues enrolled 539 smoking women in a state prison in the United States into a randomized controlled trial. The women in the treatment group participated in a 10-week, weekly group intervention focused on mood management; they also received NRT with follow-up during incarceration at 3, 6, and 12 months after treatment. Those in the control group received neither.[71] Quit rates during incarceration in the intervention group were 18% immediately after the intervention, 17% at 3 months, 14% at 6 months, and 12% at 12 months (similar to community). Quit rates among control group participants, meanwhile, were approximately 0% until rising to 2.8% at 6 months.
2. *Richmond et al., 2012*—From 2006 to 2009, Richmond and colleagues enrolled 425 smoking male prisoners in New South Wales and Queensland, Australia, in a multi-component smoking cessation intervention involving CBT, NRT in the form of the nicotine transdermal patch, access to self-help guides designed by fellow inmates, and a stress kit for particularly trying situations such as court hearings.[72] The study employed a randomized placebo-controlled design to assess the impact of adding nortriptyline to the standard intervention and found that adding nortriptyline conferred no additional benefit compared with placebo in achieving long-term abstinence (here defined as continuous abstinence at 12 months). However, both intervention groups achieved continuous abstinence rates of nearly 12% at 12-month follow-up in prison and the community. Differences in abstinence rates between those who completed follow-up in the community versus in prison were not reported.

1. Many incarcerated smokers have never thought about remaining abstinent after release.
2. Participants welcomed an intervention about their health and not an illegal behavior.
3. The ride home was an important time of relapse and focus of the intervention.
4. People with social support had better outcomes.
5. CBT focused on smelling smoke on visitors and officers, noticing triggering behaviors (drinking coffee, speaking on the phone) without cigarettes, planning for the first few weeks in the community.

3. *Clarke et al., 2013*—The WISE Study Group in Rhode Island evaluated an intervention combining MI and CBT compared with an educational video in a randomized controlled trial. Participants were individuals who reported smoking prior to incarceration and were in the last 8 weeks of incarceration in a smoke-free facility. The MI and CBT intervention comprised two sessions of MI and four sessions of CBT, with sessions lasting 30 to 60 minutes each. Intervention participants were significantly more likely than control group participants to report abstinence at 3 weeks after release (OR 4.4; 95%CI 2.0–9.7).[44] This was the only study in our review to assess the impact of interventions on post-release smoking rates. The lower abstinence rate (7%) observed in the control group at follow-up compared with the treatment group (25%) suggests that forced withdrawal alone is insufficient to address the behavioral or social motivations behind smoking. Key components and observations from the WISE intervention are presented in Box 5.1. The quit rates observed in that study are similar to quit rates in community samples; however, the high relapse rates suggest a need for ongoing support in the community.

CHALLENGES TREATING TOBACCO ADDICTION IN PRISON

Treating smoking and addiction always has its challenges, but a few issues are unique to or more pronounced in correctional settings:

1. *Socio-cultural role of tobacco smoking*—Cigarettes are ingrained in prison culture and in the prison economy as currency[73,74] or as tokens in social networks, as a way of managing the stress of the environment,[74] and for their anti-depressive properties. Because of their use as currency in correctional settings, taking away cigarettes can be akin to taking away inmates' money or means of trade. Furthermore, pro-smoking social environments (or those in which smoking is normative) are an important risk factor for both initiating and relapsing to

smoking.[29,30] In facilities that permit smoking, cigarettes may be used as a tool in managing the stresses of daily life in prison as well as other times such as court dates.[31,74-76]

2. *Comorbid illness*—Smokers in correctional settings often suffer from other comorbid illnesses, including other substance use disorders,[5] which can exacerbate the difficulties of smoking cessation.[23,77] Among inmates in a multi-component smoking cessation intervention in Australia, for example, those who did not regularly use heroin in the year before their imprisonment had more than five times greater odds of reporting continuous abstinence from smoking at 12 months, compared with those who did regularly use heroin.[23]

3. *Underestimation of the problem*—Inmates and their providers may dismiss tobacco smoking as a minor problem in comparison with violence risk, recidivism, unemployment, relapse risk to other drugs, and other pressing issues. Some research suggests that providers may be subtly reinforcing the habit by not asking prisoners whether they want to quit, possibly due to the assumption that disadvantaged people do not want to quit or that cigarette smoking is a minor problem in comparison to the other problems they face.[78] Although smoking may be a less pressing issue, this is not an adequate justification to ignore the problem.

4. *Re-entry into the community*—Re-entry poses a radical and often hectic change in setting and exposure to triggers, meaning that released individuals may relapse to smoking as a way to restore a sense of balance; because smoke-free facilities provide an artificial environment in many ways, some CBT strategies for managing smoking habits and dealing with triggers may not apply. For example, in the correctional setting, one is much less likely to encounter many real-world triggers (eg, driving, drinking, a party, being around smokers), and a coping strategy such as taking a walk may be restricted due to facility schedules. Smoke-free facilities therefore may not provide practice for dealing with real-world triggers after release. Ensuring that released smokers are familiar with how to access self-help resources or quit lines in the community and can easily do so may be particularly important.[36]

It has also been suggested that some smokers may associate smoking with freedom and see the act of smoking is a way of exerting one's independence. A survey of inmates in a smoke-free facility in Rhode Island found that those who associated smoking with freedom were more likely to have resumed smoking at two weeks post release than inmates who did not ($r = .134, p = .057$).[36] The authors point to US Department of Health data that indicate more than 90% of adult smokers begin smoking as adolescents, when they see smoking as a way of rebelling against authority, and suggest that these associations may persist into adulthood.[79-81]

5. *Lack of evidence*—With little evidence supporting the effectiveness of smoking cessation programs in prisons, administrators may be reluctant to pay for such programs. Development of evidence-based interventions targeting this population may help expand the implementation of smoking cessation programs in prisons.

REFERENCES

1. Surgeon General's Office. *The Health Consequences of Smoking—50 Years of Progress.* Atlanta, GA: Surgeon General's Office, CDC; 2014.
2. World Health Organization. *Tobacco Fact Sheet N°339.* Geneva, Switzerland: World Health Organization; 2014.
3. Chaiton M, Diemert L, Cohen JE, et al. Estimating the number of quit attempts it takes to quit smoking successfully in a longitudinal cohort of smokers. *BMJ.* 2016;6(6):e011045.
4. Ritter C, Stover H, Levy M, Etter JF, Elger B. Smoking in prisons: the need for effective and acceptable interventions. *J Public Health Policy.* 2011;32(1):32–45.
5. National Center on Addiction and Substance Abuse at Columbia University (CASA). *Behind Bars II—Substance Abuse and America's Prison Population.* New York, NY: CASA; 2010.
6. Binswanger IA, Stern MF, Deyo RA, et al. Release from prison—a high risk of death for former inmates. *N Engl J Med.* 2007;356(2):157–165.
7. Lincoln T, Tuthill RW, Roberts CA, et al. Resumption of smoking after release from a tobacco-free correctional facility. *J Correct Health Care.* 2009;15(3):190–196.
8. Max W, Rice DP, Sung HY, Zhang X, Miller L. The economic burden of smoking in California. *Tob Control.* 2004;13(3):264–267.
9. Centers for Disease Control and Prevention. Vital signs: current cigarette smoking among adults aged >/=18 years with mental illness—United States, 2009–2011. *MMWR Morb Mortal Wkly Rep.* 2013;62(5):81–87.
10. Villanti A, German D, Sifakis F, Flynn C, Holtgrave D. Smoking, HIV status, and HIV risk behaviors in a respondent-driven sample of injection drug users in Baltimore, Maryland: The BeSure Study. *AIDS Educ Prev.* 2012;24(2):132–147.
11. Marshall MM, Kirk GD, Caporaso NE, et al. Tobacco use and nicotine dependence among HIV-infected and uninfected injection drug users. *Addict Behav.* 2011;36(1–2):61–67.
12. Flint AJ, Novotny TE. Poverty status and cigarette smoking prevalence and cessation in the United States, 1983–1993: the independent risk of being poor. *Tob Control.* 1997;6(1):14–18.
13. Agaku IT KB, Dube SR. Current cigarette smoking among adults—United States, 2005–2012. *MMWR Morb Mortal Wkly Rep.* 2014;63(2).
14. Laaksonen M, Rahkonen O, Karvonen S, Lahelma E. Socioeconomic status and smoking: analysing inequalities with multiple indicators. *Eur J Pub Health.* 2005;15(3):262–269.
15. Palipudi KM, Gupta PC, Sinha DN, Andes LJ, Asma S, McAfee T. Social determinants of health and tobacco use in thirteen low and middle income countries: evidence from Global Adult Tobacco Survey. *PLos ONE.* 2012;7(3):e33466.
16. Centers for Disease Control and Prevention. Vital signs: current cigarette smoking among adults aged >or=18 years—United States, 2009. *MMWR Morb Mortal Wkly Rep.* 2010;59(35):1135–1140.
17. Aubin HJ, Rollema H, Svensson TH, Winterer G. Smoking, quitting, and psychiatric disease: a review. *Neurosci Biobehav Rev.* 2012;36(1):271–284.
18. Tidey JW, Miller ME. Smoking cessation and reduction in people with chronic mental illness. *BMJ Open.* 2015;351:1–13.
19. National Institute on Drug Abuse. *Comorbidity: Addiction and Other Mental Illnesses.* Bethesda, MD: National Institute on Drug Abuse; 2008.
20. Drobes DJ. *Concurrent Alcohol and Tobacco Dependence: Mechanisms and Treatment.* Bethesda, MD: National Institute on Alcohol Abuse and Alcoholism; 2002.
21. Falk DE, Yi, H.Y., Hiller-Sturmhofel, S. An epidemiologic analysis of co-occurring alcohol and tobacco use and disorders: findings from the National Epidemiologic Survey on Alcohol and Related Conditions. *Alcohol Res Health.* 2006;29(3):162–171.

22. Clarke JG, Stein MD, McGarry KA, Gogineni A. Interest in smoking cessation among injection drug users. *Am J Addict.* 2001;10(2):159–166.
23. Indig D, Wodak AD, Richmond RL, Butler TG, Archer VA, Wilhelm KA. Heroin use impairs smoking cessation among Australian prisoners. *BMC Public Health.* 2013;13(1200):1–8.
24. Ciapponi A, Bardach, A., Glujovsky, D., et al. *Systematic Review of the Link Between Tobacco and Poverty—2014 Update.* Geneva, Switzerland: World Health Organization; 2014.
25. Hosseinpoor AR, Parker, L.A., d'Espaignet, ET, Chatterji, S. Social determinants of smoking in low- and middle-income countries: results from the World Health Survey. *PLoS ONE.* 2011;6(5):1–7.
26. Gilman SE, Martin LT, Abrams DB, et al. Educational attainment and cigarette smoking: a causal association? *Int J Epidemiol.* 2008;37(3):615–624.
27. Giskes K, Kunst AE, Benach J, et al. Trends in smoking behaviour between 1985 and 2000 in nine European countries by education. *J Epidemiol Community Health.* 2005;59(5):395–401.
28. Degenhardt L, Hall W. *The Relationship Between Tobacco Use, Substance Use Disorders and Mental Disorders: Results from the National Survey of Mental Health and Well-Being.* Sydney, Australia: NDARC; 1999.
29. Cropsey KL, Linker JA, Waite DE. An analysis of racial and sex differences for smoking among adolescents in a juvenile correctional center. *Drug Alcohol Depend.* 2008;92(1–3):156–163.
30. Bock B, Lopes CE, van den Berg JJ, et al. Social support and smoking abstinence among incarcerated adults in the United States: a longitudinal study. *BMC Public Health.* 2013;13(859):1–9.
31. Sieminska A, Jassem E, Konopa K. Prisoners' attitudes towards cigarette smoking and smoking cessation: a questionnaire study in Poland. *BMC Public Health.* 2006;6(181):1–9.
32. Kauffman RM, Ferketich AK, Murray DM, Bellair PE, Wewers ME. Tobacco use by male prisoners under an indoor smoking ban. *Nicotine Tob Res.* 2011;13(6):449–456.
33. Malarcher A, Dube S, Shaw L, Babb S, Kaufmann R. Quitting smoking among adults—United States, 2001–2010. *MMWR Morb Mortal Wkly Rep.* 2011;60(44):1513–1519.
34. Long D. Smoking as a coping strategy. *Nursing Times.* 2003;99(33):50.
35. Taylor P, Ogeden C, Corteen K. Tobacco smoking and incarceration: expanding the "last poor smoker" thesis. *Internet J Criminol.* 2012.
36. van den Berg JJ, Bock B, Roberts MB, et al. Cigarette smoking as an expression of independence and freedom among inmates in a tobacco-free prison in the United States. *Nicotine Tob Res.* 2014;16(2):238–242.
37. White BR. Helling v. McKinney. In: Court S, ed. *509 US 25.* Vol 91-19581993.
38. Weiss LE. Note: Helling v. McKinney: creating a constitutional right to be free from environmental tobacco smoke. *Tulane Environmental Law Journal.* 1993;7(1):249–270.
39. Kennedy SM, Davis SP, Thorne SL. Smoke-free policies in U.S. prisons and jails: a review of the literature. *Nicotine Tob Res.* 2015;17(6):629–635.
40. Collinson L, Wilson N, Edwards R, Thomson G, Thornley S. New Zealand's smokefree prison policy appears to be working well: one year on. *NZ Med J.* 2012;125(1357):164–168.
41. Collier R. Prison smoking bans: clearing the air. *CMAJ.* 2013;185(10):E474.
42. Australian Institute of Health and Welfare. *The Health of Australia's Prisoners 2015.* Canberra, Australia: Australian Institute of Health and Welfare; 2015.
43. Kauffman RM, Ferketich AK, Wewers ME. Tobacco policy in American prisons, 2007. *Tob Control.* 2008;17(5):357–360.
44. Clarke JG, Stein LA, Martin RA, et al. Forced smoking abstinence: not enough for smoking cessation. *JAMA Int Med.* 2013;173(9):789–794.

45. de Andrade D, Kinner SA. Systematic review of health and behavioural outcomes of smoking cessation interventions in prisons. *Tob Control*. 2016;0:1–7.
46. Moller L, Stover H, Jurgens R, Gatherer A, Nikogosian H. *Health in Prisons: A WHO Guide to the Essentials in Prison Health*. Copenhagen, Denmark: World Health Organization Regional Office for Europe; 2007.
47. Nijhawan AE, Salloway R, Nunn AS, Poshkus M, Clarke JG. Preventive healthcare for underserved women: results of a prison survey. *J Women's Health*. 2010;19(1):17–22.
48. Indig DTL, Ross B., Mamoon H., et al. *2009 NSW Inmate Health Survey: Key Findings Report*. Sydney, Australia: Justice Health; 2010.
49. Butler TLM. *The 2001 Inmate Health Survey*. Sydney, Australia: NSW Corrections Health Service; 2003.
50. Belcher JM, Butler T, Richmond RL, Wodak AD, Wilhelm K. Smoking and its correlates in an Australian prisoner population. *Drug Alcohol Rev*. 2006;25(4):343–348.
51. Cropsey K, Eldridge GD, Ladner T. Smoking among female prisoners: an ignored public health epidemic. *Addict Beh*. 2004;29(2):425–431.
52. Cahill K, Stevens S, Perera R, Lancaster T. Pharmacological interventions for smoking cessation: an overview and network meta-analysis. *Cochrane Database of Syst Rev*. 2013;5:CD009329.
53. Fiore MC, Jaén CR, Baker TB, et al. *Treating Tobacco Use and Dependence: 2008 Update. Clinical Practice Guideline*. Rockville, MD: US Department of Health and Human Services, Public Health Service; May 2008.
54. World Health Organization. *Tools for Advancing Tobacco Control in the XXIst Century: Policy Recommendations for Smoking Cessation and Treatment of Tobacco Dependence*. Geneva, Switzerland: WHO; 2003.
55. Cropsey KL, McClure LA, Jackson DO, Villalobos GC, Weaver MF, Stitzer ML. The impact of quitting smoking on weight among women prisoners participating in a smoking cessation intervention. *Am J Public Health*. 2010;100(8):1442–1448.
56. Richmond RL, Wilhelm KA, Indig D, Butler TG, Archer VA, Wodak AD. Cardiovascular risk among Aboriginal and non-Aboriginal smoking male prisoners: inequalities compared to the wider community. *BMC Public Health*. 2011;11(783):1–7.
57. Herbert K, Plugge E, Foster C, Doll H. Prevalence of risk factors for non-communicable diseases in prison populations worldwide: a systematic review. *Lancet*. 2012;379(9830):1975–1982.
58. Mahmoudi M, Coleman CI, Sobieraj DM. Systematic review of the cost-effectiveness of varenicline vs. bupropion for smoking cessation. *Int J Clin Pract*. 2012;66(2):171–182.
59. Casey ER, Scott MG, Tang S, Mullins ME. Frequency of false positive amphetamine screens due to bupropion using the Syva EMIT II immunoassay. *J Med Toxicol*. 2011;7(2):105–108.
60. Miller WR, Benefield RG, Tonigan JS. Enhancing motivation for change in problem drinking: a controlled comparison of two therapist styles. *J Consult Clin Psychol*. 1993;61(3):455–461.
61. Project MATCH Research Group. Project MATCH secondary a priori hypotheses. *Addiction*. 1997;92(12):1671–1698.
62. Davis TM, Baer JS, Saxon AJ, Kivlahan DR. Brief motivational feedback improves post-incarceration treatment contact among veterans with substance use disorders. *Drug Alcohol Depend*. 2003;69(2):197–203.
63. Miller W. *Motivational Interviewing: Preparing People to Change Addictive Behavior*, 2nd ed. New York, NY: Guilford Press; 2002.
64. Miller W. *Motivational Interviewing: Preparing People to Change Addictive Behavior*. New York, NY: Guilford Press; 1991.

65. Lotecka L, MacWhinney M. Enhancing decision behavior in high school "smokers." *Int J Addict*. 1983;18(4):479–490.

66. McDonald P, Colwell B, Backinger CL, Husten C, Maule CO. Better practices for youth tobacco cessation: evidence of review panel. *Am J Health Behav*. 2003;27 (suppl 2):S144–158.

67. Milton MH, Maule CO, Backinger CL, Gregory DM. Recommendations and guidance for practice in youth tobacco cessation. *Am J Health Behav*. 2003;27 (suppl 2):S159–169.

68. Myers M. Cigarette smoking treatment for substance-abusing adolescents. In: Wagner E, Waldron H, eds. *Innovation in Adolescent Substance Abuse Interventions*. Oxford, England: Pergamon, Elsevier Science; 2001:263–283.

69. Chen YF, Madan J, Welton N, et al. Effectiveness and cost-effectiveness of computer and other electronic aids for smoking cessation: a systematic review and network meta-analysis. *Health Technol Assess*. 2012;16(38):1–205.

70. Task Force on Community Preventive Services. Recommendations regarding interventions to reduce tobacco use and exposure to environmental tobacco smoke. *Am J Prev Med*. 2001;20(2 suppl):10–15.

71. Cropsey K, Eldridge G, Weaver M, Villalobos G, Stitzer M, Best A. Smoking cessation intervention for female prisoners: addressing an urgent public health need. *Am J Public Health*. 2008;98(10):1894–1901.

72. Richmond R, Indig D, Butler T, Wilhelm K, Archer V, Wodak A. A randomized controlled trial of a smoking cessation intervention conducted among prisoners. *Addiction*. 2012;108(5):966–974.

73. Lankenau SE. Smoke 'em if you got 'em: cigarette black markets in US prisons and jails. *Prison Journal*. 2001;81(2):142–161.

74. Richmond R, Butler T, Wilhelm K, Wodak A, Cunningham M, Anderson I. Tobacco in prisons: a focus group study. *Tob Control*. 2009;18(3):176–182.

75. Valera P, Cook SH, Darout R, Dumont DM. "They are not taking cigarettes from me . . . I'm going to smoke my cigarettes until the day I die. I don't care if I get cancer": the smoking behaviors of men under community supervision in New York City. *Nicotine Tob Res*. 2014;16(6):800–806.

76. Richmond RL, Butler T, Belcher JM, Wodak A, Wilhelm KA, Baxter E. Promoting smoking cessation among prisoners: feasibility of a multi-component intervention. *Aust N Z J Public Health*. 2006;30(5):474–478.

77. Butler T, Richmond R, Belcher J, Wilhelm K, Wodak A. Should smoking be banned in prisons? *Tob Control*. 2007;16(5):291–293.

78. Cancel Council Victoria. *Smoking and Disadvantage: Evidence Brief*. Melbourne, Australia: Cancer Council; 2013.

79. US Department of Health and Human Services. *Preventing Tobacco Use Among Youth and Youth Adults: A Report of the Surgeon General*. Atlanta, GA: US Department of Health and Human Services; 2012.

80. Jackson C. Perceived legitimacy of parental authority and tobacco and alcohol use during early adolescence. *J Adolesc Health*. 2002;31(5):425–432.

81. Moolchan ET, Ernst M, Henningfield JE. A review of tobacco smoking in adolescents: treatment implications. *J Am Acad Child Adolesc Psychiatry*. 2000;39(6):682–693.

CHAPTER 6

Substance Use After Release From Prison

SARAH LARNEY, PhD, MARK STOOVÉ, PhD,
AND STUART A. KINNER, PhD

INTRODUCTION

As discussed in previous chapters, a considerable proportion of prisoners globally are dependent on alcohol, tobacco, and/or other drugs or experience problems related to substance use.[1] Incarceration usually represents a period of significantly reduced substance use, if not total (forced) abstinence, for these individuals. The notable exception is tobacco smoking, which remains normative in most prisons where smoking bans have not been implemented. Almost all prisoners return to the community, however, at which point substance use may resume (or, if use has continued in prison, increase in frequency). Understanding substance use in the post-release period is important for a myriad of reasons, including the risks to individual and public health (discussed in chapter 14), as well as the impact that substance use may have on further offending behavior (discussed in chapter 13).

PREVALENCE OF POST-RELEASE SUBSTANCE USE

There have been far fewer studies of substance use following release from prison than of substance use among arrestees or current prisoners. This is despite the importance of post-release substance use to individual health outcomes, public health, and risk of further offending. Table 6.1 summarizes observational cohort studies examining the prevalence of substance use after release from prison. There is considerable variation between these studies in research design, sampling, follow-up periods, and measurement of substance use, making comparison between studies difficult. Many studies have recruited convenience samples or selected high-risk subgroups (eg, people with a history of injecting drug use [IDU]), making it difficult to generalize the

Table 6.1. OBSERVATIONAL COHORT STUDIES OF SUBSTANCE USE AMONG PEOPLE RELEASED FROM PRISON [a]

Study	Sample	Pre-incarceration substance use	Timing of post-release interview	Follow-up *n* (%)	Post-release substance use
Adams, 2013[4]	542 male and female jail inmates, northern Virginia, USA	21% lifetime injecting drug use; 12% injected drugs in the 6 months prior to incarceration	12 months	297 (55%)	"less than 8%" reported injecting drugs in the year since release
Calcaterra, 2014[5]	200 ex-prisoners recruited 1–3 weeks after release, Denver, USA	Not reported	2–9 months (aim: 3 months)	155 (78%)	17% used illicit drugs in the 30 days prior to interview; 21% hazardously drinking in the 30 days prior to interview
Graffam, 2012[6]	36 ex-prisoners (56% male), recruited 1–4 weeks after release, Victoria, Australia	77% lifetime history of substance use	1–4 weeks	N/A (baseline interview)	75% using alcohol or other drugs
			3–4 months	19 (53%)	68% using alcohol or other drugs
Kinner, 2006[7]	160 prisoners (68% male) within 4 weeks of release, Queensland, Australia	53% hazardous or harmful alcohol use (3 months before incarceration); 92% any illicit drug (lifetime); 64% injecting drug use (lifetime)	1 month	91 (57%)	55% any illicit drug; 30% injecting drug use
			4 months	77 (48%)	42% hazardous or harmful alcohol use; 56% any illicit drug; 23% injecting drug use

Study	Sample	Preincarceration prevalence	Follow-up	n (%)	Postrelease outcome
Lincoln, 2009[8]	200 newly admitted inmates of a smoke-free prison with a chronic physical or mental illness, Massachusetts, USA. Only those inmates with a history of tobacco smoking (n =165) were included in postrelease follow-up	83% of total sample smoking tobacco	1 month	102 (62%)	86% of preincarceration smokers were smoking tobacco
			6 months	129 (78%)	98% of preincarceration smokers were smoking tobacco
Thibodeau, 2010[9]	49 male inmates of a smoke-free prison with a history of tobacco smoking and within 1 month of release, Wisconsin, USA	100% smoking tobacco in the month prior to incarceration	1 month	44 (90%)	39% smoking tobacco
Visher, 2004[10]	324 prisoners (73% male), Baltimore, USA	78% any illicit drug use, 61% any alcohol use	1–3 months	141 (44%)	33% any illicit drug use or alcohol consumption to intoxication
Visher, 2010[11]	1,036 male prisoners in Chicago, Cleveland, and Houston, USA	80% used illicit drugs or alcohol to intoxication in the 6 months before incarceration	2 months	652 (63%)	20% any illicit drug use or alcohol consumption to intoxication

[a]This table includes longitudinal, observational cohort studies that reported data on prevalence of substance use after release from prison. It does not include observational cohort studies of postrelease substance use that did not report prevalence data, or intervention/treatment outcome studies.

findings to the wider population of ex-prisoners. Whereas some studies have relied on self-report to ascertain post-release substance use, others have used urine screens or other biological samples. Self-report data may be subject to social desirability bias, particularly if an individual faces criminal justice sanctions for substance use. Biological specimens, on the other hand, may only provide an accurate assessment of very recent substance use. In interpreting this body of evidence, it is also important to take into account the impact of follow-up rates on the reported prevalence of post-release substance use. Maintaining high follow-up rates in studies of people involved in the criminal justice system can be challenging,[2,3] and the lower the follow-up rate, the greater the risk that the reported prevalence of post-release substance use is either an over-estimate or an under-estimate of the true prevalence.

Bearing these limitations in mind, many of the studies in Table 6.1 show substantial proportions of participants using substances after release. This is evident across alcohol, tobacco, illicit drug, and injecting drug use, and in both men and women. Most studies, however, provide little or no information on patterns of use—simply reporting that the individual had used the substance on at least one occasion. Given the varying harms associated with different patterns of substance use, more nuanced measures that take into account the type, frequency, and context of substance use are needed.

In many studies, relapse to substance use occurred soon after release.[12] Former prisoners participating in qualitative studies have reported that they used substances as soon as they were able, often on the first day after release.[13] These findings stand in stark contrast to the notion that periods of incarceration (and associated abstinence) serve to "rehabilitate" substance-using offenders.

FACTORS AFFECTING POST-RELEASE SUBSTANCE USE

Individual, interpersonal, social-environmental, and structural factors may all play a role in shaping patterns of substance use after release from prison. Although these factors are discussed separately here, in reality they often co-occur and interact. The complex interactions between drivers of substance use after release from prison are not well understood and can be difficult to address comprehensively in the clinical context.

Individual Differences

Pre-incarceration substance use can be a strong predictor of post-release substance use, although this is not always the case. In one study of 160 prisoners in Queensland, Australia, hazardous/harmful alcohol use prior to incarceration was associated with a 6.5-fold increase in the odds of this behavior after release.[7] In another Australian study involving 1,325 prisoners, 72% of those who were drinking at hazardous/harmful levels before prison (as measured by a score of 8 or more on the Alcohol Use Disorders Identification Test) were also drinking at hazardous/harmful levels

3 months after release from prison.[14] However, in a study of 210 women who were drinking hazardously before jail in Rhode Island, USA, there was no statistically significant association between frequency of alcohol use prior to incarceration and time to first alcohol consumption after release; instead, this outcome was influenced by social relationships (discussed later).[15]

Studies of the influence of pre-incarceration behavior on post-release illicit drug use have produced similarly conflicting results. Perhaps surprisingly, some studies find no significant association between pre-incarceration and post-release illicit drug use.[7] However, in a multi-site study in the United States, HIV-infected jail detainees who had used opioids in the 30 days prior to incarceration had a 30-fold increase in odds of post-release opioid use, compared with their peers with no pre-incarceration opioid use, and there was some evidence that pre-incarceration cocaine use was associated with post-release cocaine use.[16]

Several studies have focused on injecting drug use after release from prison. Injecting drug use is associated with particular risks, including acquisition and transmission of blood-borne viral infections such as HIV and hepatitis C, and fatal and non-fatal overdose. Two large cohort studies of people who inject drugs have found that incarceration is negatively associated with cessation of injecting drug use,[17,18] perhaps because it inhibits access to evidence-based drug treatment and other community-based programs that promote injecting cessation.[18]

Studies specifically examining the prevalence of injecting drug use prior to and after incarceration have reported varying levels of continuity. In one Australian study, pre-incarceration injecting drug use was strongly predictive of post-release injecting drug use, both 1 month and 4 months after release.[7] In another Australian study, 77% of 185 former prisoners who had injected drugs before prison also injected in the 3 months after release, although the proportion injecting daily fell from 66% pre-incarceration to 30% by 3 months after release.[19] In a third Australian study, 41% of a cohort of 533 former prisoners with a lifetime history of injecting drug use resumed injecting within 6 months of release; the rate of relapse was highest in the first month.[20] In a cohort study in Edinburgh, Scotland, just over one-third (37%) of participants with a lifetime history of injecting drug use were injecting shortly after release from prison, with 20% injecting on a regular (daily or almost daily) basis.[21]

Personal expectations and behavior patterns play an important role in the initiation of substance use after release from prison. Some individuals leave prison with the expectation of using substances, and such expectations are positively correlated with actual use.[14,22] For some prisoners, post-release substance use, along with sexual activity, is initiated rapidly after release as part of a desire to "make up for lost time,"[23] or as an impulsive response to substance use triggers such as being around substance-using friends or having easy access to substances.[12,24] For others, substance use is a coping mechanism used in the face of the substantial challenges many people experience after release from prison.[12,25] Former prisoners may also use substances to cope with psychological distress and serious mental health problems.[12]

There is some evidence for a period of particularly high-risk injecting drug use immediately following release from custody, with recent incarceration associated with an increased probability of needle and syringe sharing among people who inject drugs.[26,27] The reasons for this acute period of heightened risk are poorly understood; some authors have attributed post-release needle and syringe sharing to the normalization of this behavior during incarceration.[27]

Interpersonal Factors

Social support is often cited as an important factor in achieving positive post-release outcomes, including avoiding relapse to substance use.[24,28] Social support can have both positive and negative influences. From the perspective of preventing relapse to harmful substance use, social support may be considered positive when family members, close friends, and others are supportive of the former prisoner's intentions to avoid harmful substance use. Conversely, social support may be considered negative if it is likely to lead to a poor outcome (such as reoffending), or if the recipient of the support perceives it as negative.[29]

The distinction between positive and negative social support is not clear-cut, and the relationship between social support and post-release substance use is complex. People released from prison often nominate social support, particularly the support of family members who are not involved in substance use, as an important factor in avoiding relapse after release.[24,25,30] However, support from family members or close friends may be predicated on certain conditions, such as the releasee finding employment and making a financial contribution to the household. If the former prisoner is not able to meet these expectations, positive social support (eg, providing shelter) can be perceived by the former prisoner as coercive. Several qualitative studies have explored the tensions that can arise when people recently released from prison seek support from family and friends, noting that difficulties in meeting the expectations of well-intentioned family members (eg, gaining employment and contributing to the household in exchange for shelter) led to withdrawing from these relationships to avoid stress, or returning to drug selling to generate income for the family.[25,30] However, some ex-prisoners credit their relationships with family members and their children as critical to their success in avoiding substance use after release.[24]

It may be that lack of conflict with close family and friends, rather than active support from family and friends, is key to avoiding post-release relapse to substance use.[5,31,32] In a longitudinal study of 200 people recently released from prison, both illicit drug use (reported by 17% of participants) and hazardous alcohol use (21%) were associated with being moderately to extremely "bothered by family problems," although it is possible that perceived family problems were influenced by the ex-prisoner's relapse to substance use, rather than the other way around.[5] Similarly, conflict with family, but not family support, was a significant predictor of post-release substance use among 740 men released from prisons in several regions of the United States.[32]

Associating with peers who use substances or hold norms supportive of substance use is clearly linked to post-release substance use. In one study of women released from prison, alcohol consumption was predicted by having a partner with an alcohol use problem and associating with peers supportive of alcohol use.[15] In a small

(n = 50) mixed-sex sample of recent releasees, the number of "heavy drug users" in an individual's social network was associated with the percentage of days abstinent from drug use, with a higher number associated with fewer days of abstinence.[33] Formerly incarcerated men with high levels of negative social support (defined as a social network that impeded integration into the community) were more likely than their peers with positive social support to use "hard drugs" (defined as illicit drugs other than cannabis).[25] It seems that this point is self-evident to former prisoners, many of whom nominate avoiding old friends and acquaintances as an important factor in avoiding harmful substance use after release from prison.[12,24,25]

Structural and Social-Environmental Factors

Multiple structural and social-environmental factors work against former prisoners who wish to avoid harmful substance use. One critical factor in determining post-release substance use patterns is the availability of treatment for substance use disorders in prisons, with some prison systems limiting or restricting access to effective therapies,[34] and treatment demand often far exceeding availability.[30] Furthermore, the "treatment" services that are offered may not be grounded in evidence.[35] Inadequate prison-based treatment for co-occurring mental disorders may also compound poor outcomes associated with limited access to treatment for substance use disorders.[35] An important consequence of this lack of effective treatment is that prisoners may approach the end of their sentence no better equipped to avoid problematic substance use in the community than they were when they entered custody.

There can also be barriers to accessing treatment for substance-related problems after release. If prisoners are released without adequate identification documents, access to government and many non-government services can be difficult.[11,13,30] Release plans or parole conditions may require that former prisoners attend treatment for a substance use disorder, but correctional and/or parole services may not provide adequate resources or assistance to access such treatment.[36] In the United States, some states' prison systems terminate government-provided (Medicaid) health insurance when an individual is incarcerated, with coverage only restored following a lengthy bureaucratic process.[37] This may impede access to treatment for substance use disorders and other "behavioral health" services in the critical weeks after release.[30] Additionally, there may be few treatment services available to ex-prisoners returning to non-urban environments.[38,39]

In addition to limited access to treatment, the propensity for post-release substance use can be exacerbated by stresses associated with meeting basic needs, such as obtaining safe housing and finding employment or other legal income. Housing stability and income and employment stability are key predictors of cessation of substance use, with or without utilization of treatment services.[40] Unstable housing and homelessness after release from prison are associated with increased likelihood of substance use,[41] but identifying suitable, safe housing for prisoners nearing release can be a difficult task. Some prisoners may be able to return to the homes of family members, but as noted earlier, family relationships can become sources of stress and conflict that increase the risk of substance use.[32] Furthermore, in the United States, family members may be prevented from offering shelter to released ex-prisoners by regulations that prohibit people convicted of certain offenses from residing in government-subsidized housing.[30] Newly released ex-prisoners who lack other options often rely on homeless shelters for accommodation, but drug use and opportunities to buy drugs are often ubiquitous in shelters and the neighborhoods in which they are located.[24]

Finding legitimate employment can similarly create stress and place former prisoners in situations of high risk for drug use. Many ex-prisoners, understandably, place a high priority on finding a source of income as soon as possible after release.[25,30,42] Without a job and a reliable income stream, securing stable accommodation is unlikely. Additionally, employment is viewed by former prisoners as a means of finding purpose and direction in life, and an indicator of one's intentions to be a provider for family and children.[25] Finding a job is also thought by some former prisoners to be helpful in avoiding relapse because they consider that the job will keep them busy and prevent boredom or psychological distress, which can trigger substance use.[12]

Finding a job, however, often proves difficult.[30,43] Most prisoners have limited education and poor employment records prior to incarceration,[10,44] and imprisonment further decreases employability. Substance use disorders, mental illness, and physical and intellectual disability may all interfere with former prisoners' ability to get and maintain a job.[45] For some former prisoners, barriers to legitimate employment appear insurmountable, and selling drugs is perceived as the only way to generate income to meet basic survival needs.[30]

MINIMIZING POST-RELEASE SUBSTANCE USE

Although modifiable structural and social-environmental factors can increase the risk of harmful substance use after release from prison, the majority of work around reducing post-release substance use has focused on intervening at the individual level. Interventions that focus on the individual are best commenced during incarceration and should continue after release. Ideally, prisoners with substance use disorders should have access to evidence-based treatment, both in custody and after release. This should be complemented by treatment for comorbid mental and physical illnesses and by programs designed to increase the likelihood of successful community integration on release, such as literacy and vocational education.

Although there is evidence that at least some prison-based drug treatment programs can reduce reoffending in ex-prisoners,[46] there is less evidence that such programs reduce either substance use per se or substance-related harm. Furthermore, relatively few post-release programs addressing substance use in ex-prisoners have been rigorously evaluated. Some recent evaluation studies in the United States, using case management and collaborative behavioral management approaches, have produced promising results,[47,48] but these preliminary findings will require replication in other settings.

Although services in prison are important, any gains made in prison may be lost soon after release from custody without an appropriate release plan in place, followed by ongoing support to execute this plan once the individual returns to the community. Comprehensive release plans ideally take into account the diversity of pre-incarceration experiences within the prisoner population and the broad range of challenges experienced by prisoners returning to the community, and should be tailored to the needs of the individual.[49] Release plans should address basic survival needs, such as shelter and food; access to financial resources, clothing, and identification documents; longer-term housing and employment; access to health care for physical and mental illness, including substance use disorders; and strategies to build, maintain, and nurture positive social support networks.[28]

FUTURE RESEARCH DIRECTIONS

There are substantial variations globally in the epidemiology of substance use, societal responses to substance use, health and social harms associated with substance use, and the prevalence of substance use in prisoners.[50] However, most of the published literature on post-release substance use originates from the United States, and almost all is from developed, Western nations. The majority of the world's prisoners reside in low- and middle-income countries,[51] and very little is known about their health status or patterns of substance use, either in custody or after release. Lack of knowledge on substance use after release prevents the development and evaluation of evidence-based interventions to reduce harms and improve post-release outcomes. Additionally, given the high prevalence of HIV[52] and hepatitis C virus[53] in correctional populations in many countries,[54] a better understanding of the epidemiology of substance use following release from custody is critical to efforts to halt the spread of these infections.

Published research on substance use after release from prison frequently relies on convenience samples that may be biased in unknown ways, and many studies suffer from low follow-up rates and biased attrition. Poor reporting of study design and other parameters also limits the utility of some published studies, with a lack of basic detail regarding sampling, follow-up rates, and/or descriptive statistics making it almost impossible to adequately evaluate study quality or compare findings between studies. There is a substantial need for well-designed epidemiological studies of substance use and related risks among correctional populations, including longitudinal cohort studies to illustrate trajectories of use as people transition from prison or jail to the community. Such studies are essential for understanding the scale of the problem and determining the responses that are needed.

There is considerable variation across existing studies in how substance use is measured. Some studies rely on crude binary measures of use, failing to differentiate between single episodes of use and relapse to regular substance use, although the latter is considerably more likely to result in health and social harm. There may also be a failure in research to differentiate between substances, despite the very different health and offending risks associated with different substances. Researchers' decisions regarding how to define and measure post-release substance use may be affected by prevailing social attitudes and legal responses to substance use, which vary widely between and within countries, and often stand in stark contrast to the perspectives of the individuals who are being studied. There remains a need for research that examines post-release substance use in a nuanced manner, taking into account substance type, frequency and quantity of substances used over time, and specific harms related to substance use.

The significant limitations of the existing body of evidence stand in stark contrast to the substantial health, social, and economic consequences of harmful substance use in ex-prisoners. There is an urgent need for methodologically rigorous studies that assess the epidemiology of post-release substance use, particularly outside the United States and in low- and middle-income countries. To permit generalization of findings to the population of ex-prisoners, studies should attempt to recruit representative samples, either during incarceration or shortly after release from custody. Assessment of substance use should be undertaken in a detailed and nuanced manner, taking into account types of substances used, frequency of use, route of administration, and diagnostic criteria for substance use disorders. Ideally, substance use would be measured consistently or in a comparable manner across studies, to permit comparisons between different contexts and over time. To inform the development of evidence-based preventive interventions, studies should also aim to assess risk and protective factors for post-release substance use and related harm at the individual, interpersonal, social-environmental, and structural level. Given the difficulties associated with follow-up of people released from prison, researchers should consider the potential for linkage to routinely collected data to describe post-release trajectories[55] and the integration of record linkage into prospective studies.[56] More broadly, research is required to inform general principles to guide re-entry planning and post-release care for former prisoners with substance use disorders. Some questions are not amenable to quantification, and a mix of quantitative and qualitative methods will be required to fully understand the epidemiology of substance use in people recently released from prison.

CONCLUSION

A large proportion of prisoners enter custody with a history of problematic substance use. Most abstain from or reduce their use of substances in prison, but the available evidence suggests that many rapidly return to harmful substance use after release from prison. Release from prison is a distressing and challenging time for most, with individual, interpersonal, social-environmental and structural factors interacting to increase the risk of relapse. Despite the significant health, social, and economic harms associated with relapse to drug use in ex-prisoners, the epidemiology of substance use in ex-prisoners is poorly understood, with most studies suffering from significant and avoidable design limitations. Studies of risk and protective factors—which are required to inform evidence-based prevention—are similarly limited. Most published studies have been conducted in the United States or other high-income, Western countries, yet the majority of the world's prisoners are in low- and middle-income countries. There is an urgent need for rigorous, mixed-methods prospective studies to document and understand both the epidemiology and the drivers of harmful substance use in ex-prisoners. These studies are a prerequisite for the development of evidence-based programs and policies to reduce substance use and its harmful health and social consequences in ex-prisoners.

ACKNOWLEDGMENTS

Thank you to Manasa Reddy for editorial assistance. Sarah Larney is supported by National Health and Medical Research Council (NHMRC) Early Career Fellowship no. 1035149. Stuart Kinner is supported by NHMRC Senior Research Fellowship no. 1078168. The National Drug and Alcohol Research Centre at the University of New South Wales is supported by funding from the Australian Government under the Substance Misuse Prevention and Service Improvements Grants Fund.

REFERENCES

1. Fazel S, Bains P, Doll H. Substance abuse and dependence in prisoners: a systematic review. *Addiction.* 2006;101(2):181–191.
2. Crisanti AS, Case BF, Isakson BL, Steadman HJ. Understanding study attrition in the evaluation of jail diversion programs for persons with serious mental illness or co-occurring substance use disorders. *Crim Justice Behav.* 2014;41(6):772–790.
3. David MC, Alati R, Ware RS, Kinner SA. Attrition in a longitudinal study with hard-to-reach participants was reduced by ongoing contact. *J Clin Epidemiol.* 2013;66(5):575–581.
4. Adams LM, Kendall S, Smith A, Quigley E, Stuewig JB, Tangney JP. HIV risk behaviors of male and female jail inmates prior to incarceration and one year post-release. *AIDS Behav.* 2013;17(8):2685–2694.
5. Calcaterra SL, Beaty B, Mueller SR, Min S-J, Binswanger IA. The association between social stressors and drug use/hazardous drinking among former prison inmates. *J Subst Abuse Treat.* 2014;47(1):41–49.
6. Graffam J, Shinkfield AJ. The life conditions of Australian ex-prisoners: an analysis of intrapersonal, subsistence, and support conditions. *Int J Offender Ther Comp Criminol.* 2012;56(6):897–916.
7. Kinner S. Continuity of health impairment and substance misuse among adult prisoners in Queensland, Australia. *Int J Prison Health.* 2006;2(2):101–113.
8. Lincoln T, Tuthill RW, Roberts CA, et al. Resumption of smoking after release from a tobacco-free correctional facility. *J Correct Health Care.* 2009;15(3):190–196.
9. Thibodeau L, Jorenby DE, Seal DW, Kim SY, Sosman JM. Prerelease intent predicts smoking behavior postrelease following a prison smoking ban. *Nicotine Tob Res.* 2010;12(2):152–158.
10. Visher CA, Kachnowski V, La Vigne N, Travis J. *Baltimore Prisoners' Experiences Returning Home.* Washington, DC: Urban Institute; 2004.
11. Visher CA, Yahner J, La Vigne N. *Life After Prison: Tracking the Experiences of Male Prisoners Returning to Chicago, Cleveland and Houston.* Washington, DC: Urban Institute; 2010.
12. Johnson JE, Schonbrun YC, Nargiso JE, et al. "I know if I drink I won't feel anything": substance use relapse among depressed women leaving prison. *Int J Prison Health.* 2013;9(4):1–18.

13. Luther JB, Reichert ES, Holloway ED, Roth AM, Aalsma MC. An exploration of community reentry needs and services for prisoners: a focus on care to limit return to high-risk behavior. *AIDS Patient Care STDs*. 2011;25(8):475–481.

14. Thomas E, Degenhardt L, Alati R, Kinner S. Predictive validity of the AUDIT for hazardous alcohol consumption in recently released prisoners. *Drug Alcohol Depend*. 2014;134:322–329.

15. Clarke JG, Anderson BJ, Stein MD. Hazardously drinking women leaving jail: time to first drink. *J Correct Health Care*. 2011;17:61–68.

16. Krishnan A, Wickersham JA, Chitsaz E, et al. Post-release substance abuse outcomes among HIV-infected jail detainees: results from a multisite study. *AIDS Behav*. 2013;17(1):S171–S180.

17. Bruneau J, Brogly SB, Tyndall MW, Lamothe F, Franco EL. Intensity of drug injection as a determinant of sustained injection cessation among chronic drug users: the interface with social factors and service utilization. *Addiction*. 2004;99(6):727–737.

18. DeBeck K, Kerr T, Li K, Milloy M-J, Montaner J, Wood E. Incarceration and drug use patterns among a cohort of injection drug users. *Addiction*. 2009;104(1):69–76.

19. Dolan K, Wodak A, Hall W, Gaughwin M, Rae F. HIV risk behaviour of IDUs before, during and after imprisonment in New South Wales. *Addiction Res*. 1996;4(2):151–160.

20. Winter RJ, Young JT, Stoové M, et al. Resumption of injecting drug use following release from prison in Australia. *Drug Alcohol Depend*. 2016;168:104–111.

21. Shewan D, Reid M, Macpherson S, Davies JB, Greenwood J. Injecting risk behaviour among recently released prisoners in Edinburgh: the impact of in-prison and community drug treatment services. *Legal Criminol Psych*. 2001;6(1):19–28.

22. Souza KA, Lösel F, Markson L, Lanskey C. Pre-release expectations and post-release experiences of prisoners and their (ex-)partners. *Legal Criminol Psych*. 2013;20(2):306–323.

23. Adams J, Nowels C, Corsi KF, Long J, Steiner JF, Binswanger IA. HIV risk after release from prison: a qualitative study of former inmates. *J Acquir Immune Defic Syndr*. 2011;57(5):429–434.

24. Binswanger IA, Nowels C, Corsi KF, et al. Return to drug use and overdose after release from prison: a qualitative study of risk and protective factors. *Addict Sci Clin Pract*. 2012;7(3):1–9.

25. Seal DW, Eldridge G, Kacanek D, Binson D, MacGowan RJ. A longitudinal, qualitative analysis of the context of substance use and sexual behavior among 18- to 29-year-old men after their release from prison. *Soc Sci Med*. 2007;65(11):2394–2406.

26. Milloy MJ, Wood E, Small W, et al. Incarceration experiences in a cohort of active injection drug users. *Drug Alcohol Rev*. 2008;27(6):693–699.

27. Milloy MJ, Buxton J, Wood E, Li K, Montaner J, Kerr T. Elevated HIV risk behaviour among recently incarcerated injection drug users in a Canadian setting: a longitudinal analysis. *BMC Public Health*. 2009;9(156):1–7.

28. La Vigne N, Davies E, Palmer T, Halberstadt R. *Release Planning for Successful Reentry*. Washington, DC: Urban Institute; 2008.

29. Pettus-Davis C, Howard MO, Roberts-Lewis A, Scheyett AM. Naturally occurring social support in interventions for former prisoners with substance use disorders: conceptual framework and program model. *J Crim Just*. 2011;39(6):479–488.

30. van Olphen J, Freudenberg N, Fortin P, Galea S. Community reentry: perceptions of people with substance use problems returning home from New York City jails. *J Urban Health*. 2006;83(3):372–381.

31. Bahr SJ, Harris L, Fisher JK, Harker Armstrong A. Successful reentry: what differentiates successful and unsuccessful parolees? *Int J Offender Ther Comp Criminol*. 2010;54(5):667–692.

32. Mowen TJ, Visher CA. Drug use and crime after incarceration: the role of family support and family conflict. *Justice Q.* 2013;32(2):337–359.
33. Owens MD, McCrady BS. The role of the social environment in alcohol or drug relapse of probationers recently released from jail. *Addict Disor Their Treat.* 2014;13(4):179–189.
34. Larney S, Dolan K. A literature review of international implementation of opioid substitution treatment in prisons: equivalence of care? *Eur Addict Res.* 2009;15(2):107–112.
35. National Center on Addiction and Substance Abuse at Columbia University. *Behind Bars II: Substance Abuse and America's Prison Population.* New York, NY: CASA Columbia; 2010.
36. Binswanger IA, Nowels C, Corsi KF, et al. "From the prison door right to the sidewalk, everything went downhill": a qualitative study of the health experiences of recently released inmates. *Int J Law Psychiatry.* 2011;34(4):249–255.
37. Rosen DL, Dumont DM, Cislo AM, et al. Medicaid policies and practices in US state prison systems. *Amer J Public Health.* 2014;104(3):418–420.
38. Staton-Tindall M, McNees E, Leukefeld C, et al. Treatment utilization among metropolitan and nonmetropolitan participants of corrections-based substance abuse programs reentering the community. *J Soc Serv Res.* 2011;37(4):379–389.
39. Olson DE, Rozhon J, Powers M. Enhancing prisoner reentry through access to prison-based and post-incarceration aftercare treatment: experiences from the Illinois Sheridan Correctional Center therapeutic community. *J Exp Criminol.* 2009;5(3):299–321.
40. Hser Y, Longshore D, Anglin MD. The life course perspective on drug use: a conceptual framework for understanding drug use trajectories. *Eval Rev.* 2007;31(6):515–547.
41. Baldry E, McDonnell D, Maplestone P, Peeters M. Ex-prisoners, homelessness and the state in Australia. *Austr N Z J Criminol.* 2006;39(1):20–33.
42. Morozova O, Azbel L, Grishaev Y, Dvoryak S, Wickersham JA, Altice FL. Ukrainian prisoners and community reentry challenges: implications for transitional care. *Int J Prison Health.* 2013;9(1):5–19.
43. Visher CA, Debus-Sherrill SA, Yahner J. Employment after prison: a longitudinal study of former prisoners. *Justice Q.* 2011;28(5):698–718.
44. Indig D, Topp L, Ross B, et al. *2009 Inmate Health Survey: Key Findings Report.* Sydney, Australia: Justice Health; 2010.
45. Viitanen P, Vartiainen H, Aarnio J, et al. Work ability and treatment needs among Finnish female prisoners. *Int J Prison Health.* 2012;8(3):99–107.
46. Wilson DB, Bouffard LA, McKenzie DL. A quantitative review of structured, group-oriented, cognitive-behavioral programs for offenders. *Crim Justice Behav.* 2005;32(2):172–204.
47. Friedmann PD, Green TC, Taxman FS, et al. Collaborative behavioral management among parolees: drug use, crime and re-arrest in the Step'n Out randomized trial. *Addiction.* 2012;107(6):1099–1108.
48. Lattimore PK, Visher CA. *The Multi-Site Evaluation of SVORI: Summary and Synthesis.* Washington, DC: National Institute of Justice; 2009.
49. van Dooren K, Claudio F, Kinner S, Williams M. Beyond reintegration: a framework for understanding ex-prisoner health. *Int J Prison Health.* 2011;7(4):26–36.
50. UNODC. *World Drug Report 2014.* http://www.unodc.org/documents/wdr2014/World_Drug_Report_2014_web.pdf: United Nations Office on Drugs and Crime; 2014.
51. Walmsley R. *Word Prison Population List.* 10th ed. http://www.prisonstudies.org/sites/prisonstudies.org/files/resources/downloads/wppl_10.pdf: International Centre for Prison Studies; 2013.
52. Dolan K, Moazen B, Noori A, et al. People who inject drugs in prison: HIV prevalence, transmission and prevention. *Int J Drug Policy.* 2015;26(suppl 1):S12–S26.

53. Larney S, Kopinski H, Beckwith CG, et al. Incidence and prevalence of hepatitis C in prisons and other closed settings: results of a systematic review and meta-analysis. *Hepatology*. 2013;58(4):1215–1224.

54. Dolan K, Wirtz, AL, Moazen B, et al. Global burden of HIV, viral hepatitis, and tuberculosis in prisoners and detainees. *Lancet*. 2016;388(10049):1089–1102.

55. Degenhardt L, Larney S, Kimber J, et al. The impact of opioid substitution therapy on mortality post-release from prison. *Addiction*. 2014;109(8):1306–1317.

56. Kinner SA, Lennox N, Williams GM, et al. Randomised controlled trial of a service brokerage intervention for ex-prisoners in Australia. *Contemp Clin Trials*. 2013;36(1):198–206.

CHAPTER 7

Drug Use, HIV, and the High-Risk Environment of Prisons

LYUBA AZBEL, MSc AND FREDERICK L. ALTICE, MD

BACKGROUND

Globally, the intertwined epidemics of HIV and substance use disorders find their epicenter in prisons. Sentencing guidelines favoring harsh penalties concentrate marginalized populations with overlapping and complex comorbidities, including HIV, viral hepatitis, substance use disorders, mental illness, and an array of social comorbidities such as homelessness, discontinuous healthcare eligibility, and unemployment. Particularly, policies favoring punishment over decriminalization of drug use result in a disproportionate number of drug users in criminal justice settings (see also chapter 1). The increased prevalence of blood-borne infections among prisoners compared with those in community settings is, in large part, associated with the over-representation of people who inject drugs (PWID) within prisons, considering that infection through infected injection paraphernalia is a highly efficient method of HIV transmission.[1] Despite international guidelines for providing healthcare for incarcerated persons (see chapter 12),[2] HIV prevention and treatment in prisons are often sub-standard and seldom consistent with care provided in community settings.

With notable exceptions, primarily in Western Europe, internationally recommended HIV prevention services are not widely available in prisons. Very few countries provide sterile injecting equipment to PWID in prisons through needle and syringe programs (NSP), and globally, the scale and coverage of opioid agonist therapies (OAT) with methadone or buprenorphine provided in prisons vary markedly by geographical region. In many settings, HIV prevention services, if they are available at all, exist as pilot programs, insufficiently scaled to need and, in the case of OAT, often with suboptimal dosing.[3–5] Condoms are rarely available in prisons for either primary or secondary prevention. Routine HIV testing in prisons, with the ability to opt out of testing, is the most effective strategy to identify new HIV infections and to re-engage individuals estranged from care.[6–10] Any HIV testing strategy, however, should be linked to evidence-based treatment using recommended medications, including combined antiretroviral therapy (ART) and prophylaxis for opportunistic infections. There is no evidence of prisoners being provided pre-exposure prophylaxis despite its proven efficacy for serodiscordant heterosexuals, men who have sex with men, and PWID.[11-13] There are multiple potential reasons why HIV prevention and treatment services are not as widely available in prisons as in community settings, including (1) the presence of prison health services that operate distinctly from national healthcare systems; (2) legal and regulatory barriers to the provision of services in prisons; (3) limited financial and human resources for the provision of health services in prisons; and (4) challenges and/or restrictions in engaging community-based providers and non-governmental organizations (NGOs) to provide these services in prisons.

Criminal justice settings, by virtue of their structure and concentration of individuals at high risk for HIV and other comorbid conditions, present a seminal platform for HIV prevention, detection, and treatment. Many individuals who interface with the criminal justice setting are not engaged in community-based treatment and prevention. Therefore, individuals who interface with this system present an opportunity to engage patients in care that could significantly improve not only their health but also that of their community contacts. Regrettably, this potential opportunity is largely missed in most prison settings. The dearth of harm reduction programs and the high HIV prevalence, compounded by concomitant tuberculosis, viral hepatitis, and sexually transmitted infections (STIs), result in a high-risk prison environment where injection-related activities can facilitate HIV transmission.[14]

In this chapter, we consider the interdependency between two coexisting epidemics—substance use disorders and HIV—both during incarceration and at the time of community reentry. We review the evidence for the treatment of these two epidemics and examine opportunities for improving HIV treatment and prevention outcomes by incorporating evidence-based treatment of substance use disorders to reduce HIV transmission and facilitate HIV treatment. We will identify barriers and ways forward for the implementation of treatments targeting individuals with substance use disorders in order to curb HIV and other blood-borne virus transmission both within and outside of prison.

HIV PREVALENCE AND SUBSTANCE USE IN PRISON

Imprisonment is a common occurrence in the life of individuals with substance use disorders. Incarceration itself is associated with a significantly elevated risk of HIV for PWID.[15] Estimates of the prevalence of incarceration among people with substance use disorders come mainly from high-income countries; available data suggest that between 56% and 90% of PWID have transitioned through a prison setting.[16] Estimates of the prevalence of substance use disorders in prisoners vary widely between countries but appear higher among women (30% to 60%) than men (10% to 48%).[17] Together, a history of incarceration and substance use disorders create a perfect storm for HIV transmission. A recent comprehensive review provides updated data on HIV prevalence among prisoners.[18]

Methods for measuring HIV prevalence among prisoners vary considerably; one study reviewed estimates from 75 low- and middle-income countries and found that 18 of these reported HIV prevalence exceeding 10%.[15] Estimates ranged from 0% in Bulgaria and Albania to 28% in Vietnam.[15] HIV infection prevalence is particularly high among prisoners in countries of the former Soviet Union[14] and Latin America.[19] In addition, female prisoners generally have a higher HIV prevalence than their male counterparts, primarily because a higher proportion of female prisoners have substance use disorders and incarcerated women are more likely to have a history of high-risk sexual behaviors, including commercial sex work.[20]

While evidence abounds that HIV prevalence is several-fold higher in prison than in the surrounding community, obtaining accurate estimates of HIV prevalence globally among prisoners is challenging for several reasons, including (1) most estimates are derived from existing HIV reporting data rather than from scientifically rigorous methodologies; (2) few estimates are nationally representative or systematic, and many are restricted to non-representative settings or methods dictated by the criminal justice staff; (3) there is seldom political will by criminal justice agencies to allow researchers to obtain accurate estimates of disease, especially since such surveys often identify deficits in provision of evidence-based screening and treatment services; and (4) ethical constraints dissuade researchers from conducting research on a population that is often exploited.

THE PRISON RISK ENVIRONMENT

The prison environment is especially risky in relation to HIV transmission for a number of interrelated reasons, resulting in concentration of disease, further amplification of disease and deterioration of health status within prison, and dissemination of disease to the community after release (Figure 7.1). First, prisoners enter correctional facilities with markedly more risk factors for HIV infection than the general population, including underlying substance use disorders, mental illness, sexually transmitted diseases, poverty, homelessness, and limited access to healthcare.[21] Second, by virtue of these increased risk factors, there is a greater number of individuals with HIV within these settings, thus exacerbating risk when such individuals engage in injection or sexual risk behaviors. Third, healthcare provision in prison settings falls below that of community norms, resulting in deterioration in health and creating an environment where individuals are selectively deprived of access to measures that reduce the risk of HIV transmission, such as clean syringes and condoms.

The risk environment in prison is especially volatile for PWID as a consequence of both micro-level and macro-level factors that combine reciprocally to facilitate HIV transmission.[22] While individual HIV risk behaviors can result in HIV seroconversion, structural-level factors at the social, political, and environmental levels,[23] such as institutional policies contributing to the absence of effective HIV prevention

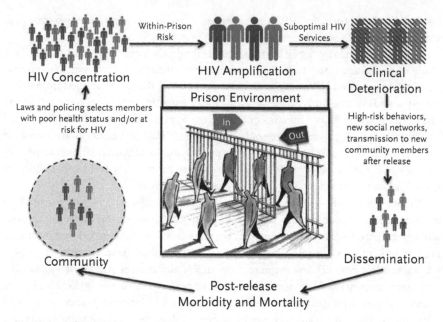

Figure 7.1: The prison environment increases HIV morbidity and mortality, both within prison and in the community after release

options, shape these behaviors.[24] In community settings, behavioral interventions alone have shown little impact on HIV incidence in the absence of structural interventions.[25-27] Similarly, prisons operate within a larger context that includes policy, community, relationship, and individual issues that need to be addressed in concert in order to curb HIV transmission (Figure 7.2). Only through an understanding of physical, social, economic, and policy influences on public health in prisons can an appropriate risk reduction strategy be applied.

On a macro level, the overcrowding of prisons with individuals most at risk for HIV[28] is a direct consequence of the scale-up of mass incarceration as the primary worldwide response to the use and supply of illegal drugs.[19] As a result of this epidemic of incarceration, inmates consistently bear a larger burden of HIV infection than the general population. This disparity is, in part, attributable to harsh drug laws and draconian penalties for substance use that explain why PWID in many countries represent half of all inmates.[15] These punitive policies therefore lead directly to an over-representation of people living with HIV (PLH) passing through the correctional system (as much as one-sixth of the 1.2 million PLH in the United States, for example).[29,30] This is especially relevant in the countries of Eastern Europe and Central and South-East Asia, which are home to HIV epidemics that are primarily driven by injection drug use.[31] In sub-Saharan African prisons, where extreme overcrowding is rampant,[32] higher HIV prevalence in prisons is a reflection of limited resources for prisoner health in a region that is already burdened by extremely high rates of HIV.[16]

PRISON RISK ENVIRONMENT				
	Micro	Macro		Mechanisms leading to HIV vulnerability
Physical	–availability of HIV testing and antiretroviral therapy –drug injecting locations	–location of drug trade routes –distance from HIV concentration –prison population mixing		–increases substance use –transmission of blood-borne infections
Social	–stigmatization of drug users –negative attitudes toward substance users from staff and inmates –social norms	–lack of social support –gender inequalities and gendered risk –ethnic inequalities	→	–increases vulnerability to violence –decreases ability to negotiate protective practices (condom use, etc.)
Economic	–economic vulnerability within prison –scarcity of employment	–economically and socially disempowered populations concentrated within prison –funding for HIV prevention and harm reduction services		–leads to recidivism –increases social vulnerability
Policy	–availability and quality of harm reduction services –cost of addiction treatment and antiretroviral therapy	–policy on within-prison substance use –health and human rights policies –laws governing prison-based harm reduction services		–increases within prison drug injection –increases risky injection practices

Figure 7.2: The role of the prison risk environment in shaping vulnerability to HIV

On a micro level, prison healthcare providers often lack the necessary training and qualifications to deal with the complex health needs of prison populations. This paradoxical observation does not adequately serve public health mandates given the more serious communicable disease burden carried by the prison population when compared with the community. There is a well-documented link between health-care providers' attitudes and the quality of healthcare clients ultimately receive. Despite authoritarian influences in prisons, when therapeutic treatment programs are made available in prisons that are not fully supported by front-line staff, inmates do not enroll in such programs, and prison officers undermine delivery of care to inmates.[33,34] Studies have, however, documented insufficient knowledge[35] and negative attitudes toward addiction treatment among prisoners[36] and prison staff.[36]

These micro-level and macro-level environmental factors conflate to influence individual risk, where PWID engage in within-prison drug-related risk behaviors. There is a paucity of information, however, evaluating prisoners' injection patterns. It is especially challenging to gather information on within-prison HIV risk behaviors, since reporting such behaviors may incriminate the respondent and result in harsh penalties. As such, post-release surveys may be more reliable for estimating such behaviors.[37] Despite the risks, however, there is growing evidence that individuals continue to use drugs while serving their sentences (also see chapters 3, 11).[38-40] Although drug use typically decreases[41] during incarceration, this reduction in frequency is offset by an increase in the risk associated with each injection because of the scarcity of equipment and reliance on sharing of contaminated injection equipment.[42,43] Evidence of within-prison drug injection occurs globally: in Latin America,[44] the Middle East,[45] North America,[38] Western Europe,[46,47] Eastern Europe,[48,49] Central Asia,[50] Australia,[51] and sub-Saharan Africa.[52] In some settings, drug injection first begins in prison,[46,53,54] often as a way of coping with the environment.[53] Within-prison equipment sharing[16,55] and HIV outbreaks have been recorded[56] throughout the world.[57-60]

COMMUNITY RE-ENTRY

For PWID, drug-related HIV risk continues beyond the confines of prison. The period after release is a particularly hazardous time for former prisoners. The risk of death from overdose in this period increases three- to eight-fold.[61] For those who had injected heroin before incarceration, there is a 1 in 200 risk of death in the first 4 weeks after release.[62] During this time, PWID relapse to risk behaviors such as syringe sharing[63] and unprotected sex that propagate HIV and other STIs.[63] A study from Ukraine documented that the most effective strategy to reduce HIV transmission in PWID who interface with prisons is to initiate OAT within prison and maintain them on it for at least a year after release.[14] Prisoners therefore need an alternative and integrated approach that would ensure that healthcare delivered in prison is effectively transitioned to the community and vice versa.

In the overwhelming majority of countries, though, the transition process from prison to the community does not meet the complex health needs of the inmate population. This is largely attributed to the fact that civic and prison health services are run by separate entities that do not effectively communicate—one is responsible for healthcare in the general population, while the other, overseen by a distinct department within criminal justice, provides treatment and prevention services for prisoners.[19] Furthermore, prisoners cycle between prison and the community—a process that is a predisposing factor for poor health outcomes.[64] In Ukraine, in 2011, approximately 600 HIV-infected individuals were released into the community each month, mostly without assistance.[65] Moreover, there is growing evidence that a history of incarceration continues to negatively impact health after release, for example, by increasing syringe-sharing events[66] or decreasing ART adherence[67] among HIV-infected former prisoners. New modeling data from Ukraine estimates that the contribution of incarceration to the spread of HIV accounts for more than half of incident HIV cases among PWID.[14] This is especially troubling given that there is often no recognition of the problem and no mechanism in place to connect the prison and community healthcare administrations and to effectively transition prisoners to effective healthcare services upon release. As a result, newly released prisoners remain in limbo about their healthcare at a time of heightened vulnerability.

When HIV-infected inmates are not linked to services in the community according to WHO standards, negative health consequences ensue. Poor retention in care leads to poor HIV treatment outcomes such as inadequate continuity of ART,[68] suboptimal ART adherence and insufficient viral suppression,[69] and low retention in care,[70] thereby increasing poor treatment outcomes and HIV transmission to others in settings of risky HIV behaviors.[71,72] Ideally, prisons should screen all inmates for substance use disorders, effectively treat symptoms of physical withdrawal, and provide relapse prevention strategies prior to release. A study in the United States comparing patients on methadone who were entering prison and were randomized either to maintain methadone or to discontinue it within prison found that those maintained on methadone were significantly less likely to relapse to drug use after release and remained engaged in treatment for longer.[73] Linkage to community services should be prioritized, especially in the absence of a connection between the structure of community and prison healthcare services.[74] Also, within prison, there are often disruptions in care during the transfer of prisoners from one facility to another from jail to prison, during court hearings, or for medical treatment. In Russia, relocating to another prison facility involves the grueling process of *etap*. Prisoners can spend months in prison cells on a train going thousands of miles in an indirect route to a new facility, often enduring unhygienic conditions and lack of food.[75] During such extended travel, patients may be without medications or adequate access to treatment for HIV or substance use disorders. Ensuring the continuity of care between prison facilities and the community is essential to implementing universal access to HIV prevention.

CURRENT PRACTICES AND STANDARD OF CARE IN HIV-RELATED PRISONER HEALTH

There are five internationally recommended, evidence-based HIV treatment and prevention strategies that should be provided to address the HIV pandemic, including in prison settings (Figure 7.3). These include expanded HIV testing, OAT with methadone (MMT) or buprenorphine (BMT) for prisoners with opioid use disorders, unfettered access to condoms and sterile injecting equipment, and universal access to ART.[76,77]

Despite the wealth of evidence supporting the key role of OAT for treating opioid use disorders, to date, it remains insufficiently implemented within prisons. OAT is the most effective treatment for opioid dependence, with a wealth of evidence from the community setting showing that it decreases criminal activity,[78] reduces opioid use[79] and injection-related risk behaviors,[80] and prevents HIV infection[81] and recidivism.[82] OAT also increases access to and improves adherence to ART,[83] and retains people in HIV care.[84] Furthermore, OAT has been shown to have positive health effects within prisons: a randomized trial showed that prisoners with a history of heroin injection before incarceration who received MMT during incarceration were retained on MMT for a longer time after release compared with those who received counseling or MMT plus a voucher to start MMT.[85] Debate remains about the most suitable dose of MMT for prisoners transitioning to the community. While one study showed that doses above 60 mg daily, uninterrupted, and for the duration of imprisonment optimized treatment,[86] another study found that HIV-infected prisoners were three-fold more likely to be retained after 1 year if their doses exceeded 80 mg per day as compared with those with lower doses.[3,87] Nonetheless, initiating OAT

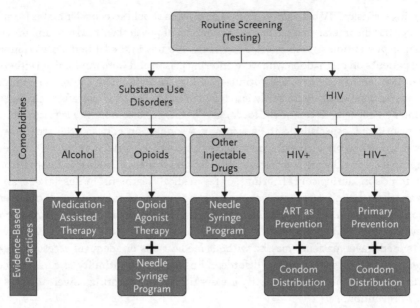

Figure 7.3: Evidence-based practices for the prevention and treatment of HIV and its comorbidities

within prison with effective transition after release is the most optimal approach to prevent HIV transmission and relapse to opioid use.[14] For opioid-dependent prisoners with HIV, being retained on buprenorphine after release for 24 weeks is associated with maximal viral suppression,[88] which not only reduces morbidity and mortality for HIV-infected persons but also may have secondary prevention benefits by harnessing HIV treatment as prevention (TasP) strategies.[89]

Affordable, properly dosed OAT is therefore necessary to optimize treatment outcomes.[3] There are some prisons that provide OAT for opioid-dependent inmates in the United States, Canada, Western and Eastern Europe, Australia, and Central and South-East Asia. If OAT is available in prison, though, it is often restrictive and inadequately scaled to need.[90] Furthermore, many countries that provide OAT in prison require supervised withdrawal before release, often because treatment in the community cannot be guaranteed. A case in point is Moldova—one of only three countries in the Commonwealth of Independent States (a group of former Soviet Republics) to provide methadone during incarceration.[91] Portugal and Spain, by contrast, have community-based programs that are adequately scaled to ensure a smooth transition from prison. HIV prevalence in Spanish prisoners reached a high of 24% in 1996 but decreased to 12% by 2003 after the introduction of within-prison harm reduction programs, including MMT and NSPs.[92] Spain and Portugal have had one of the most successfully implemented MMT programs in prisons for more than 10 years, and this can be used as a model for other countries. Prisoners are offered methadone after a full examination. It is then dispensed in set amounts for each person and monitored to make sure complete doses are taken.[93] In the United Kingdom an integrated psychosocial and clinical drug treatment program with methadone or detoxification in every prison is available, including a computer-controlled methadone dispensing device. Importantly, this program includes a large staff training component to overcome barriers to treatment.[94]

Provision of ART for all HIV-infected individuals[95] is pivotal to the TasP model,[96] proven to be effective in a randomized controlled trial[97] and through mathematical modeling.[98] The TasP strategy also has the possibility of reducing tuberculosis (TB) transmission,[99] which is particularly relevant in prisons given that the HIV epidemic has fueled the resurgence of TB in prisons, which is the primary cause of death for people living with HIV/AIDS (see chapter 8).[100] The risk of TB disease in prisons is on average 23-fold[100] to 100-fold[101] higher than in the general population. In Zambian prisons, the prevalence of HIV-TB co-infection is extremely high and exacerbated by a lack of medical care and dire conditions.[102] People who live with HIV and inject drugs have a 2- to 6-fold increased risk of developing TB compared with non-injectors.[100] Among PWID who develop TB, at least one in three will also have HIV.[100] This further underscores the benefits of high coverage of ART in the prison setting, which has been associated with improving survival for TB patients.[103]

While most prisoners who inject drugs inject opioids, and OAT effectively reduces within-prison drug injection,[104] not all prisoners inject opioids.[105] Therefore, there is a complementary need for both prison-based OAT and NSPs. NSPs reduce risky injection behaviors such as syringe sharing and substance use and limit transmission of blood-borne infections.[106] In countries where such programs are not available, the limited access to needles and syringes in prison causes prisoners to make constrained choices to address their drug dependence.[107]

Sex, either consensual or forced, between prisoners or prisoners and staff, occurs commonly. Condom distribution in prisons—although a cost-effective way of reducing HIV transmission[108]—is markedly limited in most countries,[109] although the effectiveness of condoms would be reduced when sex is not consensual. The low uptake of these evidence-based strategies in correctional settings throughout the world is often due to resistance from prison administrations, driven by unsubstantiated beliefs that these practices increase sexual activity[110,111] and a fear that adopting such strategies would be tantamount to an acknowledgment that drugs circulate and prisoners have sex within prisons. Despite the fact that these attitudes toward HIV risk reduction have been tempered with factual information about the benefits of effective public health strategies, they remain intractable.

Despite growing evidence-based support for harm reduction interventions within prisons, insufficient coverage remains. Prisoners' lack of trust in the prison administration running the healthcare services further complicates quality healthcare delivery.[112] Prisoners may reject treatment because of the associated stigma or the belief that OAT substitutes one drug for another. Discussion and information are necessary to inform all involved individuals of the benefits of MMT.[94] Moreover, even if OAT is successfully introduced, it often requires consistent education and training for both inmates and prison officers alike, since there is considerable movement both within and between prison facilities, thereby requiring booster training sessions.[3] A tele-education initiative—Project Extension for Community Healthcare Outcomes

(ECHO)—was created with the purpose of educating primary care clinicians in New Mexico about specialty hepatitis C care in rural and prison settings by linking them to university specialists.[113] Primary care physicians discuss cases with specialists, receive training, and raise the quality of care delivered. Because of the restricted access to specialists within prisons and the lack of qualified physicians who want to work there, this strategy may be adapted for an array of training—including regarding HIV—and may be an important way to overcome disparities in healthcare delivery in prisons.

Furthermore, some policies intended to curb HIV transmission are counterproductive for HIV prevention efforts. Non-consensual HIV testing remains standard in the prisons of some countries, despite the costly and inefficient[76] nature of this policy. The WHO guidelines clearly oppose involuntary testing as unethical and advocate for its prohibition. Routine and voluntary testing and counseling, on the other hand, has an evidence base in prisons and jails.[7,8,114] Voluntary opt-out testing greatly increases testing rates as compared with testing upon request.[114] This is particularly useful in settings where a large percentage of prisoners are unaware of their HIV status, such as in Ukraine.[65] The practice of segregating prisoners who undergo mandatory HIV testing has been widely debated and practiced. Inmates who test positive are secluded in a separate unit within the prison facility and sometimes made to wear identifying armbands. This was the case in the US state of Alabama until a 2012 class action lawsuit led by the American Civil Liberties Union ordered the Alabama Department of Corrections to end segregation of prisoners on the grounds that it denied them equal access to rehabilitative programs. In 2013, South Carolina became the last US state to outlaw this practice in prisons, yet it persists in many countries globally. HIV segregation can negatively influence health due to the immunosuppressant effects of HIV and thereby accelerate development of active TB in those who are co-infected.[115,116] In one US state, 71% of the prisoners residing in a separate HIV unit either newly tested positive on a tuberculin skin test or developed tuberculosis in an outbreak.[117] The prison environment is, in reality, dynamic. Individuals in the prison units where inmates are perceived to be HIV-negative are able to engage in high-risk behaviors as they shift between court hearings, jail, and other prison facilities, putting them at risk for seroconversion. Moreover, prison walls are porous and prone to drug smuggling.[118] There is strong evidence of injection within prison[119,120] and reports of HIV seroconversion during incarceration, although the exact level of disease transmission is unknown.[121] Segregation is riddled with shortcomings such as increased stigma, worsened mental health outcomes,[122] mistreatment, unequal access to services, and further spread of disease. This policy, which favors segregation as HIV prevention, therefore provides a false sense of security.

CONCLUSION

Numerous inter-related structural and individual factors have resulted in the concentration of people with HIV and substance use disorders in criminal justice settings.

Especially in the United States, but also globally due to influences endorsed by the United States, this has resulted in zero-tolerance policies toward drug use that have led to an exponentially increasing prison populations with a high concentration of PWID. As a result of this war on drug users, incarceration of PWID rather than markedly expanded and low-threshold treatment for addiction has been preferentially promoted. In settings where OAT has been markedly scaled up and treatment prioritized over incarceration, incarceration rates have markedly lowered. For example, incarceration rates are extraordinarily high in the United States, Eastern Europe, and Central Asia and in some settings in Southeast Asia (eg, Thailand, Malaysia) where large numbers of PWID are incarcerated. In contrast, many countries of Western Europe have low incarceration rates and policies that favor treatment over incarceration. In places where incarceration is high and people living with HIV and PWID are concentrated most in prisons, these policies, exacerbated by a weak public health infrastructure, have fomented an extremely high-risk environment, especially when HIV prevention and treatment services remain either unavailable or suboptimally scaled. The lack of progress globally on bringing prisoners' healthcare up to worldwide standards creates a risk environment that concentrates the most vulnerable populations and further prolongs disease both within and outside of prison.[76] Disciplinary sentencing for drug crimes must be replaced, where possible, with noncustodial measures, keeping detention as a last resort. Simultaneously, the standard of care in prison settings must be raised by shifting the framework from punitive to preventative and palliative.

HIV prevention strategies aimed exclusively at the individual will only partially reduce the incidence of disease. Such measures must also be targeted at macro-level factors to encourage greater social change, such as a reduction in the prison population to decrease crowding and the re-organization of prison health structures to allocate delivery of services to public health authorities. Individual and network-based approaches will have the greatest overall influence on disease burden. For this, a combination approach to drug treatment is necessary.[123] A strong evidence base attests to the treatments that garner the best health outcomes in prisons, such as NSP and OAT.[16] International agencies recommend equal access to HIV prevention and treatment to prisoners and those in the community, which is supported by human rights mandates.

The transmission of disease is not limited to within the prison walls: released ex-prisoners act as drivers for the community HIV epidemic. Especially where sexual transmission is rising, successful community transition programs are indispensable to limit the incidence of HIV.[124] Because the prison population is not contained but, rather, dynamic and constantly interacting with the community, it is essential to extend OAT programs to the prison environment in countries where there is ample experience running OAT in the community. Because the time after release is critical to ending the cycle of relapse and recidivism, efforts must be concentrated on the time before release to establish comprehensive harm reduction and treatment programs with linkage to community care. Funding to scale up, rigorously assess, and replicate good surveillance and evidence-based interventions in diverse environments is crucial.

In a system stuck between punitive and health-serving needs, untreated opioid dependence—a chronic and relapsing disease—poses a major barrier to HIV prevention and treatment as prisoners cycle in and out of the criminal justice system. It has long been high time to enforce policies that reflect that prison health is public health.

REFERENCES

1. Kaplan EH, Heimer R. A model-based estimate of HIV infectivity via needle sharing. *J Acquir Immune Defic Syndr*. 1992;5(11):1116–1118.
2. United Nations Office on Drugs and Crime. *HIV in Prisons: Situation and Needs Assessment Toolkit*. Geneva, Switzerland: UNODC; 2013.
3. Wickersham JA, Marcus R, Kamarulzaman A, Zahari MM, Altice FL. Implementing methadone maintenance treatment in prisons in Malaysia. *Bull World Health Organization*. 2013;91(2):124–129.
4. Vagenas P, Azbel L, Polonsky M, et al. A review of medical and substance use co-morbidities in Central Asian prisons: implications for HIV prevention and treatment. *Drug Alcohol Depend*. 2013;132(suppl 1):S25–31.
5. Stöver H, Kastelic A. *Drug Treatment and Harm Reduction in Prisons*. Geneva, Switzerland: World Health Organization; 2014.
6. Branson BM, Handsfield HH, Lampe MA, et al. Revised recommendations for HIV testing of adults, adolescents, and pregnant women in health-care settings. *MMWR Recomm Rep*. 2006;55(RR-14):1–17.
7. Kavasery R, Maru DS, Cornman-Homonoff J, Sylla LN, Smith D, Altice FL. Routine opt-out HIV testing strategies in a female jail setting: a prospective controlled trial. *PLoS ONE*. 2009;4(11):e7648.
8. Kavasery R, Maru DS, Sylla LN, Smith D, Altice FL. A prospective controlled trial of routine opt-out HIV testing in a men's jail. *PLoS ONE*. 2009;4(11):e8056.
9. Flanigan TP, Zaller N, Beckwith CG, et al. Testing for HIV, sexually transmitted infections, and viral hepatitis in jails: still a missed opportunity for public health and HIV prevention. *J Acquir Immune Defic Syndr*. 2010;55(suppl 2):S78–83.
10. de Voux A, Spaulding AC, Beckwith C, et al. Early identification of HIV: empirical support for jail-based screening. *PLoS ONE*. 2012;7(5):e37603.
11. Choopanya K, Martin M, Suntharasamai P, et al. Antiretroviral prophylaxis for HIV infection in injecting drug users in Bangkok, Thailand (the Bangkok Tenofovir Study): a randomised, double-blind, placebo-controlled phase 3 trial. *Lancet*. 2013;381(9883):2083–2090.
12. Grant RM, Lama JR, Anderson PL, et al. Preexposure chemoprophylaxis for HIV prevention in men who have sex with men. *N Engl J Med*. 2010;363(27):2587–2599.
13. Baeten JM, Donnell D, Ndase P, et al. Antiretroviral prophylaxis for HIV prevention in heterosexual men and women. *N Engl J Med*. 2012;367(5):399–410.
14. Altice FL, Azbel L, El-Bassel N, et al. The perfect storm: incarceration and multi-level contributors to perpetuating HIV and tuberculosis in Eastern Europe and Central Asia. *Lancet*. 2016;388(10050):1228–1248.
15. Dolan K, Kite B, Black E, Aceijas C, Stimson GV, Reference Group on HIV AIDS Prevention Care Among Injecting Drug Users in Developing Transitional Countries. HIV in prison in low-income and middle-income countries. *Lancet Infect Dis*. 2007;7(1):32–41.
16. Jurgens R, Ball A, Verster A. Interventions to reduce HIV transmission related to injecting drug use in prison. *Lancet Infect Dis*. 2009;9(1):57–66.
17. Fazel S, Bains P, Doll H. Substance abuse and dependence in prisoners: a systematic review. *Addiction*. 2006;101(2):181–191.

18. Dolan K, Wirtz A, Moazen B, et al. Global burden of HIV, viral hepatitis and tuberculosis among prisoners and detainees. *Lancet*. 2016;388(10049):1089–1102.
19. Jurgens R, Nowak M, Day M. HIV and incarceration: prisons and detention. *J Int AIDS Soc*. 2011;14(26):1–17.
20. Fazel S, Baillargeon J. The health of prisoners. *Lancet*. 2011;377(9769):956–965.
21. Reindollar RW. Hepatitis C and the correctional population. *Am J Med*. 1999;107(6B):100S–103S.
22. Rhodes T, Simic M. Transition and the HIV risk environment. *BMJ*. 2005;331(7510):220–223.
23. Rhodes T, Singer M, Bourgois P, Friedman SR, Strathdee SA. The social structural production of HIV risk among injecting drug users. *Soc Sci Med*. 2005;61(5):1026–1044.
24. Sarang A, Rhodes T, Sheon N, Page K. Policing drug users in Russia: risk, fear, and structural violence. *Subst Use Misuse*. 2010;45(6):813–864.
25. Adimora AA, Auerbach JD. Structural interventions for HIV prevention in the United States. *J Acquir Immune Defic Syndr*. 2010;55(suppl 2):S132–135.
26. Copenhaver MM, Johnson BT, Lee IC, Harman JJ, Carey MP, Team SR. Behavioral HIV risk reduction among people who inject drugs: meta-analytic evidence of efficacy. *J Subst Abuse Treat*. 2006;31(2):163–171.
27. Gupta GR, Parkhurst JO, Ogden JA, Aggleton P, Mahal A. Structural approaches to HIV prevention. *Lancet*. 2008;372(9640):764–775.
28. Boutwell A, Rich JD. HIV infection behind bars. *Clin Infect Dis*. 2004;38(12):1761–1763.
29. Spaulding AC, Seals RM, Page MJ, Brzozowski AK, Rhodes W, Hammett TM. HIV/AIDS among inmates of and releasees from US correctional facilities, 2006: declining share of epidemic but persistent public health opportunity. *PLoS ONE*. 2009;4(11):e7558.
30. Hammett TM, Harmon MP, Rhodes W. The burden of infectious disease among inmates of and releasees from US correctional facilities, 1997. *Am J Public Health*. 2002;92(11):1789–1794.
31. Aceijas C, Stimson GV, Hickman M, et al. Global overview of injecting drug use and HIV infection among injecting drug users. *AIDS*. 2004;18(17):2295–2303.
32. Todrys KW, Amon JJ. Criminal justice reform as HIV and TB prevention in African prisons. *PLoS Med*. 2012;9(5):e1001215.
33. Friedmann PD, Taxman FS, Henderson CE. Evidence-based treatment practices for drug-involved adults in the criminal justice system. *J Subst Abuse Treat*. 2007;32(3):267–277.
34. Taxman FS, Perdoni ML, Harrison LD. Drug treatment services for adult offenders: the state of the state. *J Subst Abuse Treat*. 2007;32(3):239–254.
35. Springer SA, Bruce RD. A pilot survey of attitudes and knowledge about opioid substitution therapy for HIV-infected prisoners. *J Opioid Manag*. 2008;4(2):81–86.
36. Polonsky M, Azbel L, Wickersham JA, et al. Challenges to implementing opioid substitution therapy in Ukrainian prisons: personnel attitudes toward addiction, treatment, and people with HIV/AIDS. *Drug Alcohol Depend*. 2015;148:47–55.
37. Izenberg J, Bachireddy C, Wickersham JA, et al. Within-prison drug injection and injection equipment sharing among HIV-infected Ukrainian prisoners: incidence and correlates of extremely high-risk behaviours. Paper presented at: 7th IAS Conference on HIV Pathogenesis, Treatment and Prevention; 30 June–3 July 2013; Kuala Lumpur, Malaysia.
38. Martin RE, Gold F, Murphy W, Remple V, Berkowitz J, Money D. Drug use and risk of bloodborne infections: a survey of female prisoners in British Columbia. *Can J Public Health*. 2005;96(2):97–101.
39. Gore SM, Bird AG, Burns SM, Goldberg DJ, Ross AJ, Macgregor J. Drug injection and HIV prevalence in inmates of Glenochil prison. *BMJ*. 1995;310(6975):293–296.

40. Plourde C, Brochu S. Drugs in prison: a break in the pathway. *Subst Use Misuse*. 2002;37(1):47–63.
41. Shewan D, Gemmell M, Davies JB. Behavioural change amongst drug injectors in Scottish prisons. *Soc Sci Med*. 1994;39(11):1585–1586.
42. Shewan D, Macpherson A, Reid MM, Davies JB. Patterns of injecting and sharing in a Scottish prison. *Drug Alcohol Depend*. 1995;39(3):237–243.
43. Darke S, Kaye S, Finlay-Jones R. Drug use and injection risk-taking among prison methadone maintenance patients. *Addiction*. 1998;93(8):1169–1175.
44. Cravioto P, Medina-Mora ME, de la Rosa B, Galvan F, Tapia-Conyer R. Patterns of heroin consumption in a jail on the northern Mexican border: barriers to treatment access. *Salud Publica Mex*. 2003;45(3):181–190.
45. Navadeh S, Mirzazadeh A, Gouya MM, Farnia M, Alasvand R, Haghdoost AA. HIV prevalence and related risk behaviours among prisoners in Iran: results of the National Biobehavioural Survey, 2009. *Sex Transm Infect*. 2013;89(suppl 3):iii33–36.
46. Bird AG, Gore SM, Cameron S, Ross AJ, Goldberg DJ. Anonymous HIV surveillance with risk factor elicitation at Scotland's largest prison, Barlinnie. *AIDS*. 1995;9(7):801–808.
47. Koulierakis G, Gnardellis C, Agrafiotis D, Power KG. HIV risk behaviour correlates among injecting drug users in Greek prisons. *Addiction*. 2000;95(8):1207–1216.
48. Frost L, Tchertkov V. Prisoner risk taking in the Russian Federation. *AIDS Educ Prev*. 2002;14(5 suppl B):7–23.
49. Drobniewski FA, Balabanova YM, Ruddy MC, et al. Tuberculosis, HIV seroprevalence and intravenous drug abuse in prisoners. *Eur Resp J*. 2005;26(2):298–304.
50. United Nations Office on Drugs and Crime. *Accessibility of HIV Prevention, Treatment and Care Services for People Who Use Drugs and Incarcerated People in Azerbaijan, Kazakhstan, Kyrgyzstan, Tajikistan, Turkmenistan and Uzbekistan: Legislative and Policy Analysis and Recommendations for Reform*. Geneva, Switzerland: United Nations Office on Drugs and Crime, Regional Office for Central Asia; 2010.
51. Kinner SA, Jenkinson R, Gouillou M, Milloy MJ. High-risk drug-use practices among a large sample of Australian prisoners. *Drug Alcohol Depend*. 2012;126(1–2):156–160.
52. Adjei AA, Armah HB, Gbagbo F, et al. Prevalence of human immunodeficiency virus, hepatitis B virus, hepatitis C virus and syphilis among prison inmates and officers at Nsawam and Accra, Ghana. *J Med Microbiol*. 2006;55(pt 5):593–597.
53. Hughes RA, Huby M. Life in prison: perspectives of drug injectors. *Deviant Behav*. 2000;21(5):451–479.
54. Chu S, Peddle K. *Under the Skin: A People's Case for Prison Needle and Syringe Programs*. Toronto, Canada: Canadian HIV/AIDS Legal Network; 2010.
55. Dufour A, Alary M, Poulin C, et al. Prevalence and risk behaviours for HIV infection among inmates of a provincial prison in Quebec City. *AIDS*. 1996;10(9):1009–1015.
56. Dolan K, Black E, Kite B, et al. *Review of Injection Drug Users and HIV Infection in Prisons in Developing and Transitional Countries*. London, England: Centre for Research on Drugs and Health Behavior; 2004.
57. Taylor A, Goldberg D, Emslie J, et al. Outbreak of HIV infection in a Scottish prison. *BMJ*. 1995;310(6975):289–292.
58. Dolan K, Wodak A, Hall W, Kaplan E. A mathematical model of HIV transmission in NSW prisons. *Drug Alcohol Depend*. 1998;50(3):197–202.
59. Dolan K, Hall W, Wodak A, Gaughwin M. Evidence of HIV transmission in an Australian prison. *Med J Austr*. 1994;160(11):734.
60. Bobrik A, Danishevski K, Eroshina K, McKee M. Prison health in Russia: the larger picture. *J Public Health Policy*. 2005;26(1):30–59.
61. Merrall EL, Kariminia A, Binswanger IA, et al. Meta-analysis of drug-related deaths soon after release from prison. *Addiction*. 2010;105(9):1545–1554.
62. Strang J, Bird SM, Parmar MK. Take-home emergency naloxone to prevent heroin overdose deaths after prison release: rationale and practicalities for the N-ALIVE randomized trial. *J Urban Health*. 2013;90(5):983–996.

63. Wood E, Li K, Small W, Montaner JS, Schechter MT, Kerr T. Recent incarceration independently associated with syringe sharing by injection drug users. *Public Health Rep*. 2005;120(2):150–156.
64. Fu JJ, Herme M, Wickersham JA, et al. Understanding the revolving door: individual and structural-level predictors of recidivism among individuals with HIV leaving jail. *AIDS Behav*. 2013;17(suppl 2):S145–155.
65. Azbel L, Wickersham JA, Grishaev Y, Dvoryak S, Altice FL. Burden of infectious diseases, substance use disorders, and mental illness among Ukrainian prisoners transitioning to the community. *PLoS ONE*. 2013;8(3):e59643.
66. Milloy MJ, Kerr T, Salters K, et al. Incarceration is associated with used syringe lending among active injection drug users with detectable plasma HIV-1 RNA: a longitudinal analysis. *BMC Infect Dis*. 2013;13(565):1–10.
67. Milloy MJ, Kerr T, Buxton J, et al. Dose-response effect of incarceration events on nonadherence to HIV antiretroviral therapy among injection drug users. *J Infect Dis*. 2011;203(9):1215–1221.
68. Baillargeon J, Giordano TP, Rich JD, et al. Accessing antiretroviral therapy following release from prison. *JAMA*. 2009;301(8):848–857.
69. Meyer JP, Cepeda J, Springer SA, Wu J, Trestman RL, Altice FL. HIV in people reincarcerated in Connecticut prisons and jails: an observational cohort study. *Lancet HIV*. 2014;1(2):e77–e84.
70. Althoff AL, Zelenev A, Meyer JP, et al. Correlates of retention in HIV care after release from jail: results from a multi-site study. *AIDS Behav*. 2013;17(suppl 2):S156–170.
71. Andrews JR, Wood R, Bekker LG, Middelkoop K, Walensky RP. Projecting the benefits of antiretroviral therapy for HIV prevention: the impact of population mobility and linkage to care. *J Infect Dis*. 2012;206(4):543–551.
72. Gardner EM, McLees MP, Steiner JF, Del Rio C, Burman WJ. The spectrum of engagement in HIV care and its relevance to test-and-treat strategies for prevention of HIV infection. *Clin Infect Dis*. 2011;52(6):793–800.
73. Rich JD, McKenzie M, Larney S, et al. Methadone continuation versus forced withdrawal on incarceration in a combined US prison and jail: a randomised, open-label trial. *Lancet*. 2015;386(9991):350–359.
74. Kothari G, Marsden J, Strang J. Opportunities and obstacles for effective treatment of drug misusers in the criminal justice system in England and Wales. *Br J Criminol*. 2002;42(2):412–432.
75. Lahusen T, Solomon P. *What Is Soviet Now? Identities, Legacies, Memories*. Berlin, Germany: LIT Verlag; 2008.
76. World Health Organization. *Interventions to Address HIV in Prisons: HIV Care, Treatment and Support*. Geneva, Switzerland: WHO; 2007.
77. Donoghoe MC, Verster A, Pervilhac C, Williams P. Setting targets for universal access to HIV prevention, treatment and care for injecting drug users (IDUs): towards consensus and improved guidance. *Int J Drug Policy*. 2008;19(suppl 1):S5–14.
78. Keen J, Rowse G, Mathers N, Campbell M, Seivewright N. Can methadone maintenance for heroin-dependent patients retained in general practice reduce criminal conviction rates and time spent in prison? *Br J Gen Pract*. 2000;50(450):48–49.
79. Mattick RP, Breen C, Kimber J, Davoli M. Methadone maintenance therapy versus no opioid replacement therapy for opioid dependence. *Cochrane Database Syst Rev*. 2009(3):CD002209.
80. Sorensen JL, Copeland AL. Drug abuse treatment as an HIV prevention strategy: a review. *Drug Alcohol Depend*. 2000;59(1):17–31.
81. Gowing LR, Farrell M, Bornemann R, Sullivan LE, Ali RL. Brief report: methadone treatment of injecting opioid users for prevention of HIV infection. *J Gen Int Med*. 2006;21(2):193–195.

82. Werb D, Kerr T, Marsh D, Li K, Montaner J, Wood E. Effect of methadone treatment on incarceration rates among injection drug users. *Eur Addict Res.* 2008;14(3):143–149.

83. Uhlmann S, Milloy MJ, Kerr T, et al. Methadone maintenance therapy promotes initiation of antiretroviral therapy among injection drug users. *Addiction.* 2010;105(5):907–913.

84. Lucas GM, Chaudhry A, Hsu J, et al. Clinic-based treatment of opioid-dependent HIV-infected patients versus referral to an opioid treatment program: a randomized trial. *Ann Intern Med.* 2010;152(11):704–711.

85. Kinlock TW, Gordon MS, Schwartz RP, Fitzgerald TT, O'Grady KE. A randomized clinical trial of methadone maintenance for prisoners: results at 12 months postrelease. *J Subst Abuse Treat.* 2009;37(3):277–285.

86. Stallwitz A, Stover H. The impact of substitution treatment in prisons—a literature review. *Int J Drug Policy.* 2007;18(6):464–474.

87. Wickersham JA, Zahari MM, Azar MM, Kamarulzaman A, Altice FL. Methadone dose at the time of release from prison significantly influences retention in treatment: implications from a pilot study of HIV-infected prisoners transitioning to the community in Malaysia. *Drug Alcohol Depend.* 2013;132(1–2):378–382.

88. Springer SA, Qiu J, Saber-Tehrani AS, Altice FL. Retention on buprenorphine is associated with high levels of maximal viral suppression among HIV-infected opioid dependent released prisoners. *PLoS ONE.* 2012;7(5):e38335.

89. Cohen MS, Chen YQ, McCauley M, et al. Prevention of HIV-1 infection with early antiretroviral therapy. *N Engl J Med.* 2011;365(6):493–505.

90. Larney S, Dolan K. A literature review of international implementation of opioid substitution treatment in prisons: equivalence of care? *Eur Addict Res.* 2009;15(2):107–112.

91. UN AIDS. *UNGASS Country Progress Report on HIV/AIDS: Republic of Moldova.* Cisinau, Moldova: UNAIDS; 2010.

92. The Lancet Infectious Diseases. HIV in prisons. *Lancet Infect Dis.* 2007;7(1):1.

93. Rincon-Moreno S. *Ten Years of Methadone Maintenance Programs in Spanish Prisons (1996–2005).* 4th International Conference on Alcohol and Harm Reduction. Barcelona, Spain; 2008.

94. Stover H, Michels, II. Drug use and opioid substitution treatment for prisoners. *Harm Reduct J.* 2010;7(17):1–7.

95. World Health Organization. *Guideline on When to Start Antiretroviral Therapy and on Pre-Exposure Prophylaxis for HIV.* Geneva, Switzerland: WHO; 2015.

96. Montaner JS. Treatment as prevention—a double hat-trick. *Lancet.* 2011;378(9787):208–209.

97. Cohen MS, Chen YQ, McCauley M, et al. Prevention of HIV-1 infection with early antiretroviral therapy. *N Engl J Med.* 2011;365(6):493–505.

98. Granich RM, Gilks CF, Dye C, De Cock KM, Williams BG. Universal voluntary HIV testing with immediate antiretroviral therapy as a strategy for elimination of HIV transmission: a mathematical model. *Lancet.* 2009;373(9657):48–57.

99. Wood R, Lawn SD. Antiretroviral treatment as prevention: impact of the "test and treat" strategy on the tuberculosis epidemic. *Curr HIV Res.* 2011;9(6):383–392.

100. Getahun H, Gunneberg C, Sculier D, Verster A, Raviglione M. Tuberculosis and HIV in people who inject drugs: evidence for action for tuberculosis, HIV, prison and harm reduction services. *Curr Opin HIV AIDS.* 2012;7(4):345–353.

101. World Health Organization. *Tuberculosis Control in Prisons: A Manual for Programme Managers.* Geneva, Switzerland: WHO; 2000.

102. Todrys KW, Amon JJ, Malembeka G, Clayton M. Imprisoned and imperiled: access to HIV and TB prevention and treatment, and denial of human rights, in Zambian prisons. *J Int AIDS Soc.* 2011;14:8.

103. Cohen K, Meintjes G. Management of individuals requiring antiretroviral therapy and TB treatment. *Curr Opin HIV AIDS.* 2010;5(1):61–69.

104. Dolan K, Hall W, Wodak A. Methadone maintenance reduces injecting in prison. *BMJ*. 1996;312(7039):1162.
105. European Monitoring Centre for Drugs and Drug Addiction. *Prisons and Drugs in Europe: The Problem and the Responses*. Lisbon, Portugal: EMCDDA; 2012.
106. Dolan K, Rutter S, Wodak AD. Prison-based syringe exchange programmes: a review of international research and development. *Addiction*. 2003;98(2):153–158.
107. Hughes RA. Drug injectors and the cleaning of needles and syringes. *Eur Addict Res*. 2000;6(1):20–30.
108. Leibowitz AA, Harawa N, Sylla M, Hallstrom CC, Kerndt PR. Condom distribution in jail to prevent HIV infection. *AIDS Behav*. 2013;17(8):2695–2702.
109. Dolan K, Lowe D, Shearer J. Evaluation of the condom distribution program in New South Wales prisons, Australia. *J Law Med Ethics*. 2004;32(1):124–128.
110. Yap L, Butler T, Richters J, et al. Do condoms cause rape and mayhem? the long-term effects of condoms in New South Wales' prisons. *Sex Transm Infect*. 2007;83(3):219–222.
111. Butler T, Richters J, Yap L, Donovan B. Condoms for prisoners: no evidence that they increase sex in prison, but they increase safe sex. *Sex Transm Infect*. 2013;89(5):377–379.
112. Jurgens R, Betteridge G. Prisoners who inject drugs: public health and human rights imperatives. *Health Hum Rights*. 2005;8(2):46–74.
113. Arora S, Thornton K, Jenkusky SM, Parish B, Scaletti JV. Project ECHO: linking university specialists with rural and prison-based clinicians to improve care for people with chronic hepatitis C in New Mexico. *Public Health Rep*. 2007;122(suppl 2):74–77.
114. Liddicoat RV, Zheng H, Internicola J, et al. Implementing a routine, voluntary HIV testing program in a Massachusetts county prison. *J Urban Health*. 2006;83(6):1127–1131.
115. Centers for Disease Control and Prevention. Drug-susceptible tuberculosis outbreak in a state correctional facility housing HIV-infected inmates—South Carolina, 1999–2000. *Morb Mortal Wkly Rep*. 2000;49(46):1041–1044.
116. Culbert GJ, Pillai V, Bick J, et al. Confronting the HIV, TB, addiction, and incarceration syndemic in Southeast Asia: lessons learned from Malaysia. *J Neuroimmune Pharmacol*. 2016;11(3):446–455.
117. United Nations Office on Drugs and Crime. *HIV and AIDS in Places of Detention: A Toolkit for Policymakers, Programme Managers, Prison Officers and Health Care Providers in Prison Settings*. New York, NY: UNODC; 2008.
118. George S, Clayton S, Namboodiri V, Boulay S. "Up yours": smuggling illicit drugs into prison. *BMJ Case Reports*. 2009.
119. Boys A, Farrell M, Bebbington P, et al. Drug use and initiation in prison: results from a national prison survey in England and Wales. *Addiction*. 2002;97(12):1551–1560.
120. Small W, Kain S, Laliberte N, Schechter MT, O'Shaughnessy MV, Spittal PM. Incarceration, addiction and harm reduction: inmates experience injecting drugs in prison. *Subst Use Misuse*. 2005;40(6):831–843.
121. Hammett TM. HIV/AIDS and other infectious diseases among correctional inmates: transmission, burden, and an appropriate response. *Am J Public Health*. 2006;96(6):974–978.
122. Dorman A, O'Connor A, Hardiman E, Freyne A, O' Neill H. Psychiatric morbidity in sentenced segregated HIV-positive prisoners. *Br J Psychiatry*. 1993;163:802–805.
123. Degenhardt L, Mathers B, Vickerman P, Rhodes T, Latkin C, Hickman M. Prevention of HIV infection for people who inject drugs: why individual, structural, and combination approaches are needed. *Lancet*. 2010;376(9737):285–301.
124. Wolitski RJ. Relative efficacy of a multisession sexual risk–reduction intervention for young men released from prisons in 4 states. *Am J Public Health*. 2006;96(10):1854–1861.

CHAPTER 8

The Perfect Storm

Tuberculosis, Substance Use Disorders, and Incarceration

HAIDER A. AL-DARRAJI, MBCHB, MSc AND
FREDERICK L. ALTICE, MD

BACKGROUND

Tuberculosis (TB), formerly known as "consumption" or "the White Plague," is a disease caused by the bacterium *Mycobacterium tuberculosis*, which primarily affects the lung but may involve any part of the body.[1] The disease causes destruction of the affected part, leading to poor health and ultimately death, if left untreated. The disease is transmitted between people through droplets disseminated in the air, and transmission is augmented by overcrowding and poor ventilation, an environment commonly seen in closed settings like prisons.[2] Most of those who are exposed to TB do not express the disease, and the bacteria go into a dormant stage, known as latent tuberculosis infection (LTBI). Those who develop the disease, also known as active TB disease, may infect others when coughing, sneezing, or even talking. Particularly infectious are those for whom, when their sputum is specially stained and examined using a microscope, bacteria are visually observed (known as smear-positive TB). Several risk factors increase the chances of development of active TB disease, including infection with HIV, malnourishment, close contact with a person who has active TB, chronic diseases like diabetes, and poor socio-economic background.

Identifying individuals suspected of having active TB disease is usually clinical (mostly due to prolonged, non-remitting cough), and confirmation of the disease is made through chest radiograph, sputum examination under light microscope, or growing the bacteria from the sputum specimen on a special medium in the laboratory.[3] The latter is the gold standard test, but it requires a minimum duration of 2 weeks to report a result. New diagnostic tools utilizing novel technologies are also emerging but are far from being 100% accurate compared with the culture examination. GeneXpert MTB/RIF is a new nucleic acid amplification test that is able to detect the bacteria and its resistance status to one of the major antibiotics (rifampicin) within 2 hours.[4] Treatment of active TB disease requires a combination of antibiotics that need to be prescribed for a minimum duration of 6 months. Diagnosis of clinically silent LTBI, however, is performed either through the injection of a tuberculin solution (derived from the bacteria itself) in the skin and measurement of the reaction after 2 to 3 days, also known as tuberculin skin test (TST), or by using blood immunological tests, such as interferon-gamma release assays (QuantiFERON and T-SPOT). To treat LTBI a single anti-TB medication, isoniazid, is usually prescribed for 6 months, but shorter combination regimens were recently introduced to minimize the duration of treatment.[5]

Globally, TB remains a major public health problem, particularly in low- and middle-income countries (LMICs).[6] Each year, it is estimated that around 9 million new TB cases occur worldwide, and more than 80% of these incident cases reside in 22 high-burden LMICs. TB also claims the lives of almost 2 million individuals each year. In 1993, the World Health Organization (WHO) declared TB a global emergency due to an unprecedented increase in TB notification, globally.[1] This was followed by the announcement of the WHO's Directly Observed Treatment—Short Course (DOTS) strategy to control TB at national levels. Additionally, the Stop TB partnership declared its goals to eliminate TB in line with the United Nations' Millennium Development Goals, and targets were set to halve the prevalence and mortality of TB by 2015 compared with 1990 figures.[7] Most LMICs failed to achieve these goals due to the modest (2%) global annual decline in TB incidence.[8,9] One factor contributing to this failure is the inability to reach a considerable number of TB cases (more than 3 million TB cases each year), which continue to fuel the TB epidemics and contribute to persistent TB-related morbidity and mortality.[10] The immunosuppressant effects of relatively recently introduced HIV infection disrupted TB control strategies in several regions, particularly in sub-Saharan Africa. HIV infection increases the risk of acquiring TB infection, progressing into the active disease form, and dying from the disease.[11] In 2014, 12% of reported active TB cases globally were HIV co-infected.[6] Interventions that improve HIV status, including antiretroviral therapy (ART), are beneficial in controlling TB in countries with high prevalence of TB/HIV co-infection,[12] but targets of improving access to ART are yet to be met, globally.[13] The spread of drug-resistant TB strains, including multidrug-resistant TB (MDR-TB), is a major hindrance to TB control in many countries, especially in Eastern Europe and Central Asia[6]; indeed, massive incarceration after the collapse of the Soviet Union gave rise to explosive TB and MDR-TB outbreaks.[2] This especially preventable problem was created by disruptions in treatment and improper use of anti-TB medications, especially in countries with weak TB control programs.[14] Even with improved access to healthcare services, poor adherence and failure to complete anti-TB treatment regimens are common among people who use drugs (PWUD), possibly due to the sedative effect of drugs or to repeated incarceration with interrupted use of treatment.[15] In a sample (N = 10,428) of TB patients in Thailand, having previously injected drugs was the primary risk factor independently associated with MDR-TB[16]; the authors of this paper referred to repeated incarceration as one of the possible causes of this association. Similarly, histories of incarceration and drug use were independently associated with MDR-TB in an analysis of nation-wide electronic TB registry over 5 years in Kazakhstan.[17] Mathematical modeling data from Ukraine suggest that incarceration itself contributes to 75% of TB cases in PWUD.[18]

TB disproportionately affects socially vulnerable populations, including the poor, ethnic minorities, homeless individuals, PWUD, and prisoners, among others.[19] This might be related to the limited access to timely healthcare services, poor housing, malnutrition, and related co-morbidities, including HIV infection and alcoholism.[20] Failure to address TB in these marginalized populations may further jeopardize TB elimination programs worldwide. Nonetheless, TB is inextricably linked to PWUD, most of whom have histories of incarceration, which acts as a source fueling onward TB transmission.[21]

TUBERCULOSIS AND DRUG USE

Having a drug use problem, especially related to incarceration of PWUD, is correlated with elevated TB risk and contributes greatly to TB transmission in many regions globally, irrespective of the country's economic status.[22] Despite the tremendous decline in TB rates in many high-income countries, TB risk remains elevated among many socially vulnerable groups, including PWUD.[23] PWUD are characterized by many TB risk factors, including an increased prevalence of HIV infection (especially among people who inject drugs [PWID]), homelessness, socioeconomic disadvantage, alcoholism, incarceration, and tobacco use.[24] TB remains a major cause of morbidity and mortality among PWUD, especially those infected with HIV.[25,26] A systematic review showed variable but generally high (10% to 59%) prevalence of LTBI among PWUD, which was independently associated with longer duration of drug use and with exposure to incarceration.[15] Two recent surveys showed a very high prevalence of LTBI among PWUD treated in methadone clinics in Malaysia (TST positivity = 86.7%)[27] and Taiwan (TST positivity = 85%).[28]

PWID have a 2-fold to 6-fold increased risk of developing active TB disease compared with those not using drugs; this risk is further increased by the presence of HIV.[21] These rates may vary based on the national TB burden. A recent case-finding study among attendees of a methadone clinic in Tanzania found that 4% of surveyed clients (N = 150) had active TB, which is 23-fold higher than the national rate.[29] Analysis of data from a national TB registry over a 15-year period (1997–2006) in the United States, where TB cases are typical among foreign-born persons, showed that 18.7% of individuals diagnosed with active TB disease were PWUD, including one third of US-born men with active TB.[22] Findings in the latter study affirmed prioritizing TB case finding among people with drug and alcohol use disorders in the United States. Also in this study, PWUD were 1.6-fold more likely to be sputum smear-positive than non–drug users, irrespective of HIV status,[22] suggesting that PWUD with TB are more likely than others to transmit TB, especially in poorly ventilated closed settings such as prisons, addiction treatment centers, and homeless shelters.[28] This may, in part, be due to delayed diagnosis because PWUD are often disenfranchised from healthcare delivery systems and may not seek care until they are incarcerated or very ill.

People living with HIV (PLWH) who acquire HIV from drug injection have poorer TB treatment outcomes (non-adherence, failure, default, and death) compared with non-drug-using PLWH.[25,30] A retrospective review of medical records of 219 PLWH diagnosed with active TB in Malaysia in 2010 showed that PWID were more likely to have unfavorable outcomes than were those who acquired HIV through sexual contact.[30] Similarly, a study of individuals diagnosed with TB in Spain found that drug use (injecting and non-injecting) was associated with increased mortality and unfavorable TB treatment outcomes among both HIV-infected and uninfected individuals.[25] A study from Ukraine, however, suggested that poor treatment outcomes among PWID with active TB can be reduced by linking individuals with opioid use disorders to methadone treatment.[31]

TB IN PRISONS

Globally, more than 11 million people are imprisoned, and 30 million people transition through closed prison settings annually.[32,33] The prevalence of HIV and TB was reported by the WHO in 2000 to be several times higher in prisons than in the general population, resulting in explosive TB outbreaks within and beyond their walls, through released inmates and prison officers.[34] Prison overcrowding and poor infection control measures contribute to increased TB risk, particularly in PLWH and PWID who already have elevated risk. Figure 8.1 depicts the effect of incarceration on the amplification of TB within prisons and the community. The prison environment is dynamic, with large numbers of people entering and leaving annually. Where laws highly criminalize PWUD, these individuals who are already at risk for TB and HIV enter prisons where the diseases are concentrated. Especially in the case of TB where individuals with HIV are housed, undiagnosed prisoners with TB transmit infection to others and further amplify disease within these settings. In the absence of adequate screening and treatment programs, health deteriorates, resulting in increasing morbidity and mortality. Those who acquire active or LTBI are released to the community at unprecedented levels and disseminate disease to other community members. Moreover, previous reports show that TB contributed largely to the mortality of prisoners before the implementation of effective control programs. In Russia, almost half (49.2%) of prison deaths were attributed to TB in 1997,[35] and the vast majority (80%) of prisoners dying in Azerbaijan prisons was attributed to TB in 1999.[36] In several LMICs, drug use, HIV, and TB are syndemic, concentrated in prisons, and require innovative and integrated programs to effectively transition prisoners with these comorbidities into the community.[37-39]

Closed settings such as prisons, jails, and compulsory drug detention centers are known amplifiers of TB, largely due to the concentration of high-risk individuals who enter them, but with the addition of the prevalent poor nutrition and ventilation in these settings, TB transmission is augmented, and further progression to active TB disease, possibly after release to the community, is facilitated.[34] Additionally, limited

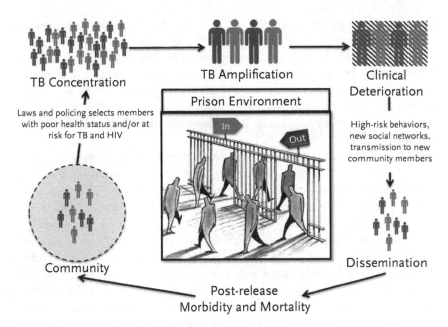

Figure 8.1: Prisons as amplifiers for tuberculosis

access to timely healthcare services in prisons, particularly in LMICs, increases the burden of the disease in such settings.[40,41] A recent intensified case-finding assessment in a Malaysian prison, where formal TB screening does not exist, showed that 12% of PLWH (nearly all were PWID) in the prison had previously undiagnosed active TB.[42] In this setting, TB-related mortality among prisoners with HIV was extraordinarily high but was markedly reduced after treating HIV with ART.[43] Undetected TB within this high-risk environment further amplifies TB transmission to other prisoners[44,45] and prison staff,[46] resulting in a high prevalence of LTBI, the main pool for subsequent development of active TB disease.[47] Moreover, overcrowding and lack of isolation facilities in many LMIC prisons compound the risk of transmission of TB and MDR-TB among prisoners.[48,49] Consequently, both active and latent TB are highly prevalent in correctional settings. LTBI was reported to be the most prevalent infection in several prison surveys, including in countries with low TB burden such as the United States and Spain, but also in intermediate- and high-burden countries (Malaysia and Pakistan),[44,50–52] and its prevalence is estimated to be several-fold higher than in the surrounding communities, globally.[34] Moreover, due to its airborne transmission dynamics, TB transmission extends beyond other prisoners to prison staff and visitors. A systematic review estimated that TB exposure in prisons contributes incrementally to 8.5% and 6.3% of active TB cases in communities of high- and low/middle-income countries, respectively.[53]

Due to harsh criminalization of drug use in many settings, incarceration rates are high, and the prevalence of both PWUD[21,54] and infectious diseases within prisons is elevated.[55–57] For example, one cross-sectional study of new entrants to a Spanish prison reported high prevalence of LTBI (44.0%) and HIV infection (43.8%) among PWID.[51] In similar settings the convergence of TB, HIV, and viral hepatitis with incarceration proved to be a major hindrance to proper healthcare service delivery owing to the pressure on healthcare systems.[21,24] Numerous studies have documented a high prevalence of incarceration among PWID.[27,28] Despite the convergence of injection drug use, HIV, and TB in prisons, adequate screening and treatment are seldom implemented, especially in LMIC settings where prisoner health is underfunded or completely ignored.[58]

The WHO provides conflicting guidance on controlling TB in PLWH as well as in closed settings such as prisons and jails. To prevent and optimize TB outcomes in PLWH, the WHO recommends the implementation of the "Three I's," namely, intensified case finding, isoniazid preventive therapy (IPT), and infection control, in addition to improving access to ART.[59] Despite the proven effectiveness of IPT in preventing TB among HIV-infected[60] and uninfected individuals,[61] and despite WHO recommendations to treat all PLWH with IPT,[5] effective use of IPT in closed settings remains limited.[62] This inadequate response may, in part, be due to existing WHO recommendations that favor deployment of resources for finding active TB disease over treatment of LTBI in resource-constrained settings,[34] despite evidence that IPT is cost-effective in controlling TB among prisoners and recommendations for urgent need to scale up IPT in prisons.[63] One of the major concerns about scaling up IPT is the fear of non-adherence during the 6 to 9 months of treatment,[64] and hence the potential promotion of isoniazid resistance in the community. WHO recommendations for prisons have not yet been updated despite evidence from a community study that an abbreviated 12-week regimen consisting of once-weekly prescription of two anti-TB medications (rifapentine plus isoniazid) was as effective as isoniazid alone in preventing active TB disease and had a significantly higher completion rate (82.1% vs. 69.0%, $p < .001$, respectively).[65] Although these results are promising, evidence for this short-course LTBI prevention strategy in detention centers and prisons has yet to be examined; this is particularly important in prisons with a high prevalence of viral hepatitis, given potential concerns about liver toxicity of the medications. Another issue with the WHO guidelines is the recommendation for prolonged (36-month) IPT in PLWH in high-burden community settings, especially those with documented LTBI.[66] Such a recommendation fails to recognize that closed settings such as prisons are high burden, and IPT is de-emphasized over case finding of active TB cases.

Despite a meta-analysis substantiating that ART reduces the risk of active TB disease by 67% (95% confidence interval: 61%–73%) in resource-constrained settings,[9] ART coverage in most prisons is inadequately scaled to need, nor has its effectiveness been examined on TB outcomes in prisons where re-infection is likely high.

Finding alternatives to incarceration for PWUD through penal reforms, including non-custodial measures and drug courts, may reduce overcrowding in prisons and is aligned with treating PWUD continuously in community settings.[67] Such measures are also likely to reduce the prevalence of TB in prisons, with flow-on benefits for the communities to which these individuals return. The observation of a significant reduction in TB burden in 27 Thai prisons was attributed to the diversion of PWID away from prison and into community-based treatment.[68]

BARRIERS AND CHALLENGES TO ACCESS TO HEALTH
Diagnosis of TB in Prisons

Unfortunately, there are no international consensus guidelines and recommendations for TB screening in prison settings, with diverse screening algorithms that often lack a strong evidence base and are tailored depending on a country's economic status or its prioritization of prisoners' healthcare.[40] Furthermore, the performance of these screening tools in prison settings may further be compromised depending on the prevalence of HIV infection,[69] which is prevalent in prisons in countries either with high incarceration rates or where drug use is harshly criminalized.[70] Most of the diagnostic tools, including symptoms and chest radiograph features, depend on the bacteria-host immunological interaction, and the immuno-suppressive effect of HIV renders these tools inaccurate (eg, PLWH with active TB may present with no symptoms and a normal chest radiograph).[3] Despite international recommendations to use symptom-based TB screening and its being the most widely utilized screening tool for TB in prisons,[40] its diagnostic performance remains persistently disappointing.[71] A cross-sectional study among 1,696 new entrants into a Brazilian prison concluded that symptom-based screening would miss 78.3% of active TB cases,[72] primarily due to underestimation of symptom reporting by inmates and to high rates of drug use, including cough-suppressing opioids, which may delay symptoms and hence care seeking.[15,73] Chest radiography has an improved diagnostic performance (higher sensitivity) compared with symptom-based screening in low HIV prevalence settings,[74] but it is limited by low specificity.[75] Mathematical modeling from a Brazilian prison with high TB prevalence found that routine chest radiography screening of all inmates was the most effective tool in reducing TB prevalence over 5 years.[76] The new WHO-endorsed GeneXpert MTB/RIF technology has revolutionized TB diagnosis by providing accurate detection of *M. tuberculosis* within 2 hours.[4] The assay was found to outperform smear microscopy examination and to improve case detection in a prison in an LMIC,[42] although its performance was influenced by the immuno-suppressive effect of HIV (production of less bacteria in sputum specimens) and number of specimens tested, being lower when a single specimen is used.[77,78] In high-TB and MDR-TB settings such as Eastern Europe, where HIV prevalence is extraordinarily high, annual GeneXpert MTB/RIF screening is the most effective tool to reduce TB and MDR-TB prevalence in the prisons,[69] yet this technology is not widely available.

Transition to the Community

One of the major challenges facing the delivery of healthcare for PWUD in prisons is the assurance of continuity of care after release.[79] Although it appears that most prisoners over-estimate their ability to access care after release from custody[80,81] post-release retention in care is particularly poor for HIV, TB, and addiction treatment.[82-87] Transitioning to the community is especially challenging for PWUD, especially with them facing several challenges including relapse to drug use, police harassment and re-incarceration, untreated mental illnesses, and difficulties in meeting the basic needs of housing, employment, and social re-integration.[84,88–90] PWUD are sometimes incorrectly perceived by healthcare providers as uncooperative, non-adherent, and undeserving of care; as a consequence, some PWUD do not seek out treatment services.[91] In addition, PWUD may be actively discriminated against by healthcare providers who withhold needed care,[92] resulting in mutual mistrust between PWUD and providers,[93] which may further reduce PWUD wanting to seek out treatment, due to real or perceived restrictions on access to healthcare services.

Adherence to Treatment

PWUD, in the absence of treatment that holistically addresses both their TB and addiction treatment needs, have suboptimal treatment outcomes compared with their counterparts without addiction. These suboptimal treatment outcomes may include missing clinic appointments (due to lack of social support, homelessness, and illicit substance and alcohol abuse); requiring more prolonged TB treatment (due to poor adherence to the long treatment regimen); and experiencing increased hospitalization.[15,94] Continuing drug and alcohol misuse contributes to suboptimal TB treatment adherence and treatment completion.[73] One clear mechanism to overcome concerns about non-adherence to TB treatment for opioid-dependent PWID is provision of opioid agonist therapy (OAT) with either methadone maintenance therapy (MMT) or buprenorphine maintenance therapy (BMT). OAT effectively reduces opioid use but remains markedly under-scaled, with only 8% of PWID enrolled globally[95] and even lower in LMICs.[96] OAT provided within prisons is available in only 29 countries and is either restricted to pilot programs or under-scaled and suboptimally dosed.[97] In the case of HIV treatment outcomes, providing BMT before release from prison markedly suppresses viral load and prevents relapse among HIV-infected prisoners compared with post-release referrals,[98] although in the case of methadone, this effect may largely depend on the pre-release MMT dose. In two prisons in Malaysia where MMT was piloted, HIV-infected prisoners who received therapeutic doses exceeding 80 mg before release were significantly more likely to be retained in treatment for 12 months after release.[99]

Patient preferences for OAT may differ regionally and contribute differentially to retention in treatment. For example, in New York[100] and Connecticut, US,[101,102] opioid-dependent prisoners preferred methadone over buprenorphine, yet in Malaysia, where there had been previously described diversion and injection of buprenorphine,[103,104] PWID preferred methadone.[105] PWID with TB in Ukraine who received methadone were significantly more likely than those who did not receive methadone to be adherent to medications and complete TB treatment.[31] Similarly, adherence to ART was reportedly higher among PLWH receiving OAT compared with those who did not, globally.[106,107] No controlled studies of OAT for transitioning prisoners with TB, including addressing their treatment preferences, have yet been conducted to improve adherence to continuity of healthcare after release, but evidence from observational studies suggests that OAT may be an important component of holistic post-release treatment of active TB or LTBI.

Several studies have found that the favorable treatment outcomes of the management of TB and HIV infections during incarceration might be lost after release from prison, largely due to failure to adhere to treatment after release, and to recidivism.[108] Though HIV differs markedly from TB in that it requires a lifetime of treatment, it can serve as a model for TB. For example, in a randomized trial involving jail detainees in the United States, those receiving intensive educational sessions about TB before release were significantly more likely than those receiving usual care to visit a TB clinic within 30 days of release to continue treatment of LTBI (24% vs. 10%), although the overall completion rate remained low in both groups (47% vs. 28%).[109] Monetary and other forms of incentives either alone or in conjunction with other outreach programs in PWUD have had conflicting outcomes.[110,111] TB directly observed therapy (DOT) administered through community outreach achieved high TB treatment success and was cost-effective among predominantly PWUD in New York.[112] Similar findings were observed with direct observation of preventive therapy (DOPT) of LTBI among PWID attending a needle and syringe exchange program in New York.[111]

Healthcare organizational factors also contribute to poor TB treatment outcomes in prisons, where treatment systems are vertically organized and managed separately without addressing other co-morbidities, which may have an impact on TB treatment, including HIV and drug use.[38,113] Several innovative models have been created to improve access to TB healthcare services among PWUD, particularly for PLWH, in the community.[110] Co-location of these services in a "one-stop shopping" model in the community was found to improve access to co-morbidity services[38,39] and is currently endorsed by the WHO.[37] OAT clinics, hence, offer ideal settings to improve TB treatment adherence[73] and deliver integrated health services,[91] including access and retention in TB screening and control programs. Recent international guidelines support integrated care for PWUD with or at risk for HIV and TB.[114] In one study comparing integrated services for PWID in Ukraine, co-located treatment settings significantly improved quality health indicators for HIV, addiction, and TB screening and treatment,[39] holding promise for new healthcare delivery strategies that can be adopted in prisons. Co-located services improved uptake of tuberculin screening among attendees of an addiction treatment clinic in New York from 55.1-70.1% to 82.6-91.1%.[91] Additionally, OAT sites may allow direct observation of TB or LTBI treatment. Combining methadone with IPT and provision of daily DOT improved IPT completion compared with routine care through the referral system in San Francisco[115] and Connecticut.[116] A randomized trial in Estonia showed that OAT clients receiving active referral (arrangement of appointments, reminders, transport provision, and incentives) were four times more likely to attend TB clinic appointments compared with those passively referred.[113] Most of these strategies, however, have not been tested for prisoners with TB. Additionally, integration of healthcare services can optimize treatment of complex patients, including drug-drug interactions, particularly between methadone and liver enzyme inducers like rifampicin (for TB treatment) and ART medications, which may induce methadone withdrawal among individuals on a stable MMT program.[108] In the case of opioid withdrawal symptoms, OAT clients may stop their anti-TB medications or supplement methadone with illicit opioids, with both having detrimental consequences.[117] Co-infection with hepatitis C virus, which is highly prevalent in both prisoners and PWID, may affect the safety profile of the treatment of TB or LTBI[118] and increase the risk of drug-induced liver damage.[119,120]

PRISONS AS SITES TO PROMOTE PUBLIC HEALTH MANDATES

Prisons can serve as sentinel sites to diagnose and treat active TB and LTBI,[121] particularly for PWUD who often have limited access to community-based healthcare services.[34] An intensified TB case finding among PLWH (predominantly PWID) in a Malaysian prison showed that despite elevated risk of TB, only one-third of participants had ever been screened for TB in their lifetime.[42] Adequate integration of treatment and prevention services in prisons, especially those that adequately support reintegration into community healthcare and society after release,[34] has been successfully deployed in several countries[110,122] and is crucial to individual and public health.

RECOMMENDATIONS

PWUD, especially those who interface with closed settings, remain at elevated risk for TB due to the convergence of adverse social circumstances, limited healthcare access and utilization, repeated detentions with exposure to TB where standardized and effective screening strategies largely remain absent, and HIV infection. Multidisciplinary interventions need to be deployed to control TB in this population, both during incarceration and during the transition back to the community. Minimally, this should include active TB case finding and treatment, screening and treatment of LTBI, improving access to HIV healthcare and therapy, and ensuring access to OAT both before and after release. Integration of TB, HIV, and OAT programs both within prisons and in the community improves management of these co-morbidities and is endorsed by WHO. Despite this endorsement, conflicting guidance remains on the most effective and cost-effective strategies for TB screening and continuity of TB care after release. There remains considerable need for research to create the evidence base for preventive TB treatment in prisoners, most of whom are PWUD, and strategies to optimize linkage to care after release.

REFERENCES

1. Zumla A, Mwaba P, Huggett J, Kapata N, Chanda D, Grange J. Reflections on the White Plague. *Lancet Infect Dis.* 2009;9(3):197–202.

2. Stuckler D, Basu S, McKee M, King L. Mass incarceration can explain population increases in TB and multidrug-resistant TB in European and central Asian countries. *Proc Natl Acad Sci USA.* 2008;105(36):13280–13285.

3. Zumla A, Raviglione M, Hafner R, von Reyn CF. Tuberculosis. *N Engl J Med.* 2013;368(8):745–755.

4. Boehme CC, Nabeta P, Hillemann D, et al. Rapid molecular detection of tuberculosis and rifampin resistance. *N Engl J Med.* 2010;363(11):1005–1015.

5. World Health Organization. *Guidelines on the Management of Latent Tuberculosis Infection.* Geneva, Switzerland: WHO; 2015.

6. World Health Organization. *Global Tuberculosis Report 2014.* Geneva, Switzerland: WHO; 2015.

7. Laserson K, Wells CD. Reaching the targets for tuberculosis control: the impact of HIV. *Bull World Heal Organ.* 2007;85(5):377–381.

8. Lönnroth K, Corbett E, Golub J, Uplekar M, Weil D, Raviglione M. Systematic screening for active tuberculosis : rationale, definitions and key considerations. *Int J Tuberc Lung Dis.* 2013;17(3):289–298.

9. Lawn SD, Wood R, De Cock KM, Kranzer K, Lewis JJ, Churchyard GJ. Antiretrovirals and isoniazid preventive therapy in the prevention of HIV-associated tuberculosis in settings with limited health-care resources. *Lancet Infect Dis.* 2010;10(7):489–498.

10. McHugh TD. World TB Day 2014: reach the three million: a TB test, treatment and cure for all. *Trans R Soc Trop Med Hyg.* 2014;108(3):119–120.

11. Corbett EL, Marston B, Churchyard GJ, De Cock KM. Tuberculosis in sub-Saharan Africa : opportunities, challenges, and change in the era of antiretroviral treatment. *Lancet.* 2006;367:926–937.

12. Lawn SD, Harries AD, Williams BG, et al. Antiretroviral therapy and the control of HIV-associated tuberculosis: will ART do it? *Int J Tuberc Lung Dis.* 2011;15(5):571–581.

13. Joint United Nations Programme on HIV/AIDS (UNAIDS). *The Gap Report.* Geneva, Switzerland: UNAIDS; 2014.

14. Chiang C-Y, Centis R, Migliori GB. Drug-resistant tuberculosis: past, present, future. *Respirology.* 2010;15(3):413–432.

15. Deiss RG, Rodwell TC, Garfein RS. Tuberculosis and illicit drug use: review and update. *Clin Infect Dis.* 2009;48(1):72–82.

16. Akksilp S, Wattanaamornkiat W, Kittikraisak W, et al. Multi-drug resistant TB and HIV in Thailand: overlapping, but not independently associated risk factors. *Southeast Asian J Trop Med Public Heal.* 2009;40(6):1264–1278.

17. Van Den Hof S, Tursynbayeva A, Abildaev T, et al. Converging risk factors but no association between HIV infection and multidrug-resistant tuberculosis in Kazakhstan. *Int J Tuberc Lung Dis.* 2013;17(4):526–531.

18. Altice FL, Azbel L, Stone J, et al. The perfect storm: incarceration and the high-risk environment perpetuating transmission of HIV, hepatitis C virus, and tuberculosis in Eastern Europe and Central Asia. *Lancet.* 2016;388(10050):1228–1248.

19. Lönnroth K, Jaramillo E, Williams BG, Dye C, Raviglione M. Drivers of tuberculosis epidemics: the role of risk factors and social determinants. *Soc Sci Med.* 2009;68(12):2240–2246.

20. Figueroa-Munoz JI, Ramon-Pardo P. Tuberculosis control in vulnerable groups. *Bull World Health Organ.* 2008;86(9):733–735.

21. Getahun H, Gunneberg C, Sculier D, Verster A, Raviglione M. Tuberculosis and HIV in people who inject drugs: evidence for action for tuberculosis, HIV, prison and harm reduction services. *Curr Opin HIV AIDS.* 2012;7(4):345–353.

22. Oeltmann JE, Kammerer JS, Pevzner ES, Moonan PK. Tuberculosis and dubstance sbuse in the United States, 1997–2006. *Arch Intern Med.* 2009;169(2):189–197.

23. Caylà JA, Orcau A. Control of tuberculosis in large cities in developed countries: an organizational problem. *BMC Med.* 2011;9(1):127.

24. Centre for Disease Control and Prevention (CDC). Integrated prevention services for HIV infection, viral hepatitis, sexually transmitted diseases, and tuberculosis

for persons who use drugs illicitly: summary guidance from CDC and the U.S. Department of Health and Human Services. *Morb Mortal Wkly Rep.* 2012;61(5).

25. Ruiz-Navarro MD, Espinosa JAH, Hernández MJB, et al. Effects of HIV status and other variables on the outcome of tuberculosis treatment in Spain. *Arch Bronconeumol.* 2005;41(7):363–370.

26. van Asten L, Langendam M, Zangerle R, et al. Tuberculosis risk varies with the duration of HIV infection: a prospective study of European drug users with known date of HIV seroconversion. *AIDS.* 2003;17(8):1201–1208.

27. Al-Darraji HAA, Wong KC, Yeow DEY, et al. Tuberculosis screening in a novel substance abuse treatment center in Malaysia: implications for a comprehensive approach for integrated care. *J Subst Abuse Treat.* 2014;46:144–149.

28. Yen Y-F, Hu B-S, Lin Y-S, et al. Latent tuberculosis among injection drug users in a methadone maintenance treatment program, Taipei, Taiwan: TSPOT.TB versus tuberculin skin test. *Scand J Infect Dis.* 2013;45(7):504–511.

29. Gupta A, Mbwambo J, Mteza I, et al. Active case finding for tuberculosis among people who inject drugs on methadone treatment in Dar es Salaam, Tanzania. *Int J Tuberc Lung Dis.* 2014;18(7):793–798.

30. Ismail I, Bulgiba A. Determinants of unsuccessful tuberculosis treatment outcomes in Malaysian HIV-infected patients. *Prev Med.* 2013;10–13.

31. Morozova O, Dvoryak S, Altice FL. Methadone treatment improves tuberculosis treatment among hospitalized opioid dependent patients in Ukraine. *Int J Drug Policy.* 2013;24(6):e91–98.

32. Dolan K, Moazen B, Noori A, Rahimzadeh S, Farzadfar F, Hariga F. People who inject drugs in prison: HIV prevalence, transmission and prevention. *Int J Drug Policy.* 2015;26:S12–S15.

33. Walmsley R. *World Prison Population List.* 11th ed. London, England: International Centre for Prison Studies; 2015.

34. World Health Organization. *Tuberculosis Control in Prisons: A Manual for Programme Managers.* Geneva, Switzerland: WHO; 2000.

35. Bobrik A, Danishevski K, Eroshina K, McKee M. Prison health in Russia: the larger picture. *J Public Health Policy.* 2005;26(1):30–59.

36. Coninx R, Eshaya-Chauvin B, Reyes H. Tuberculosis in prisons. *Lancet.* 1995;346:1238–1239.

37. World Health Organization. *Policy Guidelines for Collaborative TB and HIV Services for Injecting and Other Drug Users: An Integrated Approach.* Geneva, Switzerland: WHO; 2008.

38. Sylla L, Bruce RD, Kamarulzaman A, Altice FL. Integration and co-location of HIV/AIDS, tuberculosis and drug treatment services. *Int J Drug Policy.* 2007;18(4):306–312.

39. Bachireddy C, Soule MC, Izenberg JM, Dvoryak S, Dumchev K, Altice FL. Integration of health services improves multiple healthcare outcomes among HIV-infected people who inject drugs in Ukraine. *Drug Alcohol Depend.* 2014;1(0)106–114.

40. Vinkeles Melchers NVS, van Elsland SL, Lange JMA, Borgdorff MW, van den Hombergh J. State of affairs of tuberculosis in prison facilities: a systematic review of screening practices and recommendations for best TB control. *PLoS ONE.* 2013;8(1):e53644.

41. O'Grady J, Hoelscher M, Atun R, et al. Tuberculosis in prisons in sub-Saharan Africa—the need for improved health services, surveillance and control. *Tuberculosis.* 2011;91(2):173–178.

42. Al-Darraji HAA, Abd Razak H, Ng KP, Altice FL, Kamarulzaman A. The diagnostic performance of a single GeneXpert MTB/RIF assay in an intensified tuberculosis case finding survey among HIV-infected prisoners in Malaysia. *PLoS ONE.* 2013;8(9):e73717.

43. Culbert GJ, Pillai V, Bick J, et al. Confronting the HIV, tuberculosis, addiction, and incarceration syndemic in Southeast Asia: lessons learned from Malaysia. *J Neuroimmune Pharmacol.* 2016;11(3):446–455.

44. Al-Darraji HAA, Kamarulzaman A, Altice FL. Latent tuberculosis infection in a Malaysian prison: implications for a comprehensive integrated control program in prisons. *BMC Public Health.* 2014;14(22):1–9.

45. Margolis B, Al-Darraji HAA, Wickersham JA, Kamarulzaman A, Altice FL. Prevalence of tuberculosis symptoms and latent tuberculous infection among prisoners in northeastern Malaysia. *Int J Tuberc Lung Dis.* 2013;17(12):1538–1544.
46. Al-Darraji HAA, Tan C, Kamarulzaman A, Altice FL. Prevalence and correlates of latent tuberculosis infection among employees of a high security prison in Malaysia. *Occup Environ Med.* 2015;72(6):442–447.
47. Al-Darraji HAA, Altice FL, Kamarulzaman A. Undiagnosed pulmonary tuberculosis among prisoners in Malaysia: an overlooked risk for tuberculosis in the community. *Trop Med Int Heal.* 2016;21(8):1049–1058.
48. Stott KE, de Oliviera T, Lessells RJ. Combined antiretroviral and anti-tuberculosis drug resistance following incarceration. *South Afr J HIV Med.* 2013;14(3):135–137.
49. Johnstone-Robertson S, Lawn SD, Welte A, Bekker L, Wood R. Tuberculosis in a South African prison—a transmission modelling analysis. *S Afr Med J.* 2011;101(11):809–813.
50. Baillargeon J, Black SA, Leach CT, et al. The infectious disease profile of Texas prison inmates. *Prev Med.* 2004;38(5):607–612.
51. Martín V, Caylà JA, Bolea Á, Castilla J. *Mycobacterium tuberculosis* and human immunodeficiency virus co-infection in intravenous drug users on admission to prison. *Int J Tuberc Lung Dis.* 2000;4(1):41–46.
52. Hussain H. Prevalence of and risk factors associated with *Mycobacterium tuberculosis* infection in prisoners, North West Frontier Province, Pakistan. *Int J Epidemiol.* 2003;32(5):794–799.
53. Baussano I, Williams BG, Nunn P, Beggiato M, Fedeli U, Scano F. Tuberculosis incidence in prisons: a systematic review. *PLoS Med.* 2010;7(12):e1000381.
54. Hayashi K, Milloy M-J, Fairbairn N, et al. Incarceration experiences among a community-recruited sample of injection drug users in Bangkok, Thailand. *BMC Public Health.* 2009;9(492):1–7.
55. Azbel L, Wickersham JA, Wegman M, et al. Burden of substance use disorders, mental illness, and correlates of infectious diseases among soon-to-be released prisoners in Azerbaijan. *Drug Alcohol Depend.* 2015;151:68–75.
56. Azbel L, Wickersham JA, Grishaev Y, Dvoryak S, Altice FL. Burden of infectious diseases, substance use disorders, and mental illness among Ukrainian prisoners transitioning to the community. *PLoS ONE.* 2013;8(3):e59643.
57. Fazel S, Baillargeon J. The health of prisoners. *Lancet.* 2011;377(9769):956–965.
58. Coninx R, Maher D, Reyes H, Grzemska M. Tuberculosis in prisons in countries with high prevalence. *BMJ.* 2000;320(7232):440–442.
59. World Health Organization. *WHO Three I's Meeting: Intensified Case Finding (ICF), Isoniazid Preventive Therapy (IPT) and TB Infection Control (IC) for People Living With HIV.* Geneva, Switzerland: WHO; 2008.
60. Akolo C, Adetifa I, Shepperd S, Volmink J. Treatment of latent tuberculosis infection in HIV infected persons. *Cochrane Database Syst Rev.* 2010;(1):CD000171.
61. Smieja M, Marchetti C, Cook D, Smaill F. Isoniazid for preventing tuberculosis in non-HIV infected persons (Review). *Cochrane Database Syst Rev.* 1999;(1):CD001363.
62. Al-Darraji HAA, Kamarulzaman A, Altice FL. Isoniazid preventive therapy in correctional facilities: a systematic review. *Int J Tuberc Lung Dis.* 2012;16(7):871–879.
63. Bandyopadhyay T, Murray H, Metersky ML. Cost-effectiveness of tuberculosis prophyaxis after release from short-term correctional facilities. *Chest.* 2002;121(6):1771–1775.
64. Ngamvithayapong J, Uthaivoravit W, Yanai H, Akarasewi P, Sawanpanyalert P. Adherence to tuberculosis preventive therapy among HIV-infected persons in Chiang Rai, Thailand. *AIDS.* 1997;11(1):107–112.
65. Sterling TR, Villarino ME, Borisov AS, et al. Three months of rifapentine and isoniazid for latent tuberculosis infection. *N Engl J Med.* 2011;365(23):2155–2166.
66. World Health Organization. *Guidelines for Intensified Tuberculosis Case-Finding and Isoniazid Preventive Therapy for People Living with HIV in Resource-Constrained Settings.* Geneva, Switzerland: WHO; 2011.

67. Reid SE, Topp SM, Turnbull ER, et al. Tuberculosis and HIV control in sub-Saharan African prisons: "thinking outside the prison cell." *J Infect Dis.* 2012;205(suppl):S265–S273.
68. Jittimanee SX, Ngamtrairai N, White MC, Jittimanee S. A prevalence survey for smear-positive tuberculosis in Thai prisons. *Int J Tuberc Lung Dis.* 2007;11(5):556–561.
69. Winetsky DE, Negoescu DM, DeMarchis EH, et al. Screening and rapid molecular diagnosis of tuberculosis in prisons in Russia and Eastern Europe: a cost-effectiveness analysis. *PLoS Med.* 2012;9(11):e1001348.
70. Dolan K, Kite B, Black E, Aceijas C, Stimson GV. HIV in prison in low-income and middle-income countries. *Lancet Infect Dis.* 2007;7(1):32–41.
71. Fournet N, Sanchez A, Massari V, et al. Development and evaluation of tuberculosis screening scores in Brazilian prisons. *Public Health.* 2006;120(10):976–983.
72. Sanchez A, Larouzé B, Espinola AB, et al. Screening for tuberculosis on admission to highly endemic prisons? the case of Rio de Janeiro state prisons. *Int J Tuberc Lung Dis.* 2009;13(10):1247–1252.
73. Schluger NW, El-Bassel N, Hermosilla S, et al. Tuberculosis, drug use and HIV infection in Central Asia: an urgent need for attention. *Drug Alcohol Depend.* 2013;132(suppl):S32–S36.
74. Sanchez A, Gerhardt G, Natal S, et al. Prevalence of pulmonary tuberculosis and comparative evaluation of screening strategies in a Brazilian prison. *Int J Tuberc Lung Dis.* 2005;9(6):633–639.
75. van Cleeff MRA, Kivihya-Ndugga LE, Meme H, Odhiambo JA, Klatser PR. The role and performance of chest X-ray for the diagnosis of tuberculosis: a cost-effectiveness analysis in Nairobi, Kenya. *BMC Infect Dis.* 2005;5(111):1–9.
76. Legrand J, Sanchez A, Le Pont F, Camacho L, Larouze B. Modeling the impact of tuberculosis control strategies in highly endemic overcrowded prisons. *PLoS ONE.* 2008;3(5):e2100.
77. Lawn SD, Brooks S V, Kranzer K, et al. Screening for HIV-associated tuberculosis and rifampicin resistance before antiretroviral therapy using the Xpert MTB/RIF assay: a prospective study. *PLoS Med.* 2011;8(7):e1001067.
78. Theron G, Peter J, van Zyl-Smit R, et al. Evaluation of the Xpert MTB/RIF assay for the diagnosis of pulmonary tuberculosis in a high HIV prevalence setting. *Am J Respir Crit Care Med.* 2011;184(1):132–140.
79. Krishnan A, Wickersham JA, Chitsaz E, et al. Post-release substance abuse outcomes among HIV-infected jail detainees: results from a multisite study. *AIDS Behav.* 2013;17:S171–S180.
80. Morozova O, Azbel L, Grishaev Y, Dvoryak S, Wickersham JA, Altice FL. Ukrainian prisoners and community reentry challenges: implications for transitional care. *Int J Prison Health.* 2013;9(1):5–19.
81. Choi P, Kavasery R, Desai MM, Govindasamy S, Kamarulzaman A, Altice FL. Prevalence and correlates of community re-entry challenges faced by HIV-infected male prisoners in Malaysia. *Int J STD AIDS.* 2010;21(6):416–423.
82. Rich JD, McKenzie M, Larney S, et al. Methadone continuation versus forced withdrawal on incarceration in a combined US prison and jail: a randomised, open-label trial. *Lancet.* 2015;386(9991):350–359.
83. Meyer JP, Cepeda J, Springer SA, Wu J, Trestman RL, Altice FL. HIV in people reincarcerated in Connecticut prisons and jails: an observational cohort study. *Lancet HIV.* 2015;1(2):e77–84.
84. Meyer JP, Altice FL. Transition to the community. In: Trestman RL, Applebaum KL, Metzner JL, eds. *Oxford Textbook of Correctional Psychiatry.* New York, NY: Oxford University Press; 2015:266–274.
85. Meyer JP, Althoff AL, Altice FL. Optimizing care for HIV-infected people who use drugs: evidence-based approaches to overcoming healthcare disparities. *Clin Infect Dis.* 2013;57(9):1309–1317.

86. Springer SA, Pesanti E, Hodges J, Macura T, Doros G, Altice FL. Effectiveness of antiretroviral therapy among HIV-infected prisoners: reincarceration and the lack of sustained benefit after release to the community. *Clin Inf Dis.* 2004;38(12):1754–1760.
87. Kinlock TW, Gordon MS, Schwartz RP, Fitzgerald TT, O'Grady KE. A randomized clinical trial of methadone maintenance for prisoners: results at 12 months postrelease. *J Subst Abuse Treat.* 2015;37(3):277–285.
88. Zelenev A, Marcus R, Kopelev A, et al. Patterns of homelessness and implications for HIV health after release from jail. *AIDS Behav.* 2013;17(2):181–194.
89. Chen N, Meyer J, Avery A, et al. Adherence to HIV treatment and care among previously homeless jail detainees. *AIDS Behav.* 2013;17(8):2654–2666.
90. Althoff AL, Zelenev A, Meyer JP, et al. Correlates of retention in HIV care after release from jail: results from a multi-site study. *AIDS Behav.* 2013;17:S156–S170.
91. Rothman J, Rudnick D, Slifer M, Agins B, Heiner K, Birkhead G. Co-located substance use treatment and HIV prevention and primary care services, New York State, 1990–2002: a model for effective service delivery to a high-risk population. *J Urban Health.* 2007;84(2):226–242.
92. Westergaard RP, Ambrose BK, Mehta SH, Kirk GD. Provider and clinic-level correlates of deferring antiretroviral therapy for people who inject drugs: a survey of North American HIV providers. *J Int AIDS Soc.* 2012;15:1–10.
93. Ostertag S, Wright BRE, Broadhead RS, Altice FL. Trust and other characteristics associated with health care utilization by injection drug users. *J Drug Issues.* 2006;36(4):953–974.
94. Craig GM, Booth H, Story A, et al. The impact of social factors on tuberculosis management. *J Adv Nurs.* 2007;58(5):418–424.
95. Kermode M, Crofts N, Kumar MS, Dorabjee J. Opioid substitution therapy in resource-poor settings. *Bull World Health Organ.* 2011;89(4):243.
96. Degenhardt L, Mathers BM, Wirtz AL, et al. What has been achieved in HIV prevention, treatment and care for people who inject drugs, 2010–2012? a review of the six highest burden countries. *Int J Drug Policy.* 2015;25(1):53–60.
97. Pecoraro A, Woody GE. Medication-assisted treatment for opioid dependence: making a difference in prisons. *F1000 Med Rep.* 2011;3(1):1–3.
98. Springer SA, Spaulding AC, Meyer JP, Altice FL. Public health implications for adequate transitional care for HIV-infected prisoners: five essential components. *Clin Inf Dis.* 2011;53(5):469–479.
99. Wickersham JA, Muhsin M, Azar MM, Kamarulzaman A, Altice FL. Methadone dose at the time of release from prison significantly influences retention in treatment: implications from a pilot study of HIV-infected prisoners transitioning to the community in Malaysia. *Drug Alcohol Depend.* 2013;132(1–2):378–382.
100. Magura S, Lee JD, Hershberger J, et al. Buprenorphine and methadone maintenance in jail and post-release: a randomized clinical trial. *Drug Alcohol Depend.* 2009;99(1-3):222–230.
101. Springer SA, Qiu J, Saber-Tehrani AS, Altice FL. Retention on buprenorphine is associated with high levels of maximal viral suppression among HIV-infected opioid dependent released prisoners. *PLoS ONE.* 2012;7(5):e38335.
102. Springer S, Chen S, Altice F. Improved HIV and substance abuse treatment outcomes for released HIV-infected prisoners: the impact of buprenorphine treatment. *J Urban Health.* 2010;87(4):592–602.
103. Bruce RD, Govindasamy S, Sylla L, Haddad MS, Kamarulzaman A, Altice FL. Case series of buprenorphine injectors in Kuala Lumpur, Malaysia. *Am J Drug Alcohol Abuse.* 2008;34(4):511–517.
104. Bruce RD, Altice FL. Case series on the safe use of buprenorphine/naloxone in individuals with acute hepatitis C infection and abnormal hepatic liver transaminases. *Am J Drug Alcohol Abuse.* 2007;33(6):869–874.

105. Vijay A, Bazazi AR, Yee I, Kamarulzaman A, Altice FL. Treatment readiness, attitudes toward, and experiences with methadone and buprenorphine maintenance therapy among people who inject drugs in Malaysia. *J Subst Abuse Treat*. 2015;54:29–36.
106. Altice FL, Bruce RD, Lucas GM, et al. HIV treatment outcomes among HIV-infected, opioid-dependent patients receiving buprenorphine/naloxone treatment within HIV clinical care settings: results from a multisite study. *AIDS*. 2011;56(suppl 1):S22–S32.
107. Malta M, Magnanini MMF, Strathdee SA, Bastos FI. Adherence to antiretroviral therapy among HIV-infected drug users: a meta-analysis. *AIDS Behav*. 2010;14(4):731–747.
108. Altice FL, Kamarulzaman A, Soriano V V, Schechter M, Friedland GH. Treatment of medical, psychiatric, and substance-use comorbidities in people infected with HIV who use drugs. *Lancet*. 2010;376(9738):367–387.
109. White MC, Tulsky JP, Menendez E, Arai S, Goldenson J, Kawamura LM. Improving tuberculosis therapy completion after jail: translation of research to practice. *Health Educ Res*. 2005;20(2):163–174.
110. Grenfell P, Baptista Leite R, Garfein R, de Lussigny S, Platt L, Rhodes T. Tuberculosis, injecting drug use and integrated HIV-TB care: a review of the literature. *Drug Alcohol Depend*. 2013;129(3):180–209.
111. Perlman DC, Gourevitch MN, Trinh C, Salomon N, Horn L, Des Jarlais DC. Cost-effectiveness of tuberculosis screening and observed preventive therapy for active drug injectors at a syringe-exchange program. *J Urban Health*. 2001;78(3):550–567.
112. Schluger N, Ciotoll C, Cohen D, Johnson H, Rom WN. Comprehensive tuberculosis control for patients at high risk for noncompliance. *Am J Respir Crit Care Med*. 1995;151(5):1486–1490.
113. Rüütel K, Loit H, Sepp T, Kliiman K, McNutt L, Uusküla A. Enhanced tuberculosis case detection among substitution treatment patients: a randomized controlled trial. *BMC Res Notes*. 2011;4(192):1–6.
114. World Health Organization. *Integrating Collaborative TB and HIV Services Within a Comprehensive Package of Care for People Who Inject Drugs: Consolidated Guidelines*. Geneva, Switzerland: WHO; 2016.
115. Batki SL, Gruber VA, Bradley JM, Bradley M, Delucchi K. A controlled trial of methadone treatment combined with directly observed isoniazid for tuberculosis prevention in injection drug users. *Drug Alcohol Depend*. 2002;66(3):283–293.
116. Selwyn PA, Budner NS, Wasserman WC, Arno PS. Utilization of on site primary care services by HIV-seropositive and seronegative drug users in a methadone maintenance program. *Public Health Rep*. 1993;108(4):492–500.
117. Raistrick D, Hay A, Wolff K. Methadone maintenance and tuberculosis treatment. *BMJ*. 1996;313(7062):925–926.
118. Sadaphal P, Astemborski J, Graham NM, et al. Isoniazid preventive therapy, hepatitis C virus infection, and hepatotoxicity among injection drug users infected with *Mycobacterium tuberculosis*. *Clin Infect Dis*. 2001;33(10):1687–1691.
119. Kwon YS, Koh W-J, Suh GY, Chung MP, Kim H, Kwon OJ. Hepatitis C virus infection and hepatotoxicity during antituberculosis chemotherapy. *Chest*. 2007;131(3):803–808.
120. Bliven EE, Podewils LJ. The role of chronic hepatitis in isoniazid hepatotoxicity during treatment for latent tuberculosis infection. *Int J Tuberc Lung Dis*. 2009;13(9):1054–1060.
121. Tulsky JP, White MC, Dawson C, Hoynes TM, Goldenson J, Schecter G. Screening for tuberculosis in jail and clinic follow-up after release. *Am J Public Health*. 1998;88(2):223–226.
122. World Health Organization. *Accessibility and Integration of HIV, TB and Harm Reduction Services for People Who Inject Drugs in Portugal*. Copenhagen, Denmark: WHO; 2012.

CHAPTER 9

Drug Use in Prisoners and Hepatitis

REBECCA J. WINTER, MPH AND
MARGARET E. HELLARD, PhD, FAFPHM

INTRODUCTION

Hepatitis B and C are blood-borne viruses (BBVs); infection requires the blood of an infected individual to enter the bloodstream of another person. Hepatitis C (HCV) and hepatitis B (HBV) viruses can be transmitted through the reuse (sharing) of contaminated drug-injecting equipment, tattooing and body piercing, as well as transfusions of infected blood product before blood supply testing became available. HBV is also transmissible via the exchange of other bodily fluids such as semen and vaginal fluids, whereas HCV is rarely transmitted sexually outside the setting of male-to-male sex and HIV co-infection.[1]

In many parts of the world, particularly developed countries, injecting drug use (IDU) is the primary risk factor for HCV virus transmission.[2] Contributors to this book have described the complex relationship between IDU, imprisonment, and the risk of infectious disease transmission. Up to 50% of men and 60% of women entering prisons in developed countries meet drug dependence criteria,[3] and up to 70% of inmates are imprisoned for drug-related offending.[4]

Globally, the prevalence of BBVs is substantially higher among prisoners than in the wider population[5]; as a consequence, imprisonment has the potential to escalate onward transmission when IDU continues during incarceration. This risk is increased where prisons do not implement preventive measures. However, prisons also have the potential to play a significant role in interrupting transmission, through both prevention and treatment.[6] This chapter explores the role prisons can play in halting the epidemic of viral hepatitis among people who inject drugs (PWID).

VIRAL HEPATITIS AND AFFECTED POPULATIONS

There are five known hepatitis viruses, A through E, so called because they all cause liver inflammation. This chapter focuses on hepatitis viruses B and C, which are blood-borne and the most prevalent among PWID, and therefore highly prevalent in prison populations. HBV is also efficiently transmissible sexually.[7] Both HBV and HCV can cause fibrosis (liver scarring), cirrhosis, and hepatocellular carcinoma (HCC), the most common type of liver cancer. HBV is the leading cause of HCC worldwide, and between 520,000 and 866,000 people died as a result of HBV complications in 2013.[8] Another 350,000 to 500,000 people die each year from HCV-related liver diseases.[9] Collectively, these two viruses contribute to a significant disease burden: globally, 57% of cirrhosis and 78% of HCC is attributable to either HBV or HCV.[10] Concurrent infection with both HBV and HCV is a significant clinical concern due to the increased risk of progressive liver disease.[11]

Hepatitis C

The World Health Organization (WHO) estimates that 130 to 150 million people globally have chronic HCV infection.[9] There is considerable variation in the prevalence of HCV between countries; in countries such as Egypt and Pakistan, there is a high population prevalence that is not driven by IDU. In other countries (such as Georgia), there are mixed epidemics, and in many other countries the population most affected by HCV is PWID.[2] In countries where data are available, anti-HCV (HCV antibody, indicating exposure to HCV) prevalence is estimated to be 60% to 80% among PWID in 25 countries and 80% or higher in a further 12.[12] Between 15% and 45% of people infected spontaneously clear the virus without treatment; the remaining 55% to 85% develop chronic infection.[9] Previous infection with HCV does not confer protection from future infection; some individuals have multiple reinfections, although they may also successfully spontaneously clear the virus on multiple occasions.[13] Furthermore, individuals can be infected concurrently with multiple genotypes.[13] This makes HCV a challenging virus to control within at-risk populations, particularly where policy responses to PWID have been primarily punitive and have not adopted evidence-based preventive measures such as harm reduction programs.

Hepatitis B

Chronic active HBV infection in the general community also varies considerably between countries; the prevalence ranges from <1% in the United States, Australia, and northern European countries (low endemicity) to up to 20% in parts of the Asian and Western Pacific region and Africa (high endemicity).[14] Among PWID, the prevalence of HBV infection (assessed by the presence of HBV surface antigen in the blood, indicating current infection) ranges from <1% to 21.3%,[12] mirroring the population-wide endemicity. In most countries where data are available, the prevalence of HBV among PWID is estimated to be between 2% and 10% (42 countries), and in 10 countries it is more than 10%.[12] The high variation in HBV prevalence between countries is primarily related to high levels of mother-to-child transmission in high-endemic countries. The advent of a safe and effective vaccine, which is now administered at or soon after birth in most developed countries, has led to a marked reduction in mother-to-child HBV transmission, but it will require a number of years for vaccination efforts to achieve adequate population coverage.[14] Unlike with HCV, most adults (approximately 90%) acutely infected with HBV successfully clear the infection and are protected from future infections.[15]

EPIDEMIOLOGY OF VIRAL HEPATITIS IN PRISONS

The high proportion of PWID passing through prisons globally, coupled with the high prevalence of viral hepatitis among PWID, ongoing injecting, and the lack of harm reduction programs—and in some cases adequate healthcare—means that prisons are a particular risk environment for BBV transmission. Imprisonment is therefore a major risk factor for viral hepatitis infection.

Hepatitis C

Recent systematic reviews and meta-analyses demonstrate high prevalence and incidence of HCV in prisons worldwide. Anti-HCV prevalence among PWID in prisons is almost consistently higher than among PWID in the community in the same region,[16] suggesting an association between incarceration and HCV exposure. A meta-analysis conducted by Larney et al.[17] in 2012 pooled the results of several studies to obtain a global estimate of HCV prevalence and incidence in prisons. The researchers estimated that 26% of all prisoners and 64% of prisoners reporting a history of IDU were anti-HCV-positive, respectively.[17] Anti-HCV prevalence was higher among female than male prisoners (pooled prevalence 32% vs. 24%).[17]

Few studies have documented the transmission of viral hepatitis in prisons; those that have suggest that infections occur at a rate lower than in the comparable community.[18] HCV incidence was estimated to be 1.4 per 100 person-years (py) among all prisoners and 16.4/100 py among prisoners with a history of IDU, although only four and three studies, respectively, contributed to these pooled estimates.[17] Gough et al.[18] calculated a summary pooled HCV incidence estimate of 0.75/100 py among continuously detained prisoners in the United States.

While there is considerable variation in the pooled HCV incidence estimates in prisoners calculated by Larney et al. and Gough et al. (notwithstanding regional variation), the observed prevalence is still considerably higher than in the general population. Although Gough et al.'s results suggest that continuous imprisonment in the United States is less risky from an infectious disease perspective than cycling in and out of prison or injecting in the community, the likely explanation for this observation is that despite the increased risk from unsafe injecting while in prison per episode of IDU, the reduced frequency of injecting in prison leads to an overall decrease in HCV exposure.[19] The risk is also mediated by the proportion of PWID in prison and the background prevalence of hepatitis infection, which varies considerably between countries.

Other studies published since these meta-analyses report anti-HCV prevalence as low as 5% among prisoners in France in 2010[20] but as high as 22% in Italy in 2006,[21] 24% in England between 2005 and 2008,[22] and 60% in Ukraine in 2010.[23] Data from Ukraine reflect the extremely high prevalence of infectious diseases among people who inject drugs in Eastern Europe generally.[12]

Hepatitis B

Estimates of the prevalence of chronic HBV infection among prisoners range from 2% to 9% in developed countries,[24-26] and are as high as 14% and 25% in countries such as Iran[27] and Ghana.[28] This variation in prevalence in prisoners reflects the background prevalence of HBV in the general community; a higher prevalence of HBV in prisoners is observed in countries where HBV infection is highly endemic in the general population and vice versa.

Nevertheless, in most countries, HBV infection is higher among prisoners than in the general community and even higher among prisoners with a history of IDU.[29] In some countries, the prevalence is also higher among women than among men.[29]

There are limited data on the incidence of HBV infection in prisoners. Gough and colleagues calculated a pooled HBV incidence of <2/100 py among continuously detained prisoners in the United States.[18] This is considerably lower than was observed in a Danish study that reported an incidence of 7/100 py among prisoners and 16/100 py among PWID prisoners.[30]

Hepatitis B and C Co-infection

Despite the additional clinical complications, HBV and HCV co-infection among prisoners is rarely measured. Reports of the prevalence of active HBV and HCV co-infection among prisoners are usually less than 2%.[22,31] Exceptions to this include reports of 7% prevalence in Croatia[32] and Italy.[24]

EPIDEMIOLOGY OF HEPATITIS B AND C RISK BEHAVIORS IN PRISONS

As previously outlined, while IDU and other BBV risk behaviors occur at reduced frequency in prisons, the risk per episode may be greater due to the lack of harm reduction resources such as sterile needles and syringes, condoms, tattoo guns, and piercing implements. The sharing of needles and syringes in prison environments is well documented in many parts of the world,[5,19,33-35] and the high background prevalence of hepatitis viruses in prison populations[5] makes each injecting episode in prison a considerable risk for transmission.[34] Any increase in the frequency of IDU in prison therefore represents a considerable risk for BBV outbreaks.

In all epidemiological studies, prisoners with a history of IDU and/or those who report IDU while in prison have significantly higher prevalence of HCV infection than those without an IDU history.[16] The reported prevalence of IDU in prisons ranges between 21% to 68% in Australia,[19,35] 3% to 28% in North America,[36,37] and 61% in Mexico.[38] In Europe, 27% of 847 prisoners participating in a multicenter pilot study across six countries reported a lifetime history of IDU, and half of these reported injecting while in prison.[39]

Few studies examined the in-prison prevalence of other BBV risk behaviors such as unsterile tattooing and other body modification practices, consensual or non-consensual unprotected sexual intercourse, sharing razor blades, and violence where blood is involved. Unsterile tattooing has been identified as an independent source of viral hepatitis transmission both in prisons[40–42] and in the community.[43] Tattooing is common in prisons: between 18% and 38% of prisoners in the United Kingdom,[44,45] Australia,[40,41] United States (New Mexico),[42] and the Russian Federation[46] reported receiving a tattoo in prison. Not all of these studies assessed the correlation of in-prison tattooing with viral hepatitis infection or had the power or design to do so. However, a number of these studies found an association between HCV and/or HBV infection and in-prison tattooing. In one Australian study, 27% of 642 prisoners reported reuse of a tattoo needle, and the authors found an association between HCV infection and in-prison tattooing after adjusting for IDU and other risk factors.[41] In New Mexico, receipt of a tattoo in prison was associated with HBV infection.[42] Having a tattoo was also positively associated with anti-HCV prevalence among prisoners in Italy[24] and Taiwan,[47] although these studies did not distinguish between tattoos received in prison and in the community. Among non-injectors in Puerto Rican prisons, in-prison tattooing was positively associated with self-reported HCV status.[48]

Studies examining the prevalence of other body modification practices such as piercing, scarification, and penile implants (subcutaneous insertion of plastic beads or other objects along the shaft of the penis) in correctional settings are scarce despite evidence that the practice of penile implants is not uncommon in Asia and the Pacific.[49–51] In Fiji, one-third of prisoners leaving prison between 2011 and 2012 reported in-prison penile beading.[51] Yap et al. reported that in two states in Australia, 6% of prisoners reported penile implants.[50] Both of these studies identified the practice as a risk for BBV transmission due to making skin incisions with unsterile and potentially shared implements such as razor blades.

REDUCING THE RISK OF HEPATITIS B AND C TRANSMISSION IN PRISONS: POLICY RESPONSES

Implementing interventions to reduce drug-related harm in custodial settings has unique challenges.[37] Given the focus on security and containment in prisons, health interventions often receive comparatively limited attention and resources. Factors impacting the implementation of health services in prison settings include cost and operational and administrative procedures (providing harm reduction services is not a priority; despite being cost-effective overall, it is deemed to have a direct cost to the prison) and security level (higher levels of security lead to reduced prisoner movement and less timely access to services including healthcare).[52,53] Despite these challenges, there is a growing international body of evidence demonstrating the effectiveness of key harm reduction interventions in custodial settings.

A number of interventions to prevent the transmission of viral hepatitis are available, with varying levels of evidence for their effectiveness in correctional settings. For some interventions, there is strong evidence for their effectiveness in reducing hepatitis transmission among PWID in the community but limited or no evidence for their effectiveness in correctional settings because they either have not been implemented or have not been rigorously evaluated.

There are two main approaches to reducing HBV and HCV transmission and consequent disease burden: biomedical and behavioral interventions. These may reduce or prevent risk behaviors that lead to viral hepatitis transmission (eg, opioid substitution therapy [OST] to reduce the frequency of drug injection), reduce the level of risk associated with drug-using behaviors (eg, provision of sterile needles/syringes to prevent sharing), or reduce the possibility of disease transmission (eg, HBV vaccination to reduce the background prevalence). While it is by no means exhaustive, the following section outlines effective interventions with supporting evidence: OST, education programs, condom provision, sterile needle and syringe provision, safe tattooing/body modification kits, HBV vaccination provision and testing, and counseling. Treatment for viral hepatitis, specifically HCV, is discussed in the following section. Law enforcement (efforts to reduce drug availability and to police prisoner activity) is not discussed because these are core responsibilities of correctional authorities rather than interventions in correctional settings.

Drug Treatment: Pharmacological

Commonly used pharmacological interventions to treat drug (opiate) dependency include full opiate agonists (eg, methadone), partial agonists (eg, buprenorphine), and antagonists (eg, naltrexone). Opiate agonists mimic the effect of opiates such as heroin, preventing physical withdrawal symptoms. Conversely, opiate antagonists block the effect of opiates by binding more tightly to opioid receptor cells. The partial agonist buprenorphine essentially does both; it prevents withdrawal, similar to a full agonist, but also blocks the effect of other opiates.[54] Other, less frequently used, agonist and antagonist pharmacological interventions for the treatment of opiate dependency are not discussed here.[54]

There is strong evidence that methadone and buprenorphine (OST) reduce the frequency of drug use and the number of risky injecting episodes, both in the community and in correctional settings,[54-56] and as a consequence reduce the risk of viral hepatitis transmission among people who inject.[57,58]

The 2012 Global State of Harm Reduction report found that 41 countries (where data are available) provide OST in correctional settings.[59] A systematic review of the effectiveness of OST in prison settings reported that it was significantly associated with reduced heroin use, injecting, and syringe sharing if dosing was adequate (ie, if a sufficient amount of the drug was received).[55] Importantly, the review found that disruption to OST treatment, such as imprisonment, was associated with increased HCV incidence.[55] Another review quantified the reduction in risk behavior in prisoners receiving OST: Larney reported that injecting risk was reduced by 55% to 75% and risk of needle and syringe sharing was reduced by 47% to 73%.[60] Larney and colleagues have highlighted the need for adequate coverage of OST among drug users in prisons in order to achieve population-level effects such as BBV prevention.

There is limited evidence for the effectiveness of full opiate agonist treatment, such as naltrexone, in reducing injecting-related risk behaviors, either in the community or in custodial settings. At least two attempts to conduct randomized controlled trials in prisons comparing naltrexone to methadone treatment have encountered considerable problems, including lack of participation from prisoners.[61,62]

Education Programs

Prison education programs to improve BBV knowledge and preventive practices vary greatly in design and delivery: they may be delivered by on-site or visiting health professionals, by advocacy workers, or by trained peers (fellow prisoners and/or PWID). Despite such programs being widely recommended and practiced globally, their impact is poorly documented and evaluated. In community settings, the effectiveness of educational interventions in reducing HCV transmission or reducing injecting risk behaviors when practiced alone is limited,[63,64] but evidence suggests that, when undertaken in combination with other harm reduction interventions, the outcomes are more favorable. A meta-analysis conducted on 26 studies examining the effectiveness of single-component and multi-component interventions on HCV transmission found that HCV incidence decreased by 75% when combination interventions were applied.[63] In prisons, the effectiveness of preventive education is compromised by the unavailability of many necessary resources (eg, sterile needles and syringes, tattooing equipment) to implement preventive action.[65]

Sterile Needle and Syringe Provision

The implementation of community-based needle and syringe programs (NSPs) early in the HIV epidemic has been widely credited with keeping the prevalence of HIV very low among PWID in some countries. Providing sterile injecting equipment is known to reduce sharing of needles/syringes between PWID,[66] although to reduce BBV transmission, NSP coverage must be high and be combined with complementary strategies such as OST.[57,67] While there is some evidence for the effectiveness of NSPs in preventing HIV transmission among PWID in community settings, the evidence regarding HCV prevention is mixed.[63,66,67] Nevertheless, modeling has indicated that in countries such as the United Kingdom and Australia, where coverage of NSP is high, a considerable number of HCV infections have been averted.[67,68]

The available data show that community-based NSPs were active in 86 countries in 2012.[59] Despite evidence for their effectiveness in reducing syringe sharing and preventing some BBV transmission, the implementation of NSPs in prisons remains rare. In 2012 only 10 countries had implemented NSPs in prisons.[59] The primary barrier to the implementation of NSPs in custodial settings is political: governments and prison authorities do not want to compromise the "drug-free" ethos of the correctional system.[69] This is despite evidence that drug use in prison is common (see chapters 2 and 3) and that prison-based NSPs have been found to not increase the prevalence of drug use among prisoners.[69] A review of the evidence from prisons in 6 countries reported that prison NSPs reduced needle/syringe sharing, and no BBV seroconversions were observed.[69]

Bleach/Disinfectant Provision

A number of prison systems make bleach or other disinfectants available to prisoners to provide the means to clean used needles/syringes. The provision of bleach in prisons has been adopted in a number of countries, particularly where there has been strong opposition to the implementation of NSPs.[70]

There is insufficient evidence to evaluate the effectiveness of disinfecting needles/syringes in preventing BBV transmission; while the efficacy of using bleach has been demonstrated in laboratory studies, field studies indicate that disinfecting needles/syringes in "real-life" conditions may be less than adequate,[63] and this may be further compounded in restrictive environments such as custodial settings.[70] Additionally, the evidence surrounding the efficacy of bleach in killing viral hepatitis is mixed.[71] Bleach provision programs in prisons are therefore considered a second-line strategy, where NSPs have not been implemented.[70] Dolan and colleagues have also drawn attention to the problem of restricted access to bleach in prisons where it is available.[71]

Safe Tattooing/Body Modification Measures

Some public health experts have called for the provision of safer tattooing/body modification kits in prisons[72] or the implementation of on-site tattoo parlors[65] as part of a comprehensive preventive response to HCV in prisons. Others have argued that such measures would have minimal public health impact or cost benefit.[73] Apart from a tattooing parlor that was trialed in Canadian federal prisons for around 1 year that had some promising early results,[74] there is little evidence on how to reduce unsafe tattooing in the prison setting.

Condom Provision

Male and female condoms have been shown to reduce the incidence of HIV and other sexually transmitted infections (STIs) in community-based studies.[75] Sexual transmission of HCV virus remains uncommon, but the correct use of condoms is likely to prevent HBV transmission.[7] While sexual activity in custodial settings is probably under-reported (most studies estimate that less than 10% of prisoners engage in consensual sex while in prison),[76] there are sufficient outbreaks of STIs in prisons to provide evidence of it occurring.[77-79] No studies that assess the effectiveness of condom provision on in-prison transmission of STIs have been published; however, the strong evidence for their effectiveness in community settings supports the view that, used appropriately, condoms would have a similar protective effect in prisons.

Where prison-based condom programs have been evaluated, evidence suggests that they are both feasible and acceptable to prisoners and correctional staff.[80,81] Research also indicates that when made available in prisons, condoms do increase the prevalence of safe sexual intercourse, while not affecting the prevalence of consensual or non-consensual sexual activity.[82,83] In 2007, the WHO reported that an increasing number of countries' prison systems provide condoms.[70]

Vaccination

A safe and effective vaccine against HBV has been available since 1982.[14] Due to prisoners' heightened vulnerability to BBVs, many public health experts have called for the implementation of free HBV vaccination programs for prisoners.[84,85] Hepatitis A vaccine is also recommended for people infected with HCV. Evidence from the United Kingdom suggests that providing HBV vaccination in prisons has a substantial impact on vaccination coverage among PWID and that routine vaccination is more effective than periodic short-term campaigns.[86] Due to both the multi-dose regimen and the transient and "hidden" nature of many PWID, vaccination completion in community settings can be difficult to achieve. By routinely offering HBV vaccination at prison reception, prisons can play an important public health role in achieving high vaccination coverage among this high-risk segment of the population.[84] Accelerated and flexible dosing schedules have been successfully adopted in some prison systems,[84] enabling more people to be fully vaccinated in a short period of time, an important consideration in prisons where there is high inmate turnover. In addition, an incomplete vaccination schedule can confer substantial clinical protection.[85]

Despite strong evidence of cost-effectiveness, and WHO recommendations to offer HBV vaccination at least to prisoners with a high-risk background, program coverage in correctional settings globally remains low and inadequate to prevent viral outbreaks.[84,87] The primary barrier to implementation appears to be cost.[87]

Viral Hepatitis Testing/Diagnosis

Diagnosis of viral hepatitis infection is an important first step in the continuum of monitoring, treatment, and care. With the advent of new direct-acting antiviral

(DAA) therapies, which are highly efficacious, highly tolerable, and for the majority of people require only 8 to 12 weeks of therapy, the prospects for expanding HCV treatment in custodial settings are better than ever.[88] The new treatments also highlight the importance of testing in correctional settings. Facilitating early diagnosis and earlier access to treatment reduces the risk of future liver disease.[89] Additionally, the identification of infection provides a basis for supporting individual behavior change to reduce the risk of transmission to others.[90] Cost is a considerable barrier to the implementation of diagnostic services in prisons. The development of low-cost, point-of-care tests should help to circumvent this, simultaneously increasing testing access.

While the benefits of testing high-risk populations in the community have been well established, less information is available on the best models of care to test prisoners for BBVs. Nurse-led models of care to diagnose, manage, and treat viral hepatitis infection in prisons have been shown to be effective,[91,92] although low prisoner uptake of testing services and attrition along the testing-to-treatment pathway have been reported.[92] Prisoner uptake and attrition may improve with the advent of DAAs. Other new technologies such as rapid point-of-care testing for HCV may also reduce attrition along the testing-to-treatment pathway.[93]

TREATMENT AS PREVENTION: THE CONCEPT, THE EVIDENCE, AND IMPLEMENTING TREATMENT SERVICES IN CORRECTIONAL SETTINGS

Treatment as prevention (TasP) is the principle that, by reducing the prevalent pool of infection through treatment, onward transmission is prevented; treatment therefore becomes a core preventive public health measure, and additionally reduces burden of disease and future healthcare costs.[94] Mathematical modeling for HCV suggests that harm reduction interventions alone (NSP and OST) cannot substantially reduce the disease prevalence among PWID, but when used in combination with DAA treatment, HCV prevalence can substantially decrease (the treatment effect) and be maintained at this lower level (through harm reduction).[95]

Rapid developments in DAA therapy provide real promise for treating prisoners. Inmates with shorter prison sentences will be able to be fully treated while incarcerated, there will be fewer negative side-effects, and treatment success will be high. Similar to programs in the community, studies are underway examining the effectiveness of HCV treatment as prevention programs in prisons.[96] That said, it should be acknowledged that providing HCV treatment in prisons has many challenges, including limited resources, appropriately trained staff, and access to physicians, as well as the cost of treatment.[97] However, research indicates that treatment of active PWID[98] and prisoners[99] is cost-effective. HCV treatment in prisons holds great potential for the benefit of treated inmates and for prisoners, PWID, and public health more broadly. New treatments will enable a larger number of people to be treated in a shorter period of time. In the prison setting this has the potential to greatly reduce the proportion of prisoners infected, which, in turn, will help to protect other prisoners and staff from onward transmission. Due to the high turnover of people moving through prison for short periods of time and then back into the community, undertaking such a program in conjunction with a similar community-based program will lead to a reduction in HCV prevalence and incidence among PWID in the community.[6] Such an approach will help achieve the elimination of HCV as a public health concern by 2030, a target proposed by WHO.[100]

REFERENCES

1. Tohme RA, Holmberg SD. Is sexual contact a major mode of hepatitis C virus transmission? *Hepatology*. 2010;52(4):1497–1505.
2. Lavanchy D. The global burden of hepatitis C. *Liver Int*. 2009;29(suppl 1):74–81.
3. Fazel S, Bains P, Doll H. Substance abuse and dependence in prisoners: a systematic review. *Addiction*. 2006;101(2):181–191.
4. Center on Addiction and Substance Abuse. *Behind Bars II: Substance Abuse and America's Prison Population*. New York, NY: Columbia University; 2010: http://www. casacolumbia.org/addiction-research/reports/substance-abuse-prison-system-2010. Accessed October 28, 2014.
5. Hunt D, Saab S. Viral hepatitis in incarcerated adults: a medical and public health concern. *Am J Gastroenterol*. 2009;104(4):1024–1031.
6. Rich J, Allen S, Williams B. Responding to hepatitis C through the criminal justice system. *N Engl J Med*. 2014;370(20):1871–1874.
7. Brook M. Sexually acquired hepatitis. *Sex Transm Infect*. 2002;78(4):235–240.
8. Naghavi M, Wang H, Lozano R, et al. Global, regional, and national age-sex specific all-cause and cause-specific mortality for 240 causes of death, 1990–2013: a systematic analysis for the Global Burden of Disease Study 2013. *Lancet*. 2015;385(9963):117–171.
9. World Health Organization. *Hepatitis C Factsheet No. 164*. Geneva, Switzerland: WHO; 2014: http://www.who.int/mediacentre/factsheets/fs164/en/.
10. Perz JF, Armstrong GL, Farrington LA, Hutin YJF, Bell BP. The contributions of hepatitis B virus and hepatitis C virus infections to cirrhosis and primary liver cancer worldwide. *J Hepatol*. 2006;45(4):529–538.
11. Sterling R, Sulkowski M. Hepatitis C virus in the setting of HIV or hepatitis B coinfection. *Semin Liver Dis*. 2004;24(s2):61–68.
12. Nelson PK, Mathers BM, Cowie B, et al. Global epidemiology of hepatitis B and hepatitis C in people who inject drugs: results of systematic reviews. *Lancet*. 2011;378(9791):571–583.
13. Pham ST, Bull RA, Bennett JM, et al. Frequent multiple hepatitis C virus infections among injection drug users in a prison setting. *Hepatology*. 2010;52(5):1564–1572.
14. World Health Organization. *Hepatitis B*. Geneva, Switzerland: Department of Communicable Diseases Surveillance and Response, WHO; 2002.
15. World Health Organisation. *Hepatitis B Factsheet No. 204*. Geneva, Switzerland: WHO; 2014: http://www.who.int/mediacentre/factsheets/fs204/en/.
16. Vescio MF, Longo B, Babudieri S, et al. Correlates of hepatitis C virus seropositivity in prison inmates: a meta-analysis. *J Epidemiol Community Health*. 2008;62(4):305–313.
17. Larney S, Kopinski H, Beckwith CG, et al. Incidence and prevalence of hepatitis C in prisons and other closed settings: results of a systematic review and meta-analysis. *Hepatology*. 2013;58(4):1215–1224.
18. Gough E, Kempf MC, Graham L, et al. HIV and hepatitis B and C incidence rates in US correctional populations and high risk groups: a systematic review and meta-analysis. *BMC Public Health*. 2010;10(777):1–14.

19. Hellard M, Hocking J, Crofts N. The prevalence and the risk behaviours associated with the transmission of hepatitis C virus in Australian correctional facilities. *Epidemiol Infect*. 2004;132(3):409–415.
20. Semaille C, Le Strat Y, Chiron E, et al. Prevalence of human immunodeficiency virus and hepatitis C virus among French prison inmates in 2010: a challenge for public health policy. *Euro Surveill*. 2013;18(28):1–7.
21. Brandolini M, Novati S, De Silvestri A, et al. Prevalence and epidemiological correlates and treatment outcome of HCV infection in an Italian prison setting. *BMC Public Health*. 2013;13(1):1–6.
22. Kirwan P, Evans B, Brant L, the Sentinel Surveillance of Hepatitis Testing Study Group. Hepatitis C and B testing in English prisons is low but increasing. *J Public Health*. 2011;33(2):197–204.
23. Azbel L, Wickersham J, Grishaev Y, Dvoryak S, Altice F. Burden of infectious diseases, substance use disorders and mental illness among Ukranian prisoners transitioning to the community. *PLoS ONE*. 2013;8(3):1–9.
24. Babudieri S, Longo B, Sarmati L, et al. Correlates of HIV, HBV, and HCV infections in a prison inmate population: results from a multicentre study in Italy. *J Med Virol*. 2005;76(3):311–317.
25. Reekie J, Levy M, Richards A, et al. Trends in HIV, hepatitis B and hepatitis C prevalence among Australian prisoners—2004, 2007, 2010. *Med J Aust*. 2014;200(5):277–280.
26. Solomon L, Flynn MC, Muck MK, Vertefeuille J. Prevalence of HIV, syphilis, hepatitis B, and hepatitis C among entrants to Maryland correctional facilities. *J Urban Health*. 2004;81(1):25–37.
27. Dana D, Zary N, Peyman A, Behrooz A. Risk prison and hepatitis B virus infection among inmates with history of drug injection in Isfahan, Iran. *Scientific World J*. 2013;2013(735761):1–4.
28. Adjei AA, Armah HB, Gbagbo F, et al. Correlates of HIV, HBV, HCV and syphilis infections among prison inmates and officers in Ghana: a national multicenter study. *BMC Infect Dis*. 2008;8(33):1–12.
29. Gupta S, Altice F. Hepatitis B virus infection in US correctional facilities: a review of diagnosis, management and public health implications. *J Urban Health*. 2009;86(2):263–279.
30. Christensen P, Krarup H, Neisters H, Norder H, Georgsen J. Prevalence and incidence of blood borne viral infections among Danish prisoners. *Eur J Epidemiol*. 2001;16(11):1043–1049.
31. Hennessey KA, Kim AA, Griffin V, Collins NT, Weinbaum CM, Sabin K. Prevalence of infection with hepatitis B and C viruses and co-infection with HIV in three jails: a case for viral hepatitis prevention in jails in the United States. *J Urban Health*. 2009;86(1):93–105.
32. Burek V, Horvat J, Butorac K, Mikulic R. Viral hepatitis B, C and HIV infection in Croatian prisons. *Epidemiol Infect*. 2010;138(11):1610–1620.
33. Dolan K, Teutsch S, Scheuer N, et al. Incidence and risk for acute hepatitis C infection during imprisonment in Australia. *Eur J Epidemiol*. 2010;25(2):143–148.
34. Jürgens R, Ball A, Verster A. Interventions to reduce HIV transmission related to injecting drug use in prison. *Lancet Infect Dis*. 2009;9(1):57–66.
35. Kinner SA, Jenkinson R, Gouillou M, Milloy MJ. High-risk drug-use practices among a large sample of Australian prisoners. *Drug Alcohol Depend*. 2012;126(1–2):156–160.
36. Martin RE, Gold F, Murphy W, Remple V, Berkowitz J, Money D. Drug use and risk of bloodborne infections: a survey of female prisoners in British Columbia. *Can J Public Health*. 2005;96(2):97–101.
37. Weinbaum C, Lyerla R, Margolis HS. Prevention and control of infections with hepatitis viruses in correctional settings. *MMWR Morb Mortal Wkly Rep*. 2003;52(RR-1).

38. Pollini RA, Alvelais J, Gallardo M, et al. The harm inside: injection during incarceration among male injection drug users in Tijuana, Mexico. *Drug Alcohol Depend.* 2009;103(1):52–58.

39. Rotily M, Weilandt C, Bird SM, et al. Surveillance of HIV infection and related risk behaviour in European prisons: A multicentre pilot study. *Eur J Public Health.* 2001;11(3):243–250.

40. Butler T, Kariminia A, Levy M, Kaldor J. Prisoners are at risk for hepatitis C transmission. *Eur J Epidemiol.* 2004;19(12):1119–1122.

41. Hellard M, Aitken C, Hocking J. Tattooing in prisons—not such a pretty picture. *Am J Infect Control.* 2007;35(7):477–480.

42. Samuel MC, Doherty PM, Bulterys M, Jenison SA. Association between heroin use, needle sharing and tattoos received in prison with hepatitis B and C positivity among street-recruited injecting drug users in New Mexico, USA. *Epidemiol Infect.* 2001;127(3):475–484.

43. Jafari S, Copes R, Baharlou S, Etminan M, Buxton J. Tattooing and the risk of transmission of hepatitis C: a systematic review and meta-analysis. *Int J Infect Dis.* 2010;14(11):e928–e940.

44. Strang J, Heuston J, Whiteley C, et al. Is prison tattooing a risk behaviour for HIV and other viruses? results from a national survey of prisoners in England and Wales. *Crim Behav Ment Health.* 2000;10(1):60–65.

45. Milne D. *Tattooing in Scottish Prisons: A Healthcare Needs Assessment.* Edinburgh, Scotland: Scottish Prison Service; 2009.

46. Frost L, Tchertkov V. Prisoner risk taking in the Russian Federation. *AIDS Educ Prev.* 2002;14(5):7–23.

47. Liao K-F, Lai S-W, Chang W-L, Hsu N-Y. Screening for viral hepatitis among male non-drug-abuse prisoners. *Scand J Gastroenterol.* 2006;41(8):969–973.

48. Peña-Orellana M, Hernández-Viver A, Caraballo-Correa G, Albizu-García CEMD. Prevalence of HCV risk behaviors among prison inmates: tattooing and injection drug use. *J Health Care Poor Underserved.* 2011;22(3):962–982.

49. Thomson N, Sutcliffe C, Sirirojn B, et al. Penile modification in young Thai men: risk environments, procedures and widespread implications for HIV and sexually transmitted infections. *Sex Transm Infect.* 2008;84(3):195–197.

50. Yap L, Butler T, Richters J, et al. Penile implants among prisoners—a cause for concern? *PLoS ONE.* 2013;8(1):e53065.

51. Winter R, Saxton K, Kinner SA. *Health in Prisoners in Fiji. Research Report Prepared for the Secretariat of the Pacific Community HIV/STI Response Fund.* Melbourne, Australia: Secretariat of the Pacific Community; 2013.

52. Sylla M, Harawa N, Grinstead Reznick O. The first condom machine in a US jail: the challenge of harm reduction in a law and order environment. *Am J Public Health.* 2010;100(6):982–985.

53. Boutwell AE, Allen SA, Rich JD. Opportunities to address the hepatitis C epidemic in the correctional setting. *Clin Infect Dis.* 2005;40(suppl 5):S367–372.

54. World Health Organization. *Guidelines for the Psychosocially Assisted Pharmacological Treatment of Opioid Dependence.* Geneva, Switzerland: WHO; 2009.

55. Hedrich D, Alves P, Farrell M, Stöver H, Møller L, Mayet S. The effectiveness of opioid maintenance treatment in prison settings: a systematic review. *Addiction.* 2012;107(3):501–517.

56. Prendergast ML, Podus D, Chang E, Urada D. The effectiveness of drug abuse treatment: a meta-analysis of comparison group studies. *Drug Alcohol Depend.* 2002;67(1):53–72.

57. Turner KM, Hutchinson S, Vickerman P, et al. The impact of needle and syringe provision and opiate substitution therapy on the incidence of hepatitis C virus in injecting drug users: pooling of UK evidence. *Addiction.* 2011;106(11):1978–1988.

58. White B, Dore G, Lloyd AR, Rawlinson WD, Maher L. Opioid subsitution therapy protects against hepatitis C virus acquisition in people who inject drugs: the HITS-c study. *Med J Aust.* 2014;201(6):326–329.

59. Harm Reduction International. *The Global State of Harm Reduction 2012: Towards an Integrated Response*. London, England: Public Health, Research and Policy Programme, Harm Reduction International; 2012: http://www.ihra.net/contents/1411.
60. Larney S. Does opioid substitution treatment in prisons reduce injecting-related HIV risk behaviours? a systematic review. *Addiction*. 2010;105(2):216–223.
61. Lobmaier PP, Kunøe N, Waal H. Treatment research in prison: problems and solutions in a randomized trial. *Addiction Res Theory*. 2010;18(1):1–13.
62. Shearer J, Wodak A, Dolan K. Evaluation of a prison-based naltrexone program. *Int J Prison Health*. 2007;3(3):214–224.
63. Hagan H, Pouget ER, Des Jarlais DC. A systematic review and meta-analysis of interventions to prevent hepatitis C virus infection in people who inject drugs. *J Infect Dis*. 2011;204(1):74–83.
64. Sacks-Davis R, Horyniak D, Grebely J, Hellard M. Behavioural interventions for preventing hepatitis C infection in people who inject drugs: a global systematic review. *Int J Drug Policy*. 2012;23(3):176–184.
65. Levy MH, Treloar C, McDonald RM, Booker N. Prisons, hepatitis C and harm minimisation. *Med J Aust*. 2007;186(12):647–649.
66. MacArthur GJ, van Velzen E, Palmateer N, et al. Interventions to prevent HIV and hepatitis C in people who inject drugs: a review of reviews to assess evidence of effectiveness. *Int J Drug Policy*. 2014;25(1):34–52.
67. Vickerman P, Martin N, Turner K, Hickman M. Can needle and syringe programmes and opiate substitution therapy achieve substantial reductions in hepatitis C virus prevalence? model projections for different epidemic settings. *Addiction*. 2012;107(11):1984–1995.
68. Kwon JA, Anderson J, Kerr CC, et al. Estimating the cost-effectiveness of needle-syringe programs in Australia. *AIDS*. 2012;26(17):2201–2210.
69. Lines R, Jürgens R, Betteridge G, Stöver H. Taking action to reduce injecting drug-related harms in prisons: the evidence of effectiveness of prison needle exchange in six countries. *Int J Prison Health*. 2005;1(1):49–64.
70. World Health Organization. *Effectiveness of Interventions to Manage HIV in Prisons: Provision of Condoms and Other Measures to Decrease Sexual Transmission*. Geneva, Switzerland: WHO; 2007: http://www.who.int/hiv/idu/Prisons_condoms.pdf.
71. Dolan K, Wodak A, Hall W. HIV risk behaviour and prevention in prison: a bleach programme for inmates in NSW. *Drug Alcohol Rev*. 1999;18(2):139–143.
72. Elliott R. Deadly disregard: government refusal to implement evidence-based measures to prevent HIV and hepatitis C virus infections in prisons. [Erratum appears in CMAJ. 2007 Sep 11;177(6):606]. *Can Med Assoc J*. 2007;177(3):262–264.
73. Awofeso N. Legal prison tattooing centers: viable health policy initiative? *J Public Health Manag Pract*. 2010;16(3):240–244.
74. Correctional Service Canada. *Correctional Service Canada's Safer Tattooing Practices Pilot Initiative*. Correctional Service Canada; 2009: http://www.csc-scc.gc.ca/text/pa/ev-tattooing-394-2-39/index-eng.shtml.
75. Holmes KK, Levine R, Weaver M. Effectiveness of condoms in preventing sexually transmitted infections. *Bull World Health Organ*. 2004;82(6):454–461.
76. Hellard M, Aitken C. HIV in prison: what are the risks and what can be done. *Sex Health*. 2004;1(2):107–113.
77. Centers for Disease Control and Prevention. Hepatitis B outbreak in a state correctional facility, 2000. *MMWR Morb Mortal Wkly Rep*. 2001;50(25):529–532.
78. Centers for Disease Control and Prevention. HIV transmission among male inmates in a state prison system: Georgia, 1992–2005. *MMWR Morb Mortal Wkly Rep*. 2006;55(15):421–426.
79. Wolfe MI, Xu F, Patel P, et al. An outbreak of syphilis in Alabama prisons: correctional health policy and communicable disease control. *Am J Public Health*. 2001;91(8):1220–1225.

80. Dolan K, Lowe D, Shearer J. Evaluation of the condom distribution program in New South Wales prisons, Australia. *J Law Med Ethics*. 2004;32(1):124–128.
81. May JP, Williams EL. Acceptability of condom availability in a U.S. jail. *AIDS Educ Prev*. 2002;14(5)(suppl B):85–91.
82. Butler T, Richters J, Yap L, Donovan B. Condoms for prisoners: no evidence that they increase sex in prison, but they increase safe sex. *Sex Transm Infect*. 2013;89(5):377–379.
83. Yap L, Butler T, Richters J, et al. Do condoms cause rape and mayhem? the long-term effects of condoms in New South Wales' prisons. *Sex Transm Infect*. 2007;83(3):219–222.
84. Farrell M, Strang J, Stover H. Hepatitis B vaccination in prisons: a much-needed targeted universal intervention. *Addiction*. 2010;105(2):189–190.
85. Rich JD, Ching CG, Lally MA, et al. A review of the case for hepatitis B vaccination of high-risk adults. *Am J Med*. 2003;114(4):316–318.
86. Sutton AJ, Gay NJ, Edmunds WJ, Gill ON. Modelling alternative strategies for delivering hepatitis B vaccine in prisons: the impact on the vaccination coverage of the injecting drug user population. *Epidemiol Infect*. 2008;136(12):1644–1649.
87. Charuvastra A, Stein J, Schwartzappel B, et al. Hepatitis B vaccination practices in state and federal prisons. *Public Health Rep*. 2001;116(3):203–209.
88. Doyle JS, Aspinall E, Liew D, Thompson AJ, Hellard ME. Current and emerging antiviral treatments for hepatitis C infection. *Br J Clin Pharmacol*. 2013;75(4):931–943.
89. Aspinall E, Doyle JS, Corson S, et al. Targeted hepatitis C testing interventions: a systematic review and meta-analysis. *Eur J Epidemiol*. 2014;30(2):115–129.
90. Aspinall EJ, Weir A, Sacks-Davis R, et al. Does informing people who inject drugs of their hepatitis C status influence their injecting behaviour? analysis of the Networks II study. *Int J Drug Policy*. 2014;25(1):179–182.
91. Lloyd AR, Clegg J, Lange J, et al. Safety and effectiveness of a nurse-led outreach program for assessment and treatment of chronic hepatitis C in the custodial setting. *Clin Infect Dis*. 2013;56(8):1078–1084.
92. Skipper C, Guy JM, Parkes J, Roderick P, Rosenberg WM. Evaluation of a prison outreach clinic for the diagnosis and prevention of hepatitis C: implications for the national strategy. *Gut*. 2003;52(10):1500–1504.
93. Spaulding AC, Thomas DL. Screening for HCV infection in jails. *JAMA*. 2012;307(12):1259–1260.
94. Martin NK, Vickerman P, Foster GR, Hutchinson SJ, Goldberg DJ, Hickman M. Can antiviral therapy for hepatitis C reduce the prevalence of HCV among injecting drug user populations? a modeling analysis of its prevention utility. *J Hepatol*. 2011;54(6):1137–1144.
95. Martin NK, Hickman M, Hutchinson SJ, Goldberg DJ, Vickerman P. Combination interventions to prevent HCV transmission among people who inject drugs: modeling the impact of antiviral treatment, needle and syringe programs, and opiate substitution therapy. *Clin Infect Dis*. 2013;57(suppl 2):S39–S45.
96. Lloyd AR. STOP-C: surveillance and treatment of prisoners with hepatitis C. Presented at HIV and Hepatitis C Treatment as Prevention Colloquium, Centre for Research Excellence on Injecting Drug Use; April 16, 2014; Melbourne, Australia.
97. Mina MM, Clark PJ, Beasley HM, Herawati L, Butler TG, Lloyd AR. Enhancing hepatitis C treatment in the custodial setting: a national roadmap. *Med J Aust*. 2014;200(1):15–16.
98. Martin NK, Vickerman P, Miners A, et al. Cost-effectiveness of hepatitis C virus antiviral treatment for injection drug user populations. *Hepatology*. 2012;55(1):49–57.
99. Tan JA, Joseph TA, Saab S. Treating hepatitis C in the prison population is cost-saving. *Hepatology*. 2008;48(5):1387–1395.
100. Watts G. Hepatitis C could be virtually eliminated by 2030, experts believe. *BMJ*. 2014;348:g2700.

CHAPTER 10

Prisoners With a Substance Use Disorder and a Mental Illness

KATE DOLAN, PhD, MICHAEL FARRELL, PhD, AND
SAHAR SAEEDI MOGHADDAM, MS

INTRODUCTION

People with substance use disorders or mental illnesses are vastly overrepresented in prison populations. When these two conditions co-occur, the person is said to have a dual diagnosis.[1] It also follows that these individuals will be overrepresented within prison populations and they are, therefore, the focus of this chapter.

While the imprisonment of these persons presents additional challenges, it also provides an opportunity to detect and treat both disorders. Treatment is important not only because it relieves suffering for the individual and his or her family, but also because humane approaches to treatment within the custodial setting are likely to reduce the risk of self-harm and suicide.

For inmates with each condition and with a dual diagnosis, we examine the prevalence, incidence, effective treatments, and outcomes, including re-incarceration rates. We also examine the interplay of the two conditions to understand how one condition can affect the other. Our examination of substance use disorders focuses on the use of heroin, amphetamines, cannabis, and alcohol. The types of mental illness we focus on include post-traumatic stress disorder (PTSD), personality disorders, bipolar disorder, anxiety disorders, depression, and psychosis. We highlight gaps in our current understanding of the issues and suggest areas for future research, and for clinical practice and policy reform. We conclude with recommendations to recognize the unique risks for people in prison where there is a high concentration of psychosis, self-harm, suicide, and substance use. In particular, management of the risks for people entering and leaving prison requires proper assessment and referral for treatment, if unwanted complications are to be avoided.

THE WORLD'S PRISON POPULATION

In 2015, at least 10.3 million individuals were in prison worldwide on any given day, representing an imprisonment rate of 144 per 100,000 population. Fifteen years ago, this rate was 136 per 100,000, indicating that the world's prison population is growing faster than the world's population.[2] However, imprisonment rates vary around the world, from the very high rates found in the United States (707 per 100,000), Russia (469), and Thailand (483) to comparatively low rates in Canada (118), Egypt (80), and India (30).[3] The majority of prisoners are male, with females accounting for about 7% of all inmates.[2]

PREVALENCE OF SUBSTANCE USE DISORDERS IN PRISON POPULATIONS

Prisoners bear a major burden of substance use disorders relative to the general population. Internationally, the estimated prevalence of drug use or dependence varies from 10% to 48% in male and 30% to 60% in female prison entrants.[4] In Europe, the prevalence of lifetime use of illicit drugs prior to prison ranged from 16% in Romania to 79% in England and Wales.[5] This variation across countries broadly reflects national levels of drug use but may also be partly due to different screening and research methodologies, and to different drug laws and policies between countries (see also chapter 1).

When studies examine specific drug types, the overrepresentation of drug users in prison populations becomes readily apparent. For example, an Australian study found that approximately 40% of inmates reported a lifetime history of heroin use,[6] which is in sharp contrast with the general community level of less than 1%.[7] However, a history of drug use does not necessarily equate to a substance use disorder. A study in the United Kingdom examined drug dependence and found that 42% of inmates were classified as drug-dependent and 29% met the criteria for "severe" dependence for at least one drug.[8]

PREVALENCE OF MENTAL ILLNESS IN PRISON POPULATIONS

As early as a century ago, it was recognized that people with a mental illness are over-represented in prisons. One study of admissions to New York's Sing Sing Prison in 1918 reported on the large number of mentally ill people in custody.[9] While the overrepresentation was noted early, it would be some time before an accurate assessment of the extent would be made.

Good evidence of the prevalence of mental disorder in prison comes from two large systematic reviews. The first review examined 23,000 prisoners in 62 studies completed by 2002.[10] Common diagnoses for men and women were antisocial personality disorder (47% and 21%), major depression (10% and 12%), and psychosis (3.7% and 4.0%). This led the authors to conclude that compared with the general population, prisoners were several times more likely to have psychosis and major depression and about 10 times more likely to have antisocial personality disorder.

The same authors subsequently conducted a larger review of about 33,500 prisoners, which covered 109 studies completed by 2010. These results were almost identical: common diagnoses for men and women were major depression (10.2% and 14.1%) and psychosis (3.6% and 3.9%).[11] This review also compared levels of mental illness across countries with different income levels. It found that studies in low- to middle-income countries reported a significantly higher prevalence of psychosis (5.5% vs. 3.5%) and depression (22.5% vs. 10%) than studies from high-income countries.[11] However, it should be noted that while 72 studies came from high-income countries, just 8 came from low- to middle-income countries. With this limitation, it would be inappropriate to generalize to other low- to middle-income countries.

Much of the research in this area has come from the United States. A survey of more than 25,000 prison and jail inmates in the United States, conducted between 2002 and 2004, found that more than half had a mental health problem.[12] These inmates were found to score worse than inmates without a mental health problem on several measures. For example, the former were more likely than other inmates to have served three or more prison sentences (47% vs. 39%), to have recently used drugs before being arrested (63% vs. 49%), and to have been homeless in the year prior to arrest (13% vs. 6%). These inmates also fared worse once incarcerated. They were more likely to have been charged with breaking rules (58% vs. 43%) or assaulting an officer (24% vs. 14%), and were more likely to have been injured in a fight (20% vs. 10%) than other inmates.

Differences between male and female inmates in terms of mental illness have been observed. Among 6,982 male and female inmates in US jails, women had a higher rate of mental health problems than men (73% vs. 55%), and three-quarters of these women met criteria for substance dependence or abuse. In this study, women had a significantly higher prevalence of psychiatric conditions such as depression, bipolar disorder, psychosis, PTSD, anxiety disorder, personality disorder, and drug dependence, but not alcohol dependence, than men.[13]

Dual diagnosis, the presence of a substance use disorder and a mental health problem, was recorded for 42% of US state prisoners.[13] With a further 24% having a substance use disorder (SUD) only and 15% having a mental health problem only, this left just 19% who were free from both conditions. In terms of drugs used in the month before the offense was committed, marijuana was the most common one for those with and without a mental health problem (46% vs. 33%), followed by cocaine or crack (24% vs. 18%), methamphetamines (13% vs. 9%), and heroin (9% vs. 7%). Only one-third of the state inmates with a mental health problem had received treatment since entering prison. Treatment comprised prescribed medications (27%), therapy (23%), and an overnight stay in the hospital (5%). The proportion who received medication had increased slightly since the survey in 1997.

PREVALENCE AND INCIDENCE OF DUAL DIAGNOSIS
IN PRISON POPULATIONS

Twenty years ago, a large-scale study from the United Kingdom gave a good indication of the prevalence of dual diagnosis in that country. In 1997, a detailed and thorough study of a representative sample of more than 3,000 male and female prisoners in the United Kingdom found that 90% had some form of mental illness, drug dependence, or a personality disorder, and 70% had two or more such problems.[8] Studies such as this suggest that the scale of the dual diagnosis burden is incredibly high in prison populations, indicating a need for a broad, holistic approach to treatment to be widely available in these settings.

A study from the United States compared prisoners with a dual diagnosis (n = 436) with those who had severe mental illness only (n = 265) and found that the former were more likely to be female and to use mental health services, had more immediate service needs (eg, housing) once released, and were more likely to return to custody.[14] Similarly, in a random stratified sample of 998 prisoners in France, those with a dual diagnosis (26% of the sample) had a markedly increased risk for suicide. According to Lukasiewicz and colleagues,[15] prisoners with a dual diagnosis have a poorer prognosis and require more intense supportive care than prisoners with a single diagnosis.

Although globally there is considerable variation in the prevalence of dual diagnosis in prisons, in virtually all prisons there is a gross overrepresentation of people with substance use and mental health problems. At least in Western countries, the prevalence of psychosis, depression, personality disorders, and drug misuse is much higher among prison populations than among comparable general populations (Table 10.1).

Further evidence of the association between substance use and mental disorder in prisoners comes from an Australian study of 610 prison entrants.[16] Almost one-third (31%) of prison entrants reported having ever been told they had a mental

Table 10.1. PREVALENCE OF SUBSTANCE USE DISORDER AND
MENTAL DISORDERS IN PRISONERS AND GENERAL POPULATIONS
IN WESTERN COUNTRIES

Condition	Males (%)		Females (%)	
	Prisoners	General population	Prisoners	General population
Psychosis[11]	3–4	1	3–5	1
Major depression[11]	9–12	2–4	10–18	5–7
Any personality disorder[10]	61–68	5–10	38–45	5–10
Antisocial personality disorder[10]	46–48	5–7	19–23	0.5–1
Drug misuse/dependence[4]	10–48	4–6	30–60	2–3

illness, with 16% reporting that they were currently taking medication for a mental health–related condition. Using the Kessler psychological distress scale (K10), 14% of the sample screened positive for very high psychological distress, and illicit drug use was more common in those with very high psychological distress (81%) than in those with low psychological distress (62%).[16] Based on an audit of medication dispensing in prison, the same study found that one-third (30%) of all repeat medication was for a mental health–related condition.

Another study in New South Wales, Australia, found that 55% of inmates had a SUD and 42% had a mental disorder.[6] Women had higher rates of SUD than men, except for alcohol use disorders. The 12-month prevalence of dual diagnosis was higher for women (46%) than for men (25%). There were significant associations between cannabis use disorder and psychosis for men, and between alcohol use and affective disorder for women. The authors noted the very high rates of comorbidity and self-harm among incarcerated women and concluded that there was therefore a high need for intervention and support.

Mortality in Prison

The prison environment itself can influence the mental health of inmates. Factors in many prison systems that are likely to have negative effects on mental health include overcrowding, various forms of violence, enforced solitude or, conversely, lack of privacy, lack of meaningful activity, isolation from social networks, insecurity about future prospects (work and relationships), and inadequate health services, especially mental health services. The increased risk of suicide in prisons, which is often related to depression,[15] is unfortunately one common manifestation of the cumulative effects of these factors. Suicide is the leading cause of death among inmates and accounts for about half of all unnatural deaths in prisons.[15] Across 12 Western countries, one study found that the suicide rate ranged from 50 to 150 deaths per 100,000 male prisoners annually. Although research on the phenomenon of suicide in prison is limited, the existing evidence points to a growing problem; in France, for example, the rate of suicide in prison has doubled in the past decade.[15] Factors associated with suicide in custody include suicide ideation, previous attempts, current psychosis or depression, and alcohol misuse. Careful assessment and case management in the early period of imprisonment followed by proper treatment and care, in particular withdrawal management, are critical to reduce risk.

IMPACT OF IMPRISONMENT ON DRUG USE AND MENTAL HEALTH

The prison setting can also be one where some inmates commence drug use or injection (see chapter 3). Surveys from Scotland found that 6% and 25% of drug-injecting prisoners in two prisons, respectively,[17] had started injecting inside. Similarly, in Ireland, 20% of a sample of incarcerated people who inject drugs reported that their first injection occurred in prison.[18] A survey of more than 3,000 prisoners in the United Kingdom found that 4% of all prisoners had started injecting in prison.[19]

Certain aspects of prison life appear to exacerbate symptoms of mental illness. Solitary confinement is one such aspect, with recommendations being made to avoid its use in those with pre-existing psychiatric disorders.[20] Walker's systematic review found evidence that entering prison results in poorer mental state compared with that just prior to entry, but this improves with time in custody.[21] Isolation, overcrowding, and larger prisons are associated with poorer mental health, which carries implications for prison staff, clinicians, and policymakers and for the provision of mental health services where these conditions exist.[21]

An indication of the impact of imprisonment on mental health disorders comes from Wright and colleagues.[22] They estimated the prevalence of psychiatric morbidity and/or substance use disorders among a 10% sample of Irish female prison entrants and prison residents in 2002. While the prevalence of substance use disorders (65.6 and 65.2) and psychotic illnesses (5.4 and 5.4) was almost identical in entrants and residents, respectively, there was an increase in major depressive disorder (8.5 and 16.3) and anxiety disorder (8.6 and 15.2) in the resident prisoners compared with entrants, which is suggestive of in-prison acquisition.

A recent UK study found that while the prevalence of psychiatric symptoms was highest during the first week after reception into custody, there was a linear decline among male and sentenced prisoners, but not among female or remand prisoners.[23] This decline was apparent in prisoners with depression but not in those with other mental illnesses.[23] These findings suggest that the impact of incarceration on mental health may differ not only by disorder but also among subgroups of prisoners.

TREATMENT FOR PRISONERS WITH A SUBSTANCE USE DISORDER OR MENTAL ILLNESS

Untreated substance use disorders can result in adverse outcomes for those with the disorder; in prison settings, this can have significant implications for other prisoners and for prison staff. For example, inmates who continue to or start to inject while imprisoned risk acquiring infections such as HIV, hepatitis B, and hepatitis C.[24] Another more serious outcome is overdose in prison[25] or immediately after release.[26] For a detailed description of treatment for prisoners with a substance use disorder, see chapter 16.

According to Fazel and Seewald,[11] around one in seven inmates has a treatable mental illness. The main challenge in providing treatment for mental illness in prison in most countries is the lack of adequate health budgets and the employment of specialists.[11] In most countries, mental health services in prison are not provided at a level proportionate to need. For example, a national survey of prison and jail inmates in the United States from 2002 to 2004 found that a third of those with diagnoses of schizophrenia and bipolar disorder were not treated with psychiatric drugs.[27]

It is a basic right of prisoners and a responsibility of prison health staff to ensure that there is continuity of psychiatric medication for those who enter prison, yet this does not always occur. Similarly, despite the importance of continuing mental health treatment after release from prison, continuity of care for those with a mental illness is often suboptimal. In a study of 80 jails in North Carolina, none used evidence-based screening tools for mental illness, 35% had never contacted mental health services when mentally ill prisoners were released, and 42% had to transport prisoners to a community provider for mental health assessments.[28] These examples show how treatment coverage for prisoners in the United States is inadequate both during and after release from custody. There is also the challenge of inappropriate use of medication within custodial settings to achieve a suitably sedated population. It is important that medication be matched to the condition.

Nevertheless, prison represents an important opportunity to identify untreated mental illness and to initiate appropriate care. In one study of prisoners with a mental health condition who had previously been treated with a psychiatric medication in the United States, only 26% of federal and 30% of state inmates were taking a psychiatric medication at the time of arrest, but these figures increased to 69% and 69% after admission.[27]

TREATMENT FOR PRISONERS WITH DUAL DIAGNOSIS

Compliance with treatment can be difficult for many with a single condition, and especially so for those with a dual diagnosis. In the United States, Brady and colleagues reviewed data from five jail-based substance abuse treatment programs and found that inmates with a dual diagnosis were nearly three times more likely than inmates with a substance use disorder only to terminate a drug treatment episode.[29] For prisoners with a psychotic disorder, appropriate anti-psychotic medication is a key part of treatment. In order to promote continuity of care between custodial and community settings, there is a need for dedicated teams with a mental health in-reach function and links to community-based services, as well as properly resourced substance misuse teams, to assess and manage alcohol and drug withdrawal in custody, and to institute appropriate opiate maintenance treatment for those who require it.[29]

When a dual diagnosis is left untreated, people have poorer clinical outcomes than people with one type of disorder. They are also more likely to be criminally involved, hospitalized, and imprisoned. Effective treatments for dual diagnosis focus equally on both types of disorders and deliver services in a fully integrated model of care.[30] Those with a stable pattern of treatment have better outcomes than others.[31]

A key challenge for treatment of people with a dual diagnosis in prison settings is that the scale and complexity of the problem necessitate multiple teams and careful coordination with external agencies to ensure continuity of care after the prisoner returns to the community. In many countries, more needs to be done to meet this challenge adequately: Sung found that one-third of the US jail population met criteria for dual diagnosis, but 64% of these individuals received no treatment while incarcerated.[32]

MENTAL DISORDER, REOFFENDING AND REINCARCERATION

There is good evidence that mental illness increases the risk of crime and repeat offending in prisoners.[33-35] Appropriate treatment may ameliorate this risk. A study in Florida followed 4,056 individuals with schizophrenia or bipolar disorder for 7 years following their discharge from psychiatric hospitalization.[36] Those who remained on medication were significantly less likely to be arrested and cost the state 40% less in total healthcare costs over the 7-year period than were others who stopped taking medication. Studies such as this highlight the benefits of efforts to promote adherence to psychotropic medication after release from prison, to reduce both incarceration and associated healthcare and criminal justice costs.

RECOMMENDATIONS
Policy Reform

A recent survey by the World Health Organization (WHO) found that nearly 40% of countries do not have a mental health policy *for the community*. There is a significant association between the existence of a mental health policy and having a national mental health program, primary care training facilities in mental health, community care facilities in mental health, and the presence of non-governmental organization activities in mental health.[37] Accordingly, given the significant dual diagnosis treatment need in custodial settings, it would be most beneficial for countries to have a national prisoner health strategy that encompasses substance use disorders, mental health, and other issues to guide healthcare for inmates. In terms of lines of authority, the WHO recommends that prison health services should come under the broader health department and not the prison department, in order to remove the potential conflict of interest for custodial staff when it comes to decisions around healthcare. An independent healthcare delivery system should ideally put the interests of the individual patient/prisoner ahead of all else and ensure that full and appropriate treatment is delivered.[38]

Without quality, evidence-based care that spans custodial and community settings, when people with a dual diagnosis are released from prison, they are at high risk of relapsing to drug use and mental illness, and subsequently offending and return to prison. Effective responses to the needs of dually diagnosed prisoners will accrue benefits for both the individual and the community, the latter through reduced healthcare and criminal justice costs and reduced crime. The challenge in realizing these benefits lies not only within the prison setting but also within community-based services that deal with substance use and mental health before people are imprisoned. Effective interagency cooperation to implement a comprehensive continuum of integrated treatment services from community, to incarceration, and back to community is critical.

Clinical Practice

All prison entrants should be assessed to determine if they have a SUD or a mental illness, and appropriate treatment should be provided to all who need it. Methadone is safe and effective and reduces opioid use, HIV transmission, overdose deaths, crime, and re-imprisonment (see chapter 16). Imprisonment usually results in a decrease in drug availability, which lowers inmates' tolerance, such that upon release these inmates are at increased risk of overdose (see chapters 6 and 18). As such, it is recommended that inmates with a history of heroin use be treated with methadone during the period of incarceration and that they be released on methadone.

Screening for mental illness on prison entry will identify suicidal and severely mentally ill individuals who are in urgent need of intervention. Screening for high-prevalence disorders such as anxiety and depression is also important, particularly for remand prisoners who are less likely to experience improvements in mental health associated with a period of relative stability and low-threshold treatment in custody. Treating mental illness will improve the health and quality of life of both prisoners with mental disorders and the prison population as a whole. By promoting a better understanding of mental disorders, stigma and discrimination can be reduced.

While good evidence exists on the prevalence of substance use disorders, mental illness, and dual diagnosis in prisons in the developed world, the same cannot be said for the developing world. Large-scale epidemiological studies are required to understand the size of the problem among prison inmates in low- and middle-income countries.

All prisoners, including those with mental disorders, have the right to be treated humanely, and conditions of confinement in prisons must conform to international human rights standards (see chapter 12). The option to divert the mentally ill to community-based mental health services rather than to prisons should be available in all countries. While some individuals will still need to be imprisoned, they should be provided with access to appropriate mental health treatment and care. Access to assessment, treatment, and (when necessary) referral of people with mental disorders, including substance abuse, to specialist care should be an integral part of general health services available to all prisoners.

Health services provided to prisoners should be equivalent to those in the community. Prisoners should have the same access to psychotropic medication and psychosocial support for the treatment of mental disorders as do people in the general community. Providing training to custodial staff to improve their understanding of and capacity to respond appropriately to mental disorders, raise awareness of human rights, and challenge stigmatizing attitudes is also important. Custodial staff can be trained to recognize risk and prevent suicides. Solitary confinement should be avoided, especially for inmates with pre-existing psychiatric disorders. There is evidence that such confinement exacerbates symptoms of mental illness. Very little is known about the prognosis for dually diagnosed inmates once they leave prison. There is an urgent need for longitudinal studies that follow ex-prisoners after release from custody, to investigate their mental health and drug use and associated outcomes after imprisonment. Inmates with serious mental illness can be treated successfully in the community, if appropriate steps are taken to manage this care transition, and if both custodial and community services are adequately resourced. One important area for future research is to explore patterns of engagement with community mental health services before and at the time of arrest, and to consider alternatives to incarceration for arrestees with co-occurring substance use and mental health problems. Relapse prevention courses developed specifically for dually diagnosed inmates nearing release, coupled with good links to community programs, may reduce the re-incarceration of inmates with substance use disorders and mental illness.

Several countries have incorporated prison health services into national health departments, as recommended by the WHO. This organizational structure can lead to an improvement in the quality of prison healthcare to be closer to the standard of community care. It also separates healthcare from the prison management, thus removing the potential for role conflict to compromise healthcare for inmates.

A critical approach to handling mental health problems within the prison system is to ensure that staff members are well trained as a core part of the prison healthcare service. Established links between prison services and community services are needed. There is a need to have good models of service with good channels that enable mental health *in*-reach services to work within prisons and to link back into community-based services.

CONCLUSION

More than two decades ago it was recognized that the largest concentration of institutionalized persons with a mental illness was to be found in correctional centers. The disproportionate representation of people with substance use disorders and mental disorders among prison populations presents enormous challenges, but also provides opportunities for diagnosis and treatment. As prison populations continue to grow, prisoner health becomes increasingly important to address worldwide. Yet, despite a long-standing recognition that people with substance use disorders and mental illness are over-represented in prisons,[4,10] treatment services for these conditions remain inadequate in most settings. It is unsurprising that more than one in three prisoners is reconvicted within 2 years.[39]

An effective response to this crisis will require alternative sentencing, coupled with effective and scaled-up treatment services for SUD and mental illness. Even when strong evidence exists, such as is the case for opioid substitution treatment, many countries prohibit or severely restrict its implementation in prison. Data from the developing world are severely limited, and research of the nature presented here is desperately needed to ascertain the situation in non-Western prison populations.

Most prisoners with mental health or drug abuse problems return to their home communities, and treatment of their illnesses is therefore an important public health opportunity because treatment can decrease rates of repeat offending.

Further research is needed to identify risk factors for recidivism in prisoners with a dual diagnosis.

REFERENCES

1. Ogloff JR, Lemphers A, Dwyer C. Dual diagnosis in an Australian forensic psychiatric hospital: prevalence and implications for services. *Behav Sci Law.* 2004;22(4):543–562.
2. Walmsley R. *World Prison Briefs.* London, England: International Centre for Prison Studies; 2015.
3. Walmsley R. *World Prison Briefs.* London, England: International Centre for Prison Studies; 2011.
4. Fazel S, Bains P, Doll H. Substance abuse and dependence in prisoners: a systematic review. *Addiction.* 2006;101(2):181–191.
5. EMCDDA. *Prisons and Drugs in Europe: Problems and Responses.* Luxembourg City, Luxembourg: Publications Office of the European Union; 2012.
6. Butler T, Indig D, Allnutt S, Mamoon H. Co-occurring mental illness and substance use disorder among Australian prisoners. *Drug Alcohol Rev.* 2011;30(2):188–194.
7. Australian Institute of Health and Welfare. *National Drug Strategy Household Survey Detailed Report: 2013.* Canberra, Australia: AIHW; 2014.
8. Singleton N, Gatward R, Meltzer H. *Psychiatric Morbidity Among Prisoners in England and Wales.* London, England: Stationery Office; 1998.
9. Glueck B. A study of 608 admissions to Sing Sing prison. *Mental Hygiene.* 1918;2(1):85–151.
10. Fazel S, Danesh J. Serious mental disorder in 23 000 prisoners: a systematic review of 62 surveys. *Lancet.* 2002;359(9306):545–550.
11. Fazel S, Seewald K. Severe mental illness in 33 588 prisoners worldwide: systematic review and meta-regression analysis. *Br J Psychiatry.* 2012;200(5):364–373.
12. James D, Glaze L. *Bureau of Justice Statistics Special Report: Mental Health Problems of Prison and Jail Inmates.* Washington, DC: US Department of Justice; 2012.
13. Binswanger IA, Merrill JO, Krueger PM, White MC, Booth RE, Elmore JG. Gender differences in chronic medical, psychiatric, and substance-dependence disorders among jail inmates. *Am J Public Health.* 2010;100(3):476–482.
14. Hartwell S. Triple stigma: persons with mental illness and substance abuse problems in the criminal justice system. *Crim Justice Pol Rev.* 2004;15(1):84–99.
15. Lukasiewicz M, Blecha L, Falissard B, et al. Dual diagnosis: prevalence, risk factors, and relationship with suicide risk in a nationwide sample of French prisoners. *Alcohol Clin Exp Res.* 2009;33(1):160–168.
16. Australian Institute of Health and Welfare. *The Mental Health of Prison Entrants in Australia: 2010.* Canberra, Australia: AIHW; 2012.
17. Gore SM, Bird AG, Ross AJ. Prison rites: starting to inject inside. *BMJ.* 1995;311(7013):1135–1136.
18. Allwright S, Bradley F, Long J, Barry J, Thornton L, Parry JV. Prevalence of antibodies to hepatitis B, hepatitis C, and HIV and risk factors in Irish prisoners: results of a national cross sectional survey. *BMJ.* 2000;321(7253):78–82.
19. Boys A, Farrell M, Bebbington P, et al. Drug use and initiation in prison: results from a national prison survey in England and Wales. *Addiction.* 2002;97(12):1551–1560.
20. Arrigo BA, Bullock JL. The psychological effects of solitary confinement on prisoners in supermax units: reviewing what we know and recommending what should change. *Int J Offender Ther Comp Criminol.* 2008;52(6):622–640.
21. Walker J, Illingworth C, Canning A, et al. Changes in mental state associated with prison environments: a systematic review. *Acta Psychiat Scand.* 2014;129(6):427–436.

22. Wright B, Duffy D, Curtin K, Linehan S, Monks S, Kennedy HG. Psychiatric morbidity among women prisoners newly committed and amongst remanded and sentenced women in the Irish prison system. *Ir J Psychol Med*. 2006;23(2):47–53.
23. Hassan L, Birmingham L, Harty MA, et al. Prospective cohort study of mental health during imprisonment. *Br J Psychiatry*. 2011;198(1):37–42.
24. Dolan K, Wirtz AL, Moazen B, et al. Global burden of HIV, viral hepatitis, and tuberculosis in prisoners and detainees. *Lancet*. 2016;388(10049):1089–1102.
25. Albizu-García CE, Hernández-Viver A, Feal J, Rodríguez-Orengo JF. Characteristics of inmates witnessing overdose events in prison: implications for prevention in the correctional setting. *Harm Reduct J*. 2009;6(15):1–8.
26. Farrell M, Marsden J. Acute risk of drug-related death among newly released prisoners in England and Wales. *Addiction*. 2008;103(2):251–255.
27. Wilper AP, Woolhandler S, Boyd JW, et al. The health and health care of US prisoners: results of a nationwide survey. *Am J Public Health*. 2009;99(4):666–672.
28. Scheyett A, Vaughn J, Taylor MF. Screening and access to services for individuals with serious mental illnesses in jails. *Community Ment Health J*. 2009;45(6):439–446.
29. Brady TM, Krebs CP, Laird G. Psychiatric comorbidity and not completing jail-based substance abuse treatment. *Am J Addictions*. 2004;13(1):83–101.
30. Lurigio AJ. People with serious mental illness in the criminal justice system: causes, consequences, and correctives. *Prison J*. 2011;91(suppl 3):S66–S86.
31. Alm C, Eriksson Å, Palmstierna T, Kristiansson M, Berman AH, Gumpert CH. Treatment patterns among offenders with mental health problems and substance use problems. *J Behav Health Serv Res*. 2011;38(4):497–509.
32. Sung H-E. Nonfatal violence-related and accident-related injuries among jail inmates in the United States. *Prison J*. 2010;90(3):353–368.
33. Wallace C, Mullen P, Burgess P, Palmer S, Ruschena D, Browne C. Serious criminal offending and mental disorder: case linkage study. *Br J Psychiatry*. 1998;172(6):477–484.
34. Fazel S, Gulati G, Linsell L, Geddes JR, Grann M. Schizophrenia and violence: systematic review and meta-analysis. *PLoS Med*. 2009;6(8):e1000120.
35. Fazel S, Yu R. Psychotic disorders and repeat offending: systematic review and meta-analysis. *Schizophr Bull*. 2009;37(4):800–810.
36. Van Dorn RA, Desmarais SL, Petrila J, Haynes D, Singh JP. Effects of outpatient treatment on risk of arrest of adults with serious mental illness and associated costs. *Psych Serv*. 2013;64(9):856–862.
37. World Health Organization. *Mental Health Atlas 2011*. Geneva, Switzerland: WHO; 2011.
38. Enggist S. *Good Governance for Prison Health in the 21st Century: A Policy Brief on the Organization of Prison Health*. Copenhagen, Denmark: World Health Organization; 2013.
39. Fazel S, Baillargeon J. The health of prisoners. *Lancet*. 2011;377(9769):956–965.

CHAPTER 11

Understanding the Risk Environment Surrounding Drug Use in Prisons

The Unique Contributions of Qualitative Research

WILL SMALL, PhD AND RYAN McNEIL, PhD

INTRODUCTION

Increased attention to *why* and *how* people use drugs in prisons is critical to understanding the individual, social, and structural forces that drive in-prison drug use and associated risks and harms, and to inform the development and implementation of effective responses. Qualitative studies are uniquely positioned to provide a vivid picture of drug use in prison environments, and they illustrate how the motivations of prisoners and features of the prison risk environment shape the character of drug use and, in turn, impact on policies and interventions intended to mitigate drug-related risks and harms.[1]

Qualitative research methods are well-suited to understanding individuals' experiences and actions, and are useful for illustrating how social and structural contexts shape individual behavior,[2] including drug use.[3] Contemporary public health perspectives on substance use underscore the importance of understanding drug use in context and emphasize how individual behavior is shaped by a variety of social-, structural-, and physical-environmental factors.[4,5] Rhodes's Risk Environment framework has proven particularly influential in focusing attention on the role of extra-individual factors in producing drug-related harm.[5,6] As a heuristic, the Risk Environment framework illuminates how economic, social, structural, and environmental forces operating within particular settings or situations (eg, "shooting galleries") interact to increase or decrease vulnerability to drug-related risks and harms.[5,6] This social-ecological approach not only serves as a corrective to the emphasis on "individual risk" in drug use research and interventions but also generates insights critical to informing the development of environmental interventions aimed at reducing risks and harm.[5,7] The concept of "situated rationality" has also been employed by qualitative researchers to explain how cultural logics operating within specific risk environments make behaviors that are "risky" from a public health perspective (eg, syringe sharing) adaptive from the perspective of marginalized drug users,[4,8] and further illustrates the context-specific nature of behavior and decision-making.

While previous research drawing on the Risk Environment framework has underscored how contextual influences shape drug-related risks in street-based drug scenes,[5,9] prisons represent drug use risk environments that are distinct from these settings and yet remain poorly understood.[10] Moreover, attention to the situated risk perceptions of people who use drugs (PWUD) within prison settings has the potential to illuminate how they manage intersecting forms of risk within an environment characterized by highly constrained choices. Qualitative methods are well suited to understanding and documenting behavior within these settings, including the beliefs, social norms, and motivations underlying behavior, as well as the influence of differing aspects of the prison environment. In addition, designing and refining interventions to address the harms stemming from drug use in prisons requires highly detailed knowledge of prison environments and in-prison drug use activities and practices. For all these reasons, qualitative research is well positioned to generate knowledge and improved understandings of prison-based drug use.

While the qualitative research literature examining drug use is relatively well-recognized and has been reviewed previously,[11] qualitative studies examining in-prison drug use are less well known and have not previously been critically reviewed. The lack of awareness of this body of research stems from the fact that qualitative research is often less mainstream than quantitative health research, and many qualitative studies of prisoners' drug use may appear in relatively obscure journals. For these reasons, a scoping review of this literature is much needed to summarize existing knowledge produced through qualitative studies and provide insight into prison-based drug use that can help inform the development of appropriate interventions. In this chapter, we critically review the qualitative literature examining drug use within the prison risk environment and following release in order to highlight the contributions of these studies, while also identifying research gaps and directions for future inquiry.

METHODS

We undertook this scoping review to map key contributions of qualitative research to understandings of drug use among prisoners, and sought to examine articles reporting on qualitative studies into the experiences of PWUD within the prison risk environment and immediately following release. Building upon social-ecological approaches to drug-related risks and harm, we were particularly concerned with how contextual forces operating within prison settings and during the period following release impacted drug use and related risks.

While scoping reviews conventionally rely on systematic searches of academic databases, a more comprehensive strategy was needed to capture qualitative articles on drug use, which often appear in journals that are poorly indexed. We undertook the following steps: first, we used relevant keywords (Table 11.1) to execute searches of academic databases, including Medline, the Cumulative Index to Nursing and Allied Health Literature (CINAHL), and Scopus. Second, we hand-searched journals known to publish qualitative research focused on drug use and prisons, including the *International Journal of Drug Policy* and the *International Journal of Prisoner Health*. Third, we utilized the "related articles" function within Google Scholar to find additional articles related to key articles already identified during the earlier stages of the literature search, as well as using the "cited by" functions to find relevant articles citing these works. Finally, we reviewed the reference lists of included articles to identify any additional articles that had been overlooked. We excluded gray literature (eg, reports) to ensure that included studies had undergone peer review.

We imported citations and abstracts retrieved during the literature search into Endnote, a citation management software package, to manage the scoping review activities. A total of 25 articles remained after we removed duplicate citations and applied the following inclusion criteria: (1) qualitative methods; (2) publication in an English-language peer-reviewed journal; and (3) exploration of perspectives and experiences of prisoners in relation to in-prison or post-release drug use. We reviewed the remaining articles to map concepts and themes occurring across studies in relation to the prison and post-release drug use risk environments, as well as to document gaps in the literature. This process led to the identification of the five thematic areas outlined in the following section, as well as the limitations of the existing literature and opportunities for future research discussed at the end of this chapter.

RESULTS
Drug Use, Drug-Related Risks, and Harm

Previous qualitative studies have underscored how drug use in prisons is shaped by a number of considerations, including which drugs are available, their pharmacological effects, and correctional policies specific to the institution or jurisdiction. Importantly, while qualitative studies have suggested that drugs are as widely available in prison as in community settings,[12] and particular drugs (eg, heroin) might be

Table 11.1. SEARCH VARIABLES

Context		Method		Population
Prison		Qualitative interviews		Drug user
Penitentiary		Focus groups		Drug use
Jail		Case study		Use drugs
Incarcerat*	AND	Ethnography	AND	Inject drugs
		Ethnographic		
		Participant observation		
		Naturalistic observation		

even more accessible,[13] most studies have indicated that drugs are less accessible in prison environments and cost considerably more.[13-16] The availability of particular drugs in any given prison setting is shaped not only by local demand but also by the routes through which they enter prisons (eg, visits from family and friends, correctional personnel).[1,12,17,18]

Although prior drug use, drug dependency, and withdrawal experiences are important in shaping drug use in prison settings, studies have documented how prisoners are often motivated to use drugs to relieve stress and overcome boredom,[12] as well as enhance their ability to cope with living in prison environments.[17,18] Within the situated rationality of prisoners, the risks of adverse drug-related outcomes (eg, disease transmission) or being caught in possession of drugs are often weighed against the potential pleasures or perceived benefit (eg, reduced stress) associated with drug use.[17] In this regard, cannabis is often considered to be well suited to use within prison due to its perceived ability to relieve stress and pain, facilitate sleep, and assist in coping with incarceration.[17,19] Negative consequences of cannabis use (including sleepiness, potential for social isolation, and decreased perception of risk of injury when working with animals or machines) are recognized by inmates, and these may mitigate against continued or ongoing cannabis use.[19] A study undertaken in Swiss prison facilities, which did not at the time punish prisoners for cannabis use, suggested that the widespread consumption of cannabis and its perceived benefits (eg, improved sleep, decreased potential for conflict and violence) positively impacted the prison environment and that the enforcement of penalties for cannabis use might lead to transitions to other drugs (eg, heroin).[19]

Similar to cannabis, prisoners perceived heroin to be well-suited to use while incarcerated due to its potential to induce a sense of escape and release, as well as relieve boredom.[18] Heroin use (including initiation) can potentially be facilitated by correctional policies that enact punishment for positive drug tests (mandatory or random), as heroin is detectable for a shorter period than other drugs (eg, cannabis).[17-19] While research into the injection of stimulants in prison is limited, several studies have underscored how prison environments play a critical role in shaping decisions to continue or initiate heroin injection. These studies have outlined how the high cost and limited availability of heroin function to encourage the adoption of injection,[13,14,16] with participants in these studies noting that injecting heroin is the preferred route of administration because it is more efficient and cost-effective than other modes of consumption (eg, snorting, smoking).[1,18] Social, structural, and psychological factors may also shape the adoption of injecting behavior, such as previous experience of injection drug use, availability of drugs and syringes, and fatalism among those who feel they have "nothing to lose."[18] Meanwhile, opiate dependency and experiences of withdrawal symptoms have been found to also drive injection drug use among prisoners and, in some cases, facilitate injection initiation.[1,14]

Injection-Related Risk and Syringe Sharing

Because syringes are prohibited in most prison settings, prisoners commonly lack access to sterile injecting equipment. Previous qualitative studies have underscored how prisoners commonly share syringes or other injection-related paraphernalia and perceive this to be the "norm" in prison settings.[1,12,14-16] The culture surrounding syringe sharing in prisons is distinct from community settings in which injection routines rarely involve sharing.[16] Moreover, the environmental conditions within prison settings (eg, scarcity of syringes) function to drive syringe-sharing practices that foster HIV and hepatitis C (HCV) risks as large groups of prisoners within the same network may use the same syringe.[1,16,18] In addition, due to the high value of syringes in prisons, a prisoner who possesses a syringe will sometimes "rent" it to another prisoner in exchange for drugs, which potentially leads to large numbers of prisoners sharing a single syringe in a serial manner.[14,15,20] While studies have suggested that inmates will attempt to restrict syringe sharing to members of their immediate social group to limit potential exposure to blood-borne infections,[1,18] prisoners are often reluctant to disclose their HIV status to peers due to the stigma and discrimination that function to exclude HIV-positive inmates from drug-sharing and syringe-sharing networks.[16] In settings where mandatory HIV and HCV testing occurs upon intake, HIV-positive and HCV-positive inmates are sometimes segregated from the general prisoner population, which provides a sense of relative safety when sharing syringes due to assumption that others do not have blood-borne infections.[1] However, inmates recognize the limits of prisoner segregation insofar as the window period for blood-borne virus seroconversion (eg, HIV infection) means that some infections are not detected upon intake testing, and syringes sometimes circulate across HIV-negative and HIV-positive cellblocks.[1]

Policies prohibiting injection equipment and enacting punishment for syringe possession are fundamental barriers to reducing syringe sharing and promoting syringe sterilization among inmates.[1,15,16] While some inmates may sterilize syringes prior to injection (ie, boil syringes or clean them with bleach), studies have suggested that these practices are undermined due to fear of detection and punishment.[1,12,14-16,18] In turn, efforts to sterilize syringes are often rushed, less than thorough, and likely inadequate to reduce the potential for blood-borne infection. Within the situated risk perception of prisoners, concerns about injection-related health risks are overshadowed by the fear of punishment or violence stemming from being caught in possession of a syringe.[1,16] In addition, syringes commonly circulate for long periods of time and are frequently repaired to prolong their use, while makeshift syringes may be assembled out of available materials and parts from syringes that are no longer functional.[1,16] This also increases the number of individuals who may use a particular syringe during its lifetime, and thus the potential for infectious disease transmission and injection-related injuries. Inmate perspectives regarding the potential and implementation of prison-based syringe exchange have received considerable attention in qualitative research.[12,14,16,18] While there is support for such programs among some inmates,[12,18] who point to the need to operate the same interventions that exist for PWID in community settings and the potential of programs to reduce blood-borne infections,[14,16] others express concern regarding the potential for increased prevalence of injecting, the use of syringes as weapons, and the viability of such programs given opposition from guards and prison officials.[14]

Forces perceived to mitigate injecting in prison have been described, as the prevalence of injection drug use is noted to vary by institution or facility within a correctional system.[18] Social influences deterring injecting behavior, including "anti-injecting culture," are driven in part by recognition of health risks given the necessity of syringe sharing.[18] Stigmatization of injectors within the prisoner community may reduce the occurrence of injecting when such behavior is discouraged within peer networks.[18] Active discouragement of injecting by inmates may be motivated by the fact that the presence of syringes attracts unwanted attention from guards (eg, cell searches to confiscate injection equipment), which may disrupt drug use practices or drug-dealing activities.[18] A qualitative study in Scottish prisons reported that some inmates surrendered injection equipment to prison authorities or shared information regarding injecting activities with correctional staff.[18] However, it was noted that these individuals likely sought to reduce the likelihood of prison cell searches in order to better protect drug-dealing enterprises rather than being motivated by altruism or health concerns.[18] At the individual level, perception of health risks and concerns regarding the loss of health, family, and appearance may discourage injecting behavior.[18] A reported decline in the prevalence of injection drug use in particular Scottish prisons was attributed to decreased desire to inject among inmates, stemming from increased difficulty accessing syringes coupled with heightened awareness of the health risks associated with syringe sharing.[18]

Withdrawal and Detoxification in Prison

Studies exploring drug use among prisoners have drawn attention to how experiences of withdrawal and detoxification while incarcerated produce severe suffering and contribute to high-risk injecting practices (eg, syringe sharing).[21 24] Even in prison settings where detoxification services (including substitution treatments) were available, inconsistencies in these services (eg, inequities in prescribing practices), themselves shaped by views of who was and was not deserving of support, produced withdrawal symptoms among opiate-dependent prisoners.[21,22,24] Meanwhile, the complete lack of availability of detoxification and substitution treatment services in most prison settings was a structural-environmental barrier to withdrawal management for many prisoners. This meant that opiate-dependent prisoners were left to manage withdrawal symptoms on their own.[21] Multiple studies have documented how withdrawal symptoms thus led many prisoners to seek out and inject drugs to alleviate their suffering,[21,22,25] as well as share drugs with fellow prisoners experiencing withdrawal in order to gain access to shared drugs later in time.[23] In turn, the absence of readily available harm reduction supplies in prison settings meant that prisoners commonly shared injecting equipment despite concerns regarding HIV and HCV risks.[21,25] Within this context, the sharing of injecting equipment was characterized as a "rational choice" given the more urgent need to alleviate withdrawal symptoms, illustrating the importance of situated risk perceptions in driving injection-related risk. In some cases, prisoners loaned out syringes to people experiencing withdrawal symptoms because they understood the hardships associated with withdrawal.[21,23]

While the interplay of contextual forces and withdrawal symptoms fosters participation in high-risk injecting practices, concerns regarding the impacts of drug use have also been documented to lead many prisoners to pursue abstinence.[26,27] There is evidence that these decisions to pursue abstinence are heavily influenced by concerns regarding low or inconsistent drug availability in prison settings.[27] However, while pursuing drug abstinence meant that prisoners experienced intense withdrawal symptoms upon incarceration, which lasted from several days (heroin or opiates) to several weeks (methadone), studies have outlined how some prisoners viewed their experience positively because it enabled them to reduce or discontinue problematic drug use.[26,27] In this regard, previous studies have outlined steps taken by prisoners to moderate withdrawal. For example, Mitchell and colleagues noted that some prisoners tapered their drug use or methadone dosage prior to being incarcerated to mitigate withdrawal symptoms and the need to inject drugs in prison.[26] However, prisoners unable to "self-detox" in advance reported other illnesses to prison staff or injured themselves in order to receive medical support.[26]

Prison-Based Methadone Maintenance Therapy and Other Forms of Pharmacotherapy

Several studies examining prison-based methadone maintenance therapy (MMT) dispensation have documented inmate and staff perspectives regarding these programs, experiences of those receiving treatment, and barriers to providing and scaling up MMT provision.[13,14,28] Prison-based MMT provision produces benefits similar to those seen in programs in community settings (eg, reduced opioid use) and is perceived to reduce and prevent injection drug use and, in turn, HIV and HCV transmission within prison environments.[13,14] A study within an Iranian prison described how MMT provision reduced levels of injection drug use and sharing of injection equipment, and these benefits were attributed to the reduced prevalence of withdrawal symptoms among opioid-dependent inmates.[13] Financial and social benefits of the program extended to recipients' families, who no longer had to provide prisoners with money to obtain drugs, reducing the financial burden stemming from the extremely high cost of drugs and dependency and the associated strain on relationships with spouses and other family members.[13] This study also documented considerable stigma experienced by those receiving MMT. This was largely due to the fact that the original treatment criteria for this program gave priority to groups often subjected to discrimination and harassment in prison environments, including people living with HIV, people who inject drugs, and men who have sex with men.[13] Concerns regarding the side effects of MMT (specifically, the potential for liver damage) were documented, primarily among those waiting for MMT and those who had not yet received treatment, and were thought to be propagated by heroin dealers concerned about MMT eroding the number of heroin-dependent inmates.[13]

There is evidence that barriers to scaling up MMT within prison include a lack of capacity within prison facilities as well as inadequate continuity of MMT upon release and transition back to the community.[13,28] Challenges stemming from a shortage of prison health staff (including administrative and healthcare staff) functioned to produce long wait lists (≥100 prisoners) seeking or awaiting treatment in the Iranian program.[13] While "some" methadone diversion was documented and acknowledged by prison managers and staff in the Iranian program, due to relatively lax supervision of administration resulting from the shortage of healthcare staff,[13] such problems did not exist in relation to a MMT pilot project in Puerto Rico that was deemed an overall success and recommended for expansion.[28] Barriers to scaling up the Puerto Rican program included the need to increase staffing levels (including correctional officers and psychosocial support workers) and expand the space and facilities devoted to the program.[28] There was no formal referral system for inmates returning to the community from the Iranian prison-based MMT program, although information about MMT in the community was provided prior to release, and geographical variation in community availability of MMT resulted in long wait lists for those seeking to continue treatment outside of prison.[13] Similarly, a lack of MMT in the community was a serious concern for the Puerto Rican program as inadequate treatment capacity in the community and a lack of continuity of care posed problems for former prisoners enrolled in MMT.[28]

Other forms of pharmacotherapy provided to inmates have also been examined in qualitative studies, including methadone detoxification programs and substitution prescribing involving medications other than methadone.[14,22] Methadone detoxification involving a tapered methadone dose was largely seen to be inadequate by inmates and was reported to lead to withdrawal symptoms.[14] Substitution prescribing practices as experienced by English inmates resulted in dissatisfaction stemming from a lack of consistency between prison and community programs (where methadone maintenance is provided).[22] Restrictive prescribing practices often deviated from inmates' self-identified treatment needs and provided an inadequate level of medication to meet individual needs, which was reported to result in illicit drug use and syringe sharing.[22]

While the studies described in this section examined settings where pharmacotherapy for substance use is provided to inmates, in many settings there is a complete lack of substance use treatment, particularly evidence-based treatments and substitution therapy, even in specialized prison facilities for drug-dependent individuals.[1] Extant studies have documented great demand and desire for such programs on the part of prisoners.[1,12,14]

Understanding the Post-Release Drug Use Risk Environment

While qualitative research into the post-release risk environment is limited, and based primarily upon articles drawn from a study of 29 recently released prisoners in Denver, Colorado,[29–31] it has generated preliminary insights into contextual forces that increase the potential for drug-related harm during this critical transitional period. This research has illustrated how social, structural, and environmental forces shape the drug and health harms experienced by ex-prisoners following release, such as re-initiation of drug use,[30-34] syringe sharing,[29] and overdose risks.[30] It has underscored how individual-level vulnerabilities (eg, lowered tolerance to opiates, mental illness) are amplified by the extreme poverty, homelessness, and social isolation common among ex-prisoners following release and the critical lack of support services (eg, housing services, harm reduction supports).[29-32,35] For example, publications from the Denver study emphasized how the limited availability of harm reduction supplies (eg, injecting equipment, condoms) in some community settings fueled HIV and HCV risks by increasing the potential for syringe sharing and sex without a condom.[29,31]

This body of research has also underscored social and structural influences that increase overdose risks immediately following release from prison. For example, Binswanger and colleagues and Burgess-Allen and colleagues have outlined how recently released ex-prisoners exposed to other PWUD in emergency shelters or street-based settings reinitiated drug use despite wishing to remain abstinent.[30,32] These recently released ex-prisoners articulated how injecting drugs following extended periods of drug use cessation, resulting in decreased tolerance, increased their risk of overdose, and some noted that friends had died in these situations.[30,32] Meanwhile, multiple studies have documented how worsening mental health outcomes stemming from interruptions in access to health services and compounded by homelessness, housing vulnerability, and social exclusion following release further increased the potential for risks among those experiencing suicidal ideation.[30,33]

Previous research has also emphasized how social dynamics, particularly gendered power relations, shape post-release drug use and associated harms.[29,33] Multiple studies of post-release experiences have emphasized how social norms and problematic or exploitive social relationships surrounding drug use contribute to harm.[29,33] For instance, Adams and colleagues found that the social contexts in which women released from prison generated money to purchase drugs (ie, sex work) or consumed drugs undermined their capacity to enact drug use or sexual risk reduction practices.[29] Participants in this study reported that women had exchanged sex without using condoms and shared drug use equipment with clients due to impaired capacity stemming from intoxication and gendered power inequities (eg, coercion by sex work clients).[29]

DISCUSSION

The studies included in this review chapter make a unique contribution to understandings of drug use in prison and drug-related risks among prisoners. They have documented and identified forces and influences that shape the character of drug use practices within prison, and the associated harms. Importantly, this chapter illustrates why prisoners commonly share syringes and perceive this to be the "norm" in prison, partially due to policies that prohibit syringe possession in most settings and impede efforts to decontaminate syringes. Experiences of withdrawal and detoxification while incarcerated also function to drive syringe sharing and high-risk injecting practices, which highlights the potential of MMT programs to address injection-related risks. However, this chapter outlined how barriers to providing and scaling up MMT provision, as well as social considerations regarding the acceptability of MMT (eg, stigma, negative attitudes toward methadone), may pose important barriers to program operation, uptake, and retention. This chapter also underscored how contextual forces increase the potential for drug and health harms experienced by ex-prisoners following release, including re-initiation of drug use, syringe sharing, and fatal and non-fatal overdose. Collectively, the studies included in this review help us to understand the prison drug use risk environment and the interaction of forces that function to produce drug-related risks and harms experienced by prisoners in custody and subsequent to release.

These qualitative studies help to explain the findings generated by epidemiological and quantitative studies examining drug-related risk among prisoners and former prisoners by documenting how prison environments shape drug and health harms among PWUD. While numerous quantitative studies have documented elevated levels of injection-related risks among prisoners and people who inject drugs with a history of incarceration,[36-38] the qualitative studies reviewed here illustrate the importance of correctional policies that restrict access to sterile syringes in driving injection-related HIV risks within prison settings.[20] These findings underscore the importance of situated risk perceptions and rationality in explaining why prisoners engage in risk behaviors that might seem irrational, but which are adaptive given the constrained options in managing in-prison drug dependency. Similarly, the risk of overdose (including fatal overdose) among people recently released from prison has been documented to be greatly elevated,[36,39-41] and qualitative studies illustrate how the reduction or cessation of drug use within prison leads to reduced tolerance, which functions to exacerbate overdose risk upon release, particularly in the context of inadequate access to harm reduction supports and in relation to unintended re-initiation of opioid use. This illustrates the importance of qualitative research focused on prison environments, but also the potential of combining qualitative and quantitative methods (eg, mixed-methods or ethno-epidemiological approaches) to better document and understand drug-related harms experienced by prisoners and former prisoners.[42,43]

The findings of this review also point to promising directions for efforts to address drug-related risk among prisoners and former prisoners by identifying features of prison and postrelease risk environments amenable to modification. These include policies restricting access to syringes, poor continuity of care after release, and a lack of access to MMT programs that could be addressed through program enhancement, policy reform and modification, and targeted interventions. For example, prison-based syringe exchange programs, which operate in a considerable number of prisons and correctional systems, have been documented to have a positive impact upon injection-related risk where they have been implemented, although there is a lack of English-language evaluation of these programs.[44] In addition to policy modification and risk-reduction interventions, efforts to address social dynamics that restrict access to existing programs may also help reduce drug-related harm. For example, social considerations that undermine the acceptability of MMT (eg, stigma, negative attitudes toward methadone) pose important barriers to uptake and could potentially be addressed through targeted educational programs or social marketing among prisoners. The insights generated by qualitative research provide helpful cues for the development of efforts to minimize drug-related risk, although it is important to note that social-structural forces impeding the uptake of risk-reduction programs and the implementation of new interventions are often context-specific, which highlights the need for local research to understand relevant forces particular to a specific setting.

The relatively small body of qualitative studies identified in this review, in comparison to the larger number of quantitative studies, highlights the urgent need to scale up qualitative studies of prison and post-release risk environments and experiences. Given the recognized potential for qualitative research to help inform the development of targeted public health interventions,[3,4] future research should attempt to address documented gaps in the literature and limitations of existing studies. Further studies of drug policies in prison and their impacts are merited, particularly those examining whether correctional policies (whether they are oriented toward abstinence or harm reduction) meet their objectives. This may be particularly necessary to ensure that these policies do not have unintended effects that exacerbate drug-related risks and harms. Existing and emerging interventions should similarly be examined using qualitative approaches in a diversity of facilities and jurisdictions to more fully document their operation and impact, as context-specific forces related to these interventions often shape the associated outcomes.

Prison-based syringe exchange has not yet been examined or evaluated through a qualitative study, although perspectives regarding their implementation and operation require thorough examination due to the prevalence of within-prison syringe sharing and the importance of syringe exchange in community settings.[7,44] One limitation evident within existing studies was the reliance on retrospective examination of in-prison behavior and prison environments with former inmates subsequent to their return to the community. Post-release studies are sometimes the only research design that is feasible when correctional authorities and governments are not supportive of research with prisoners and within prisons. The considerable practical and ethical barriers to conducting research within prison environments, particularly when the research focuses on prohibited behaviors such as injecting drug use, further complicates this dynamic. Although some researchers have managed to negotiate research access with correctional systems to conduct high-quality in-prison studies, there is a need for more qualitative studies employing similar research designs in order to enrich the evidence base regarding in-prison drug use. Such approaches are also likely to generate insights into overlooked dynamics surrounding in-prison drug use that would prove instrumental in informing directions for future research.

In conclusion, the qualitative studies reviewed here afford deeper insight into the prison drug use risk environment, illustrate the situated risk perceptions of PWUD in relation to prison and post-release environments, and complement quantitative and epidemiological studies examining drug-related risks and harms among prisoners and former prisoners.

REFERENCES

1. Sarang A, Rhodes T, Platt L, et al. Drug injecting and syringe use in the HIV risk environment of Russian penitentiary institutions: qualitative study. *Addiction.* 2006;101(12):1787–1796.
2. Snape D, Spencer L. The foundations of qualitative research. In: Ritchie J, Lewis J, McNaughton Nicolls C, Ormston, R, eds. *Qualitative Research Practice: A Guide for Social Science Students and Researchers.* London, England: Sage; 2003:1–23.
3. Neale J, Allen D, Coombes L. Qualitative research methods within the addictions. *Addiction.* 2005;100(11):1584–1593.
4. Moore D. Key moments in the ethnography of drug-related harm: reality checks for policy makers? In: Stockwell TR, Gruenewald P, Toumbourou J, Loxley W, eds. *Preventing Harmful Substance Use: The Evidence Base for Policy and Practice.* Chichester, England: Wiley; 2005:433–442.
5. Rhodes T, Singer M, Bourgois P, Friedman SR, Strathdee S. The social structural production of HIV risk among injecting drug users. *Soc Sci Med.* 2005;61(5):1026–1044.
6. Rhodes T. The "risk environment": a framework for understanding and reducing drug-related harm. *Int J Drug Policy.* 2002;13(2):85–94.
7. McNeil R, Small W. "Safer environment interventions": a qualitative synthesis of the experiences and perceptions of people who inject drugs. *Soc Sci Med.* 2014;106:151–158.
8. Bourgois P. The moral economies of homeless heroin addicts: confronting ethnography, HIV risk, and everyday violence in San Francisco shooting encampments. *Subst Use Misuse.* 1998;33(11):2323–2351.
9. Strathdee SA, Hallett TB, Bobrova N, et al. HIV and risk environment for injecting drug users: the past, present, and future. *Lancet.* 2010;376(9737):268–284.
10. Strathdee SA, West BS, Reed E, Moazan B, Azim T, Dolan K. Substance use and HIV among female sex workers and female prisoners: risk environments and implications for prevention, treatment, and policies. *J Acquir Immune Defic Syndr.* 2015;69(suppl 2):S110–117.
11. Carlson RG, Singer M, Stephens RC, Sterk C. Reflections on 40 years of ethnographic drug abuse research: implications for the future. *J Drug Issues.* 2009;39(1):57–70.
12. Seal DW, Belcher L, Morrow K, et al. A qualitative study of substance use and sexual behavior among 18- to 29-year-old men while incarcerated in the United States. *Health Educ Behav.* 2004;31(6):775–789.
13. Zamani S, Farnia M, Tavakoli S, et al. A qualitative inquiry into methadone maintenance treatment for opioid-dependent prisoners in Tehran, Iran. *Int J Drug Policy.* 2010;21(3):167–172.
14. Long J, Allwright S, Begley C. Prisoners' views of injecting drug use and harm reduction in Irish prions. *Int J Drug Policy.* 2004;15(2):139–149.
15. Mahon N. New York inmates' HIV risk behaviors: the implications for prevention policy and programs. *Am J Public Health.* 1996;86(9):1211–1215.
16. Small W, Kain S, Laliberte N, Schechter MT, O'Shaughnessy MV, Spittal PM. Incarceration, addiction and harm reduction: inmates experience injecting drugs in prison. *Subst Use Misuse.* 2005;40(6):831–843.
17. Cope N. Drug use in Prison: the experience of young offenders. *Drug-Educ Prev Polic.* 2000;7(4):355–366.
18. Wilson GB, Galloway J, Shewan D, Marshall L, Vojt G, Marley C. "Phewww, bingoed!": motivations and variations of methods for using heroin in Scottish prisons. *Addict Res Theory.* 2007;15(2):205–224.
19. Ritter C, Broers B, Elger BS. Cannabis use in a Swiss male prison: qualitative study exploring detainees' and staffs' perspectives. *Int J Drug Policy.* 2013;24(6):573–578.
20. Small W, Wood E, Jurgens R, Kerr T. Injection drug use, HIV/AIDS and incarceration: evidence from the Vancouver Injection Drug Users Study. *HIV AIDS Policy Law Rev.* 2005;10(3):1, 5–10.

21. Hughes RA. Assessing the influence of need to inject and drug withdrawal on drug injectors' perceptions of HIV risk behavior. *J Psychoactive Drugs*. 2001;33(2):185–189.
22. Hughes RA. "It's like having half a sugar when you were used to three"—drug injectors' views and experiences of substitute drug prescribing inside English prisons. *Int J Drug Policy*. 2000;10(6):455–466.
23. Mjåland K. "A culture of sharing": drug exchange in a Norwegian prison. *Punishm Soc*. 2014;16(3):336–352.
24. Tompkins CNE, Neale J, Sheard L, Wright NMJ. Experiences of prison among injecting drug users in England: a qualitative study. *Int J Prison Health*. 2007;3(3):189–203.
25. Keene J. Drug use among prisoners before, during and after custody. *Addiction Res Theory*. 1997;4(4):343–353.
26. Mitchell SG, Kelly SM, Brown BS, et al. Incarceration and opioid withdrawal: the experiences of methadone patients and out-of-treatment heroin users. *J Psychoactive Drugs*. 2009;41(2):145–152.
27. Tompkins CNE. Exploring motivations to stop injecting in English prisons: qualitative research with former male prisoner. *Int J Prison Health*. 2013;9(2):68–81.
28. Heimer R, Catania H, Newman RG, Zambrano J, Brunet A, Ortiz AM. Methadone maintenance in prison: evaluation of a pilot program in Puerto Rico. *Drug Alcohol Depend*. 2006;83(2):122–129.
29. Adams J, Nowels C, Corsi K, Long J, Steiner JF, Binswanger IA. HIV risk after release from prison: a qualitative study of former inmates. *J Acquir Immune Defic Syndr*. 2011;57(5):429–434.
30. Binswanger IA, Nowels C, Corsi KF, et al. Return to drug use and overdose after release from prison: a qualitative study of risk and protective factors. *Addict Sci Clin Pract*. 2012;7(3):1–9.
31. Binswanger IA, Nowels C, Corsi KF, et al. "From the prison door right to the sidewalk, everything went downhill," A qualitative study of the health experiences of recently released inmates. *Int J Law Psychiatry*. 2011;34(4):249–255.
32. Burgess-Allen J, Langlois M, Whittaker P. The health needs of ex-prisoners, implications for successful resettlement: a qualitative study. *Int J Prison Health*. 2006;2(4):291–301.
33. Johnson JE, Schonbrun YC, Nargiso JE, et al. "I know if I drink I won't feel anything": substance use relapse among depressed women leaving prison. *Int J Prison Health*. 2013;9(4):169–186.
34. Fox AD, Maradiaga J, Weiss L, Sanchez J, Starrels JL, Cunningham CO. Release from incarceration, relapse to opioid use and the potential for buprenorphine maintenance treatment: a qualitative study of the perceptions of former inmates with opioid use disorder. *Addic Sci Clin Pract*. 2015;10(2):1–9.
35. O'Brien P. Maximizing success for drug-affected women after release from prison. *Women Crim Justice*. 2006;17(2–3):95–113.
36. Kinner SA, Milloy MJ, Wood E, Qi J, Zhang R, Kerr T. Incidence and risk factors for non-fatal overdose among a cohort of recently incarcerated illicit drug users. *Addict Behav*. 2012;37(6):691–696.
37. Milloy MJ, Buxton J, Wood E, Li K, Montaner JS, Kerr T. Elevated HIV risk behaviour among recently incarcerated injection drug users in a Canadian setting: a longitudinal analysis. *BMC Public Health*. 2009;9(156):1–7.
38. Wood E, Li K, Small W, Montaner JS, Schechter MT, Kerr T. Recent incarceration independently associated with syringe sharing by injection drug users. *Public Health Rep*. 2005;120(2):150–156.
39. Andrews JY, Kinner SA. Understanding drug-related mortality in released prisoners: a review of national coronial records. *BMC Public Health*. 2012;12(270):1–7.

40. Binswanger IA, Blatchford PJ, Mueller SR, Stern MF. Mortality after prison release: opioid overdose and other causes of death, risk factors, and time trends from 1999 to 2009. *Ann Intern Med*. 2013;159(9):592–600.

41. Winter RJ, Stoove M, Degenhardt L, et al. Incidence and predictors of non-fatal drug overdose after release from prison among people who inject drugs in Queensland, Australia. *Drug Alcohol Depend*. 2015;153:43–49.

42. Imbert G. Towards the development of an ethno-epidemiological study of type-2 diabetes and its complications. *Sante Publique*. 2008;20(2):113–124.

43. Lopez AM, Bourgois P, Wenger LD, Lorvick J, Martinez AN, Kral AH. Interdisciplinary mixed methods research with structurally vulnerable populations: case studies of injection drug users in San Francisco. *Int J Drug Policy*. 2013;24(2):101–109.

44. Canadian HIV/AIDS Legal Network. *Prison Needle Exchange: Lessons From a Comprehensive Review of International Evidence and Experience*. Canadian HIV/AIDS Legal Network: Montreal, Canada; 2006.

CHAPTER 12

Drug Use and Prison

The Challenge of Making Human

Rights Protections a Reality

JOANNE CSETE, PhD, RICK LINES, PhD, AND
RALF JÜRGENS, PhD

INTRODUCTION

For people who use drugs or who live with drug dependence, being in state custody
is a condition of high vulnerability to health problems, as noted in other chapters
in this book. For these persons, it is also a time of heightened vulnerability to violations of their human rights, including but not limited to the right to health. As
noted in chapter 1 of this volume, because of harsh drug laws in many countries
that impose custodial sentences for drug consumption, possession of quantities
of drugs for personal use and other minor, non-violent drug infractions, people
who use drugs may face a high likelihood of being in state custody at some point—
perhaps several points—in their lives. High rates of drug use have also been
documented among detainees in many countries, regardless of their reason for
detention. In addition, in some countries people convicted of minor drug infractions may be involuntarily detained in facilities that purport to provide treatment
but in reality keep people in squalor and subject them to punitive measures with
no scientific merit.

This chapter summarizes from both international and national law and guidelines the human rights protections enjoyed by prisoners, including those that are
especially relevant to people who use drugs. It describes the reality of how those
protections are often flouted and makes recommendations for policy and practice that would be conducive to protecting the human rights of this vulnerable
population.

People in state custody—whether convicted and imprisoned or in pre-adjudication remand, police lock-up, or other detention—are usually completely dependent on the state for the protection and fulfillment of their human rights. In this unique relationship between the state as "detainor" and individual as "detainee," "international law subordinates to the state a legally enforceable duty of care,"[1] meaning that the government has the responsibility for ensuring the well-being of persons it deprives of liberty. This relationship exists regardless of the reason for detention or the individual's behavior while in custody. Both of these principles are significant in the case of people who use drugs in detention, who are often in positions of increased health vulnerability due to their drug use, yet also in breach of institutional rules because of this behavior.[2]

The importance of protecting the rights of persons deprived of liberty has been clear from the beginning of the modern human rights regime. The Universal Declaration of Human Rights includes several articles on people's right to the due process of law, including protection from arbitrary arrest, presumption of innocence, protection from conviction based on laws not in force at the time of the alleged offense, and the right to a fair and public trial. Similar guarantees also feature prominently in regional human rights treaties.[3,4]

Central to the issue of drug use in prisons is the health response. In international law, the right to health is articulated within economic, social, and cultural rights, under which the right is universal and non-discriminatory in application.[5] The right is therefore understood to pertain to persons deprived of liberty, just as it does to all people. This right is articulated in a number of international and regional human rights treaties and has been interpreted in detail by the United Nations (UN) Committee on Economic, Social and Cultural Rights, which notes that the right is made meaningful when health services are (1) physicially and economically accessible without discrimination, (2) available in sufficient quantity, (3) scientifically sound and of good quality, and (4) respectful of medical ethics and the dignity of people.[6] The committee stresses that states have an affirmative responsibility to fulfill (or provide) a right when "individuals or a group are unable . . . to realize that right themselves by the means at their disposal" (para 37).[6] The right of "prisoners and other detainees" to all services of prevention, cure, and palliative care are explicitly recognized. The committee also specifies a few "core" obligations of states, including ensuring availability of the medicines designated as essential medicines by the World Health Organization (WHO).[6]

In the context of detention, the right to health also finds expression in civil and political rights instruments. The UN Human Rights Committee has stated, for example, that although there is no specific right to health provision within the International Covenant on Civil and Political Rights, questions of health in detention could be raised under the right to life (Article 6)[7] or the right to humane treatment (Article 10).[7,8] Indeed both the right to life and the right to humane treatment impose positive obligations to protect the lives and/or well-being of persons in custody, which has often been interpreted to require government authorities to take positive action to safeguard the health and well-being of detainees. With respect to prison health, these positive obligations create a powerful complement to the state's negative obligations to prevent state agents from inflicting torture or other forms of cruel, inhuman, or degrading treatment or punishment. For example, it has been argued that these positive obligations entitle persons in detention to access to needle and syringe programs.[2,9]

Drawing from these international legal principles, several core international instruments have been developed that focus exclusively, and elaborate in detail, on the rights of people in custody of the state. The UN Standard Minimum Rules for the Treatment of Prisoners (SMR)[10] cover a wide range of issues, including the following:

- The separation of women from men in state custody, and of young people from adults;
- Adequate health services and sleeping quarters, water and sanitation, food, clothing and bedding, exercise and sports activities;
- The importance of protecting the independence and autonomy of medical professionals working in prisons; and
- Protections from cruel and arbitrary punishment.[10]

It has been argued that many of these non-binding guidelines in the SMR have attained the status of international legal standards, based on their use and application by key international human rights courts and other bodies.[11] In 2015, the UN completed updated SMR to be known as the Mandela Rules, which embody the main provisions in the SMR and reinforce a number of provisions.[12] The UN has urged incorporation of these provisions into national law.

Following the original SMR, there was international agreement on the Basic Principles for the Treatment of Prisoners,[13] a concise statement that underscored two important ideas:

- That people in prison retain all human rights articulated in international treaties "except for those limitations that are demonstrably necessitated by the fact of incarceration," and
- That people in prison must "have access to the health services available in the country without discrimination on the grounds of their legal situation." That is, health services for prisoners should be the equivalent of what is offered to the general population outside prison.[13]

In 1990, the UN General Assembly also adopted rules for the protection of juveniles (persons under age 18) in state custody.[14] These include, most importantly, the use of imprisonment only as a last resort, and for those who are incarcerated the right to "meaningful activities and programmes which would serve to promote and sustain their health and self-respect."[14] Medical care standards are enumerated, including the right to be examined by a medical officer upon admission. In addition, juvenile detention facilities "should adopt specialized drug abuse prevention and rehabilitation programmes administered by qualified personnel" and "adapted to the age, sex and other requirements" of young people.[14]

The emergence of HIV/AIDS epidemics has highlighted the need for attention to the rights of people who use drugs who are in state custody to protect themselves and to be protected from this illness (see also chapter 7). The International Guidelines on HIV/AIDS and Human Rights, an expert consensus endorsed by the Joint United Nations Programme on HIV/AIDS (UNAIDS) and the High Commissioner on Human Rights, recognizes "prisoners and other detained persons," as well as people who use illicit drugs, as particularly in need of human rights protections related to HIV.[15] It enjoins prison authorities to "provide prisoners . . . with access to HIV-related prevention information, education, voluntary testing and counselling, means of prevention (condoms, bleach and clean injection equipment), treatment and care" (para 30).[15] Though it does not mention prisoners explicitly, the unanimous declaration from the first major UN General Assembly Special Session on HIV in 2001 committed UN member states to ensure access for all people to comprehensive HIV prevention, including "sterile injecting equipment" and "harm reduction measures related to drug use."[16] The letter and spirit of both these documents embody the idea of access to comprehensive and good-quality HIV services as a human right for people in and outside the custody of the state.

These ideas have been developed in practical program and policy guidance by UN agencies, all such guidance emphasizing that these services are not just good health practice but part of human rights obligations of states. The recommendations of the UN Office on Drugs and Crime (UNODC), UNAIDS, and WHO for a package of 15 comprehensive interventions to ensure HIV prevention, treatment, and care in closed settings (see chapter 16) emphasize the principle of equivalence with services in the community.[17] The guidelines also note that people have a right to care that is continuous from the time of arrest or detention until after release, when people may struggle to find care in the community, an idea also emphasized in the Mandela Rules. The UN agencies also assert that "incarceration is not a treatment for mentally ill people or for drug-dependent people" and underscore the need to protect the independence of health professionals working in closed settings.[17]

UNODC and WHO have issued principles to inform standards for the treatment of drug dependence that pertain to prisons and other closed settings, as well as to care in the community.[18] As noted in these principles, not only do people in state custody have a right to treatment for drug dependence on a par with what is offered outside prisons, but this is also an important public health investment for the state because it can help reduce drug dependence and associated harms in the community. Among the principles promoted by the UN agencies for treatment of drug dependence are the following:

- That treatment must always be voluntary;
- That treatment approaches should be chosen and implemented with meaningful involvement of the patient;
- That treatment must be scientifically sound, humane, and low-threshold (ie, without significant admission requirements) and be overseen by qualified health professionals;

- That people with drug dependence should have access to several kinds of treatment, since there is no "one size fits all" approach;
- That treatment programs must not exclude people because of criminal records;
- That women, especially pregnant women, and people with psychiatric co-morbidities should be given priority in treatment; and
- That "treatment as an alternative to imprisonment or other penal sanctions should be made available to drug-dependent offenders."[18]

THE HUMAN RIGHTS REALITY: RIGHTS HONORED IN THE BREACH

Although the right to health of prisoners is broadly protected under human rights norms, ensuring these guarantees is in practice rare. In reality, the rights of people who use drugs—and of prisoners more broadly—are flagrantly violated in prisons in many countries with no opportunity for complaint or redress.[19] As described by Rieter: "'Apart from being especially vulnerable by virtue of being detained, detainees generally are an unpopular political cause. . . . Consideration of their rights is not normally included in the political process.'"[20] As noted in chapter 1 of this volume, drug-dependent persons are over-represented in prisons and detention facilities, where they are often denied adequate treatment that might be available to them in the community. This denial of care is compounded by the particular vulnerability of people with drug dependence to mistreatment while in the custody of the state. Manfred Nowak, the former UN Special Rapporteur on Torture, denounced as a form of torture police interrogation of people in a state of withdrawal from drugs, including exploitation of that state to coerce confessions or incriminating testimony.[21]

The Special Rapporteur also noted as an infringement of human rights the denial to prisoners of proven medications for treating drug dependence, such as methadone and buprenorphine for opiate dependence.[21] In 2012 an estimated 41 countries provided opioid substitution therapy (OST) in prison, a figure that represents some progress but is much lower than the number of countries that make OST available in the community.[22] Even in countries where this proven therapy is offered in prison, programs may exist in only a few prisons or may screen out some prisoners who need it most.[23]

Where drug use and minor infractions are criminalized, people who use drugs are likely to be over-represented in pre-trial detention as well as prison. Pre-trial settings may be especially overcrowded as admissions may swell in unplanned ways linked to police crackdowns or raids. They are unlikely to offer drug treatment services, often on the excuse that turnover is high, even though in some countries people are detained awaiting trial for months or even years.[24] Drug-related education or peer support programs that may exist in prisons are very rare in pretrial settings. Pretrial facilities are also less likely than prisons to have the sports and education programs that may help people turn away from drugs.

The human rights of incarcerated women who use drugs are particularly vulnerable to abuse. In some countries, a higher percentage of women than men are imprisoned for drug offenses, though the relatively small number of women in custody compared with men is often used as an excuse for not offering drug-related services.[25] Women in prison also often have higher HIV prevalence than men, frequently facing the multiple risks of sexual violence, injection with contaminated equipment, and lack of condoms and other prevention services.[25] Women who use drugs, in prison and in the community, are highly stigmatized as "fallen" women in the public mind, a barrier to giving due priority to funding for services for them.[26] Lesbian, gay, transgender, and bisexual persons who use drugs, who may be overrepresented in prison and pre-trial detention where homosexuality and transgenderism are criminalized, also face multiple human rights risks, especially the risk of physical and sexual violence.[27]

In addition to prisons and pretrial detention facilities, numerous countries have detention facilities that are purportedly for treatment and rehabilitation of people who use drugs and sometimes sex workers. These are not prisons but are prison-like in many ways. As noted in a 2012 UN statement, compulsory drug "treatment" facilities rarely offer scientifically sound treatment but rather impose punishment in the form of forced labor or punitive exercises.[28] Even more than in the criminal justice system, people may be detained in these facilities without due process of law or any means of complaint or restitution for the rights that have been abused. The UN agencies called for closing these centers and strengthening treatment services in the community for the persons detained there.

RIGHTS-BASED ALTERNATIVES: CONCLUSIONS AND RECOMMENDATIONS

Some countries have made meaningful reforms in policies and practices that reflect a concern for the human rights of people who use drugs who are imprisoned or in remand. Some member states of the European Union, for example, as well as several Latin American countries, have removed drug use and some minor possession offenses from the penal code and manage them instead through the health and social service sectors.[29,30] Reforms of this nature are consistent with UN recommendations[31] and with expert recommendations for rights-directed action.[32]

A few countries, including some middle-income countries, have made particular efforts to ensure access to a broad range of services for people who use drugs in prison. Several Western European countries such as Switzerland and Spain have for years made sterile injection equipment available in at least some prisons, as have, for example, Moldova and the Kyrgyz Republic.[33,34] All of these programs reduced HIV transmission in prisons. As Swiss officials have noted, if policy-makers can get past a state of denial about drug use in prison, syringe programs embody both respect for human rights of people in prison and a pragmatic commitment to cost-effective health programs.[35] A few countries, but not nearly enough, have made efforts to offer a range of drug treatment services to people in detention and to ensure links to services in the community for those who are released.[33] Peer-based programs in prisons in several countries demonstrate that respecting the rights of people who use drugs to participate meaningfully in programs affecting them contributes to good public health as well as human rights outcomes.[33]

In our view, the following actions are essential to ensure that the human rights of incarcerated people who use drugs are respected, protected, and fulfilled.

Take Drug-Related Health Problems Out of the Hands of Law Enforcement

The use of drugs should not be subject to criminal sanctions, nor should minor non-violent offenses. Decriminalization of drug use and minor possession have been shown to have excellent outcomes for the health of people who use drugs, including reduction of HIV risk, without adding to insecurity or increasing crime.[36,37] UNODC asserts that decriminalization of minor offenses is not in conflict with the international treaties that govern drug control.[31] Decriminalization of minor offenses enables the police to keep their focus on higher-level trafficking offenses and would dramatically reduce overcrowding in prisons and pre-trial detention.

More Than Equivalence of Care

While there is still a long way to go to respect the human rights idea of health services in prison that are the equivalent of what is offered in the community, equivalence may not be enough. As Lines notes, equivalence of objectives may be a more relevant and human rights–centered goal than equivalence of services in view of the "numerous public health crises that are concentrated and exacerbated by the fact of incarceration."[11] Equivalent services, even if achieved, may not address the health impact of overcrowding, poor ventilation and sanitation, violence, and—of particular concern here—unsafe injection. The UN comprehensive package on HIV services, including treatment for drug addiction, access to sterile injection equipment, prevention of violence, peer-based programs, and continuity of care after release is an excellent guide to services that address the rights and needs of people who use drugs.[17] But those services and related support measures must at times be intensified beyond the level of care and support in the community to ensure that the same objectives met in the community can be met among detained persons.

Independent Monitoring and Independence of Health Professionals

Independent monitoring of prisons and remand facilities is fundamental to human rights and is particularly necessary to ensure the realization of human rights for marginalized persons within prisons such as those who use drugs. International and civil society bodies that conduct prison visits do not always focus on the situation of people who use drugs, the services for them, and the human rights abuses they face.

There is a need for training and sharing of experiences among independent monitors in this regard. In addition, it is essential that health professionals working in prison systems, whose work is often not valued even by other health professionals, be guaranteed the independence to report and act on health problems associated with human rights abuses. Their work and initiatives should not be stifled under the guise of security or order.

Closing Compulsory Treatment and Rehabilitation Facilities

The United Nations' call for closure of compulsory drug "treatment" centers was an important step in a human rights–based direction, but much remains to be done. Political pressure for closure of these centers is needed; technical guidance on implementing community-based alternatives should also be a priority. Compulsory "treatment" is a heinous repudiation of the human rights and personhood of people who use drugs and contributes to a culture of criminalization. Rights-based approaches to health services for drug users in the community or in prison are unlikely to emerge in places where people who use drugs can be hauled off and detained for "rehabilitation" without due process.

Rights of Women, Young People, and LGBT People

The positive obligation of states to go beyond equivalent services to address health and human rights challenges faced by people who use drugs is especially urgent for women, young people, and LGBT persons who may face risks associated not only with unsafe drug use but also with violence, stigma, marginalization, and the absence of peer support. Intensified action is required to overcome the barriers these persons face to being able to enjoy equivalence of care if it exists.

The situation of incarcerated people who use drugs is an avoidable public health and human rights crisis. Excessive application of criminal law to drug use and minor drug infractions is abusive in itself and compounds the health problems of people who use drugs in the community with the violence, poor living conditions, and stigma of incarceration. The human rights norms that should oblige states to address this crisis are widely ratified in international law. The HIV pandemic has highlighted the health and human rights vulnerabilities of people who use drugs who are in conflict with the law, but too little has been done to make the rights of these people a central part of HIV responses as well as of human rights commitments.

CONCLUSION

The consensus statement resulting from the UN General Assembly Special Session (UNGASS) on the "world drug problem" in 2016 called for treatment of drug dependence to be available to people in state custody and encouraged states, within the bounds of their legal frameworks and the drug conventions, to develop and implement "alternative or additional measures with regard to conviction or punishment in cases of an appropriate nature."[38] These points represent a step forward, though it is somewhat offset by the member states' refusal to name and call for harm reduction services for prisoners or anyone else in the UNGASS statement. UN member states should continue to be called on to answer for the neglect of essential health services for these persons and the failure to ensure conditions in which they can live in dignity.

REFERENCES

1. United Nations Office on Drugs and Crime, World Health Organisation. *Good Governance for Prison Health in the 21st Century: A Policy Brief on the Organization of Prison Health*. Copenhagen, Denmark: WHO European Regional Office; 2013.
2. Lines R. Injecting reason: prison syringe exchange and Article 3 of the European Convention on Human Rights. *Eur Human Rights Law Rev*. 2007;1:66–80.
3. Organization of American States. *American Convention on Human Rights*. Washington, DC: Organization of American States; 1969.
4. Council of Europe. *European Convention on Human Rights, Articles 5,6,7*. Strasbourg, France: European Court of Human Rights; 1950.
5. United Nations Human Rights Office of the High Commissioner. *International Covenant on Economic, Social and Cultural Rights*. Geneva, Switzerland: United Nations Human Rights Office of the High Commissioner; 1966.
6. United Nations Committee on Economic Social and Cultural Rights. *General Comment 14: The Right to the Highest Attainable Standard of Health*. Geneva, Switzerland: United Nations; 2000.
7. United Nations Human Rights Committee. *General Comment 6, Article 6 (Right to Life)*. Geneva, Switzerland: United Nations; 1982.
8. United Nations Human Rights Committee. *General Comment 9, Article 10 (Humane Treatment of Persons Deprived of Liberty)*. Geneva, Switzerland: United Nations; 1982.
9. Irish Penal Reform Trust. *Shelley v. the United Kingdom: Submissions of the Intervenors the Irish Penal Reform Trust and the Canadian HIV/AIDS Legal Network to the European Court of Human Rights*. Strasbourg, Germany: Irish Penal Reform Trust; 2007.
10. United Nations Economic and Social Council. *United Nations Standard Minimum Rules for the Treatment of Prisoners*. Geneva, Switzerland: United Nations; 1957.
11. Lines R. From equivalence of standards to equivalence of objectives: the entitlement of prisoners to health care standards higher than those outside prisons. *Int J Prison Health*. 2006;2(4):269–280.
12. United Nations Economic and Social Council. *United Nations Standard Minimum Rules for the Treatment of Prisoners (the Mandela Rules)*. Geneva, Switzerland: United Nations; 2015.
13. United Nations General Assembly. *Basic Principles for the Treatment of Prisoners*. Geneva, Switzerland: United Nations; 1990.
14. United Nations General Assembly. *UN Rules for the Protection of Juveniles Deprived of Their Liberty*. Geneva, Switzerland: United Nations; 1990.
15. Joint United Nations Programme on HIV/AIDS, Office of the UN High Commissioner on Human Rights. *International Guidelines on HIV/AIDS and Human Rights*. Geneva, Switzerland: United Nations; 2006.
16. United Nations General Assembly. *Declaration of Commitment on HIV/AIDS*. Geneva, Switzerland: United Nations; 2001.
17. United Nations Office on Drugs and Crime, UNAIDS, World Health Organization. *Policy Brief. HIV Prevention, Treatment and Care in Prisons and Other Closed Settings: A Comprehensive Package of Interventions*. Vienna, Austria: United Nations; 2013.

18. United Nations Office on Drugs and Crime, World Health Organization. *Principles of Drug Dependence Treatment: Discussion Paper*. Vienna, Austria: United Nations; 2008.
19. Jurgens R, Betteridge G. Prisoners who inject drugs: public health and human rights imperatives. *Health Hum Rights*. 2005;8(2):46–74.
20. Rieter E. ICCPR case law on detention, the prohibition of cruel treatment and some issues pertaining to the death row phenomenon. *J Institute Just Int Studies*. 2002;1:83–111.
21. Nowak M. *Report of the Special Rapporteur on Torture and Other Cruel, Inhuman and Degrading Punishment to the UN Human Rights Council*. Geneva, Switzerland: United Nations; 2009.
22. Harm Reduction International. *Global State of Harm Reduction 2014*. London, England: Harm Reduction International; 2014.
23. Larney S, Dolan K. A literature review of international implementation of opioid substitution treatment in prisons: equivalence of care? *Eur Addict Res*. 2009;15(2):107–112.
24. Csete J. Consequences of injustice: Pre-trial detention and health. *Int J Prison Health*. 2010;6(1):3–14.
25. United Nations Office on Drugs and Crime. *Women and HIV in Prison Settings*. Vienna, Austria: UNODC; 2008.
26. van Olphen J, Eliason MJ, Freudenberg N, Barnes M. Nowhere to go: how stigma limits the options of female drug users after release from jail. *Subst Abuse Treat Prev Policy*. 2009;4(10):1–10.
27. United Nations Office on Drugs and Crime. *Handbook on Prisoners With Special Needs*. Vienna, Austria: UNODC; 2009.
28. International Labour Organization, UN Office on Drugs and Crime, Office of the UN High Commissioner of Human Rights. *Joint Statement: Compulsory Drug Detention and Rehabilitation Centres*. Geneva, Switzerland: United Nations; 2012.
29. European Monitoring Centre for Drugs and Drug Addiction. *Annual Report 2005— Selected Issues; Alternatives to Imprisonment—Targeting Offending Problem Drug Users in the EU*. Lisbon, Portugal: European Community; 2005.
30. Youngers C, Perez Correa C. *In Search of Rights: Drug Users and State Responses in Latin America*. Bogotá, Colombia: CEDD/CIDE; 2014.
31. Fedotov Y. *Contribution of the Executive Director of UNODC to the High-Level Review of the Implementation of the Political Declaration and Plan of Action on International Cooperation Towards an Integrated and Balanced Strategy to Counter the World Drug Problem*. Vienna, Austria: Commission on Narcotic Drugs, 57th Session; 2014.
32. Global Commission on HIV and the Law. *HIV and the Law: Risks, Rights and Health*. New York, NY: UN Development Programme; 2010.
33. Jurgens R, Ball A, Verster A. Interventions to reduce HIV transmission related to injecting drug use in prison. *Lancet Infect Dis*. 2009;9(1):57–66.
34. Wolfe D, Elovich R, Boltaev A, Pulatov D. HIV in Central Asia: Tajikistan, Uzbekistan and Kyrgyzstan. In: Celentano D, Beyrer C, eds. *Public Health Aspects of HIV/AIDS in Low and Middle Income Countries*. New York, NY: Springer Nature; 2008:557–581.
35. Csete J. *From the Mountaintops: What the World Can Learn From Drug Policy Change in Switzerland*. New York, NY: Open Society Foundations; 2016.
36. Rosmarin A, Eastwood N. *A Quiet Revolution: Drug Decriminalisation Policies in Practice Across the Globe*. London, England: Release; 2012.
37. Hughes CE, Stevens A. A resounding success or a disastrous failure: re-examining the interpretation of evidence on the Portuguese decriminalisation of illicit drugs. *Drug and Alcohol Review*. 2012;31(1):101–113.
38. United Nations General Assembly. *Our Joint Commitment to Effectively Addressing and Countering the World Drug Problem*. Geneva, Switzerland: United Nations; 2016.

CHAPTER 13

Recidivism

The Impact of Substance Abuse on Continued
Involvement in the Justice System

FAYE S. TAXMAN, PhD AND MARY MUN, BSc

INTRODUCTION

With more than 10.2 million people detained or incarcerated in prisons around the world on any given day,[1] one challenge facing many nations is the high recidivism rate. Regardless of geography, culture, or sentencing practices, countries that report recidivism rates cite rates of 60% to 70% for rearrests within 3 to 5 years of release from prison or being on supervision. The high rate of rearrest translates into very high rates of reconviction and/or reincarceration, or further involvement with the justice system.[2-5] These high recidivism rates highlight deficiencies in crime control efforts and have resulted in a worldwide concern for more effective policies, practices, and programs for reducing recidivism. The unintended and negative consequences of incarceration—such as the impact on quality of life, the ability to resume citizenship as a contributing member of the community, and health and psychosocial deficits arising from the incarceration period—are well established.[6] Individuals who use illicit drugs present a particular challenge for reducing the recidivism rate given that use of illicit drugs is tied to failure on parole (or probation) supervision due to continued substance use, and given that drug-seeking behavior frequently results in a criminal justice response (see chapter 1). The lack of sufficient treatment programs, as well as the unavailability of effective substance abuse treatment programs, in prison and community settings[7] contributes to recidivism among those who use illicit substances.

In this chapter we consider the literature on the factors that affect the recidivism rate for substance-involved individuals in the justice system. Even though the last 40 years have seen a declaration of a "war on drugs" in many countries, with increasing penalties, it does not appear that the efforts to combat drugs in this "war" have reduced the recidivism rates for substance users. Furthermore, as shown in this chapter, recidivism rates are affected by social determinants, health conditions, and other factors affecting the substance use behaviors of individuals. Understanding how to reduce recidivism among drug users will require more research to better understand how to improve client-level outcomes after release from prison.

UNDERSTANDING THE MEASUREMENT OF RECIDIVISM

Part of the challenge in identifying effective policies, practices, and programs is the inconsistent nature of the concept and measurement of recidivism. Sechrest noted that:

> There is no consistent definition of recidivism. One program may use a follow-up time of 1 year, another of 6 months. Follow-up time may be computed starting with release from prison or with release from parole. The recidivating event may be a technical violation of the conditions of parole, or it may be a return to prison. There are so many possible variations in the method of computing recidivism that one doubts if more than a handful of the hundreds of correctional evaluations are truly comparable. Nor is there any way of deciding which of the many variations is most applicable for a given situation.[8]

The measurement of recidivism can be affected by (1) the population or sample being studied; (2) the number and type of events (ie, offense type, arrest, conviction, or incarceration) considered within the definition of recidivism; and (3) the time frame of the follow-up period. For those who use illicit substances, this is complicated by divergent views regarding whether substance use should or should not be included in the definition of recidivism (since it is an illicit behavior in many countries). In most studies the population of interest is illicit substance users, which may or may not be indicative of diagnoses of substance abuse disorder. An ongoing debate in the field concerns the number and type of events that should be included in the measurement of recidivism. For example, when recidivism among sexual offenders solely reports sexual recidivism, the rate is much lower than when overall recidivism is considered (13.4% and 36.3%, respectively).[9]

The measurement of recidivism for substance-involved ex-prisoners is equally complex. First, there are issues related to the definition of substance-involved individuals in the justice system. "Drug offense" is a broad category that often relates to both a certain type of behavior and a set of legal offenses. The behavior is the use of substances, namely, drugs that are considered illicit by the law. However, penalties vary considerably depending on the country and the type of substance in possession.[10] That is, the nature of the substance-involved behavior is often affected by other factors—illicit substances that the individual uses, how frequently the person engages in drug use, and whether there are comorbid risky behaviors—and these factors may affect whether one is considered a recidivist. Second, there are measurement issues related to recidivism, specifically the types of offenses that are included and the timing of the events. The type of substance-using behavior that is included in the definition of recidivism affects the resulting rate of recidivism. If results from drug testing are included, then there is a likelihood that there will be greater recidivism rates than when measures focus on criminal acts such as possession of illicit drugs. The definition of recidivism is an area where more work is needed to better understand what we are measuring and how (or to what extent) criminal behavior defines the outcome.

SUBSTANCE USERS IN THE JUSTICE SYSTEM: UNDERSTANDING OF THE CONCEPT

Substance users are a heterogeneous population with tremendous variations in lifestyle, drugs of choice, and severity of substance use problems. These variations influence how their substance use affects their offending behavior and how their offending behavior affects their substance use (the drug-crime nexus[11]; see chapter 1). However, the general criminal justice literature treats drug offenders as a homogeneous group of individuals involved in using drugs, either as a user, an addict, or someone who sells drugs. Often, the literature does not distinguish between individuals based on how they administer substances (eg, injecting or smoking), the relationship between substance use and offending behaviors, and how substance use influences other behaviors.

Systems for monitoring drug use among police detainees in the United States,[12] United Kingdom,[13] Australia,[14] and other countries define any arrestees who test positive for substances as "substance-involved offenders." Regardless of the offense charge, these programs test a sample of arrestees to identify those who have recently used a substance.[12] Most of these drug testing programs assume that if substance use occurred prior to committing an offense, then the substance use is linked to the offending behavior. Yet, some substances remain present in the body for up to 72 hours (with the exception of marijuana, which has an average life of 15 days for males and up to 30 days for females). Definitions based on who has substance(s) in the body leave many questions unanswered, such as whether the offense is related to substance use, whether the person has been clinically diagnosed with a substance use disorder, or whether the person exhibits tolerance to substances. The 2012 US Arrestee Drug Abuse Monitoring Program found that 67% of arrestees had substances in their system at the time of arrest, with the most prevalent being cannabis; the prevalence of positive tests for other drugs varied by jurisdiction.[15] Similarly, the Drug Use Monitoring in Australia (DUMA) program found that the drug most commonly identified through urine testing was cannabis (48%), followed by opioids (16%). Overall, 48% of arrestees tested positive for at least one illicit substance.[14] In the United Kingdom, the Drug Use Forecasting system found that 69% of arrestees tested positive for one substance, and 36% tested positive for two or more substances.[13] These programs collect biological data on drug use among arrestees, but they do not consider patterns of drug use, drug-related harm, what role substance use plays in criminal behavior, or how criminal behavior could be influencing the use of substances.

TYPE OF SUBSTANCE USE AND RECIDIVISM

A recent meta-analysis of the association between substance use and recidivism assessed more than 30 primary studies that specified the drug of choice and measured recidivism. Bennett and colleagues[16] found that the odds of reoffending were three to four times greater among substance-involved individuals than among individuals who were not substance-involved. Drug of choice was also important. The odds of reoffending were about 6 times greater for individuals who used crack cocaine (odds ratio [OR] = 6.09) than for those who did not; about 3 times greater for those who used heroin (OR = 3.08) as opposed to those who did not; about two and a half times greater for individuals who used powder cocaine (OR = 2.56) than for those who did not; and about one and a half times greater for individuals who used marijuana (OR = 1.46) than for those who did not.[16] This study has three major limitations. The first is that each drug was examined separately, and therefore polydrug users were not identified; second, the study did not include alcohol use; and third, the study did not consider the odds of reoffending according to severity of substance use, polydrug use, or what proportion of individuals had a substance use disorder.

In a more recent study of 4,152 inmates with a substance use disorder in Sweden, 69% returned to prison within 2.7 years of being released.[17] Using data from the Addiction Severity Index (ASI), a tool to measure severity of substance use, recidivism rates were found to be higher for those who used amphetamines and heroin, had prior psychiatric in-patient treatment, had a history of violent behavior, or had a history of poly-substance use prior to incarceration. Substance users who had committed property offences also tended to have a higher recidivism rate in this study of Swedish ex-prisoners,[17] a finding that is consistent with other research from the United States.[2] Using DUMA data, Payne[4] found that earlier age of onset of substance use predicted an increased likelihood of involvement in property offenses, regardless of the drug of choice. Individuals who used opioids at an earlier age tended to have more criminal behavior.

COMPLEX NEEDS AND RECIDIVISM

A few more contemporary studies have focused on the comorbid factors that might affect recidivism. A 5-year prospective study in Canada examined the lifetime history of substance abuse disorders for 397 individuals who were treated for sex offenses.[18] The study found that history of alcohol abuse, more so than illicit drug abuse, was a serious risk factor for sexual recidivism.[18] A study of 379 individuals charged with drug-related crimes and undergoing psychiatric evaluation in Switzerland revealed that the recidivism rate was 41.4%; the subgroup with comorbid personality disorders and substance abuse (22%) had elevated recidivism rates compared with those with other psychiatric disorders. Most recidivism for individuals with co-occurring personality disorders and substance use disorders occurred within 1 year. In the United States, a study of recidivism for those in jail found that those with co-occurring disorders of mental illness and substance abuse had higher recidivism rates than those with a mental disorder alone.[19]

In a unique study of health-related factors that affect recidivism among 1,325 ex-prisoners in Queensland, Australia, Thomas and colleagues (2015)[20] found that risk for recidivism was elevated for those who used cannabis (hazard ratio [HR] = 1.27), amphetamines (HR = 1.28), or opioids (HR = 1.33) before incarceration, used medications for mental health problems in prison (HR = 1.52), and reported poverty prior to incarceration (HR = 1.24). The study also identified a number of protective factors that reduced the likelihood of reincarceration, including sedentary lifestyle, obesity, multiple lifetime chronic diseases, and a history of self-harm. This study lays the groundwork for considering that other health-related factors may shape recidivism risk, over and above demographic and criminal justice variables.

These limited studies illustrate that there is a need to better understand how different factors affect recidivism, particularly for substance users in the justice system. There is a need to further expand research to understand how comorbid conditions and social/environmental factors interact with substance use disorders to shape recidivism risk.

LOCATION AND RECIDIVISM

Emerging research has highlighted the role of proximity to drug treatment facilities and illicit drug markets as predictors of recidivism for ex-prisoners with a history of risky substance use. In a recent study of parolees in California, researchers found that participants who lived within a 2-mile radius of a drug treatment facility were less likely to recidivate,[21] suggesting that community drug treatment may be protective against reoffending for previously incarcerated drug users. Conversely, Wooditch and colleagues[22] found that probationers living in an area with active drug markets had higher relapse rates, potentially contributing to more antisocial behavior and to recidivism. Previous research has shown that individuals under correctional control who live in communities with a high concentration of individuals under correctional control have higher recidivism rates.[22] Whether these findings are mediated by proximity to drug-using peers is a matter for future research.

BREAKING THE CYCLE BETWEEN SUBSTANCE USE DISORDERS AND RECIDIVISM: DRUG TREATMENT

Quality drug treatment programs and drug courts have been shown to affect recidivism rates. The range of quality drug treatment programs includes cognitive behavioral therapy, in-prison therapeutic communities with aftercare, and drug treatment courts, each of which has been shown to be effective in reducing recidivism[23] (see chapter 16). There is also evidence that drug treatment courts reduce recidivism compared with traditional supervision, although the effectiveness differs according to characteristics of the program (eg, type of treatment services provided, use of different sanctions and incentives, amount of drug testing) and by type of drug court (eg, adult, juvenile).[24] Recent studies also demonstrate that participation in medication-assisted treatments reduces recidivism and prolongs relapse.[25] There is growing evidence that it is important to begin medication-assisted treatments prior to release from prison, which serves to increase engagement and retention and can serve as a conduit to participation in counseling after release—all found to reduce recidivism.[26]

DISCUSSION AND FUTURE RESEARCH AGENDA

While it is well established that substance-involved individuals have an increased risk of recidivism,[2,23] the current literature is incomplete regarding factors that can have a positive effect on reducing recidivism, other than the benefits from evidence-based substance abuse treatment. It is outside the scope of this chapter to consider the limitations of the substance abuse treatment literature as it relates to drug users in the justice system; we still have much to understand about the factors that affect recidivism for this group.

This review illustrates the need for a greater understanding of the relationship between substance use disorders and recidivism. To begin with, excluding drug-specific, medication-assisted intervention studies, few studies have examined the relationship between drug(s) of choice and recidivism. For example, in the meta-analysis by Bennett and colleagues,[16] only 30 out of 60 studies reported on the association between specific drugs and recidivism (a total of 536 studies were found, but most did not examine the association between specific drugs and recidivism). This was partly because relatively few of the included studies reported drug of choice, and many studies failed to adequately characterize polydrug use (including alcohol use) or compare illicit drug use with alcohol use. Surprisingly few studies have examined how behavior and recidivism vary as a function of either which drugs are used or how they are used. Filling this gap in the literature will assist in understanding the links between substance use and recidivism. In the early 1980s, many studies focused on opioid addicts and the role of treatment in reducing the number of drug-use days.[27] Fewer studies have considered other specific subsets of the substance-involved population, such that our knowledge of the association between substance use and recidivism is for the most part unhelpfully generic. Accordingly, the extant evidence is not sufficiently granular to provide an understanding of potential drug-specific mechanisms linking substance use to recidivism; it is thus difficult to develop targeted, evidence-based programs to disrupt the pathways between particular patterns of substance use and recidivism.

The same is true for the literature on co-occurring mental illness and substance use disorders: comparatively few studies have explored the association between specific types of mental disorder and recidivism, or considered how particular patterns of substance use may interact with specific mental disorders to increase or decrease recidivism risk. A meta-analysis by Bonta and colleagues[28] found only a handful of studies that examined a specific mental health disorder. Instead, the literature tends to treat most mental health disorders similarly, without differentiating between internalizing and externalizing disorders, or specific disorders that might be related to criminal behavior. The evidence regarding the association between mental disorders and recidivism is complex: some studies have found that mental disorders are a contributing factor in recidivism for women,[28] while others have failed to identify any direct relationship between mental disorders and criminal behavior.[29] Few studies have explored the association between co-occurring substance use and mental health disorders and recidivism; the available evidence suggests that individuals with co-occurring disorders have higher recidivism rates, although this risk varies depending on the type of mental illness.

This review has highlighted both the striking lack of studies examining factors that affect recidivism among substance users and the failure of most studies to distinguish between substances or patterns of use of those substances. Many studies also suffer from important methodological weaknesses such as small sample sizes and cross-sectional designs; the literature is heavily skewed toward North American studies. More detailed, high-quality studies will be required to inform targeted, evidence-based recidivism reduction programs. Longitudinal studies are needed to test hypotheses regarding the associations between patterns of substance use, concurrent health and psychosocial needs, and recidivism. Because substance use disorders vary in severity over time, and many criminogenic and non-criminogenic factors are dynamic, time-varying models would be most useful in testing new models to further our knowledge in this area. In a longitudinal study, it would be useful to examine how changes in substance use (such as frequency of use or a combination of behaviors related to substance use) affect involvement in criminal behavior, by accounting for changes in various criminogenic and non-criminogenic factors. This could help to isolate the effects of substance use on recidivism, and identify potential mediating and moderating factors. For example, while housing status is reported to be related to pathways of offending,[30] the state of homelessness varies over time; chronic homelessness is an extreme pattern, but more often there are cyclical patterns of unstable housing. The same is true for food security. Wang and colleagues[31] reported that more than one-third of prison releasees experience food insecurity (ie, did not have a meal for one day) at least once a month, and during these periods of deprivation, the releasees engaged in riskier behaviors. Wooditch and colleagues[32] examined a series of time-varying models to assess which criminogenic needs affect recidivism outcomes for substance-involved probationers. Further research is required to gain insight into theories of recidivism reduction and to explore how changes in dynamic factors affect substance use–recidivism pathways.

A FINAL NOTE ON RECIDIVISM

The nature of the dependent or outcome variable (ie, recidivism) is critically important, since it defines the behavior that we are trying to alter. Many studies examine only one type of recidivism (eg, arrest, conviction, reincarceration) but either implicitly or explicitly assume that similar mechanisms and factors affect any type of recidivism. There is a need for more research to explore how various substance use behaviors, individual traits and demographic factors, comorbid conditions, and so on impact different types of recidivism. In addition, it is important to be explicit about the types of criminal behavior that substance-involved individuals engage in. As noted by Morgan,[33] some opioid addicts engage in property offenses, but others engage in drug-related offenses such as selling drugs. If we are going to measure the nexus between substance use and crime, we will need to ensure that we are measuring all relevant types of criminal behavior. Rather than relying on a generic measure of recidivism, a clearer specification of the relevant offending behaviors will allow us to more meaningfully characterize the criminal conduct of different types of drug users; for example, examining whether different combinations of needs, drug of choice, and substance use severity create pathways to different types of offenses. Further, violations of parole conditions for substance use might be included in the recidivism models, since they reflect upon further engagement in substance-using behaviors while other violations, such as breaching curfews, changing addresses, or attending meetings, may not be considered indicators of continuation of substance-using behavior.

REFERENCES

1. Walmsley R. *World Prison Population List*. 10th ed. London, England: International Centre for Prison Studies; 2013.
2. Durose M, Cooper A, Snyder H. *Recidivism of Prisoners Released in 30 States in 2005: Patterns From 2005 to 2010*. Washington, DC: US Department of Justice Bureau of Justice Statistics; 2014.
3. Ministry of Justice. *Breaking the Cycle: Effective Punishment, Rehabilitation and Sentencing of Offenders*. London, England: Ministry of Justice; 2010.
4. Payne J. *Recidivism in Australia: Findings and Future Research*. Canberra, Australia: Australian Institute of Criminology; 2007.
5. Scottish Centre of Crime and Justice Research. *Reducing Reoffending in Scotland*. Glasgow, Scotland: Auditor General for Scotland and the Accounts Commission; 2012.
6. Travis J, Western B, Redburn S. *The Growth of Incarceration in the United States: Exploring Causes and Consequences*. Washington, DC: National Academy Press; 2014.
7. Taxman FS, Perdoni ML, Caudy M. The plight of providing appropriate substance abuse treatment services to offenders: modeling the gaps in service delivery. *Vict Offender*. 2013;8(1):70–93.
8. Maltz MD. *Recidivism*. Orlando, FL: Academic Press; 1984.
9. Hanson RK, Bussière MT. Predicting relapse: a meta-analysis of sexual offender recidivism studies. *J Consult Clin Psychol*. 1998;66(2):348–362.
10. Meier KJ. The politics of drug abuse: laws, implementation, and consequences. *West Polit Q*. 1992;45(1):41.
11. Newcomb MD, Galaif ER, Carmona JV. The drug-crime nexus in a community sample of adults. *Psychol Addict Behav*. 2001;15(3):185–193.
12. Taylor B. *I-ADAM in Eight Countries: Approaches and Challenges*. Rockville, MD: National Institute of Justice; 2002.
13. Bennett T, Holloway K. *Understanding Drugs, Alcohol and Crime*. Berkshire, UK: McGraw-Hill International; 2005.
14. Sweeney J, Payne J. *Drug Use Monitoring in Australia: 2009–2010 Report on Drug Use Among Police Detainees*. Canberra, Australia: Australian Institute of Criminology; 2012.

15. Arrestee Drug Abuse Monitoring Program II. *ADAM II 2013 Annual Report*. Washington, DC: Office of National Drug Control Policy; 2013.
16. Bennett T, Holloway K, Farrington D. The statistical association between drug misuse and crime: a meta-analysis. *Aggress Violent Behav*. 2008;13(2):107–118.
17. Håkansson A, Berglund M. Risk factors for criminal recidivism—a prospective follow-up study in prisoners with substance abuse. *BMC Psychiatry*. 2012;12(111):1–8.
18. Looman J, Abracen J. Substance abuse among high-risk sexual offenders: do measures of lifetime history of substance abuse add to the prediction of recidivism over actuarial risk assessment instruments? *J Interpers Violence*. 2011;26(4):683–700.
19. Wilson AB, Draine J, Hadley T, Metraux S, Evans A. Examining the impact of mental illness and substance use on recidivism in a county jail. *Int J Law Psychiatry*. 2011;34(4):264–268.
20. Thomas EG, Spittal MJ, Taxman FS, Kinner SA. Health-related factors predict return to custody in a large cohort of ex-prisoners: new approaches to predicting re-incarceration. *Health Justice*. 2015;3(10):1–13.
21. Hipp JR, Petersilia J, Turner S. Parolee recidivism in California: the effect of neighborhood context and social service agency characteristics. *Criminology*. 2010;48(4):947–979.
22. Wooditch A, Lawton B, Taxman FS. The Geography of Drug Abuse Epidemiology among probationers in Baltimore. *J Drug Issues*. 2013;43(2):231–249.
23. Mitchell O, Wilson DB, MacKenzie DL. Does incarceration-based drug treatment reduce recidivism? a meta-analytic synthesis of the research. *J Exp Criminol*. 2007;3(4):353–375.
24. Mitchell O, Wilson DB, Eggers A, MacKenzie DL. Assessing the effectiveness of drug courts on recidivism: a meta-analytic review of traditional and non-traditional drug courts. *J Crim Justice*. 2012;40(1):60–71.
25. Lee JD, Friedmann PD, Kinlock TW, et al. Extended-release naltrexone to prevent opioid relapse in criminal justice offenders. *N Engl J Med*. 2016;374(13):1232–1242.
26. Gordon MS, Kinlock TW, Schwartz RP, Fitzgerald TT, O'Grady KE, Vocci FJ. A randomized controlled trial of prison-initiated buprenorphine: prison outcomes and community treatment entry. *Drug Alcohol Depend*. 2014;142:33–40.
27. Nurco DN, Shaffer JW, Ball JC, Kinlock TW. Trends in the commission of crime among narcotic addicts over successive periods of addiction and nonaddiction. *Am J Drug Alcohol Abuse*. 1984;10(4):481–489.
28. Bonta J, Blais J, Wilson HA. A theoretically informed meta-analysis of the risk for general and violent recidivism for mentally disordered offenders. *Aggress Violent Behav*. 2014;19(3):278–287.
29. Skeem JL, Winter E, Kennealy PJ, Louden JE, Tatar JR. Offenders with mental illness have criminogenic needs, too: toward recidivism reduction. *Law Hum Behav*. 2014;38(3):212–224.
30. Huebner BM, Pleggenkuhle B. Residential location, household composition, and recidivism: an analysis by gender. *Justice Q*. 2013;32(5):818–844.
31. Wang EA, Zhu GA, Evans L, Carroll-Scott A, Desai R, Fiellin LE. A pilot study examining food insecurity and HIV risk behaviors among individuals recently released from prison. *AIDS Educ Prev*. 2013;25(2):112–123.
32. Wooditch A, Tang LL, Taxman FS. Which criminogenic need changes are most important in promoting desistance from crime and substance use? *Crim Justice Behav*. 2014;41(3):276–299.
33. Morgan N. *The Heroin Epidemic of the 1980s and 1990s and Its Effect on Crime Trends—Then and Now*. London, England: Home Office; 2014.

CHAPTER 14

Substance Use and Consequences Among People Who Have Been Incarcerated

A Public Health Issue

INGRID A. BINSWANGER, MD AND ANDREA K. FINLAY, PhD

INTRODUCTION

People released from incarceration are at high risk of poor health outcomes that negatively impact public health. A significant proportion of these poor health outcomes are related to substance use. As discussed in chapter 6, post-release substance use occurs in a complex social, policy, and economic context. In this chapter, we explore the public health consequences of substance use among individuals transitioning from incarceration to the community. First, we discuss four mechanisms that lead to poor substance use–related outcomes and their public health impacts: (1) toxic effects of substances; (2) health behaviors and self-management; (3) consequences of addiction; and (4) institutional, policy, environmental, and social contexts. Next, we consider needs during the transition from prison to the community and highlight promising strategies to address these needs. Finally, we identify opportunities to develop further knowledge on substance use and its consequences among people leaving prison.

SUBSTANCE-RELATED CONTRIBUTORS TO POOR HEALTH OUTCOMES

In this chapter, we highlight four major mechanisms by which substance use contributes to poor health outcomes among people leaving correctional facilities

> ## BOX 14.1 SUBSTANCE-RELATED CONTRIBUTORS TO POOR HEALTH OUTCOMES AMONG PEOPLE EXITING INCARCERATION
>
> 1. Toxic effects of substance use: immediate and cumulative
> 2. Health behaviors leading to new health conditions and outcomes, and suboptimal self-management of chronic conditions
> 3. Consequences of substance use disorders: social, occupational, and economic
> 4. Transitional context: institutional, policy, environmental, and social factors

(Box 14.1). These mechanisms are not exhaustive, as other social, economic, environmental, and policy issues contribute to poor outcomes (discussed in other chapters). Further, individual medical and mental health conditions may fall into more than one mechanistic category. For instance, chronic, active hepatitis C may be acquired due to health behaviors associated with drug use, such as injection drug use (category 2); subsequent liver cancer may develop due to toxic effects of alcohol (category 1) in the context of chronic, active hepatitis C; finally, the transitional context (category 4) may contribute to inadequate care for hepatitis C, alcohol use disorders, and/or liver cancer, leading to worse outcomes. In addition, people who have been incarcerated may have multiple risk factors for each health outcome. For example, human papilloma virus (HPV) infection and tobacco use are both risk factors for cervical cancer,[1] and both are common among women who have been in prison. Furthermore, some health outcomes (eg, suicide after release from prison) may be multi-factorial and involve both direct toxic effects of a substance (eg, alcohol, category 1) and underlying pathophysiological conditions (eg, depression) that have more complex roots. Despite their limitations, these conceptual categorizations may help practitioners, policy-makers, and public health officials design appropriately targeted preventive strategies and measure their effects.

Toxic Effects of Substance Use

The first mechanism by which substance use contributes to the development of new health conditions and poor outcomes is *direct exposure to toxic physiological effects of alcohol, tobacco, and other drugs*. Exposures occur prior to, during, or after incarceration, or at all three time points. Effects may be immediate (eg, overdose) or cumulative, occurring after years of exposure (eg, liver cancer). Conditions caused by substance exposure include unintentional poisoning from opioids, cocaine, or other psychostimulants; hepatitis, cirrhosis, and liver cancer from alcohol; chest pain from cocaine; and chronic obstructive pulmonary disease, coronary artery disease, and lung cancer from tobacco use. There is also evidence that tobacco and some other drugs (eg, opioids and marijuana) have immunomodulation effects that increase susceptibility to infectious diseases.[2] People may experience multiple, synergistic toxic effects due to poly-substance use. Some conditions occur in individuals who have used or currently use substances but do not necessarily meet diagnostic criteria for substance use disorders.

Among people released from incarceration, fatal and non-fatal unintentional poisoning (ie, overdose) is a well-described outcome due to toxic exposure. Drug-related mortality in the early post-release period has been documented in studies from Australia,[3-5] Finland,[6] Sweden,[7] the United Kingdom,[8,9] and the United States[10] and in an international meta-analysis[11] (see chapter 18 for more in-depth discussion of post-release mortality). Combinations of drugs, medications, and alcohol contribute to these events.[10,12] Most studies of post-release mortality have suggested an elevated risk of death among people who have been incarcerated relative to the general population, using standardized mortality ratios.[13,14] There is also a risk for non-fatal overdose in the post-release period, as demonstrated in studies from Australia,[15,16] Canada,[17] and the United States.[18]

From a public health perspective, mortality among people who have been previously incarcerated is an important contributor to overall mortality from overdose in the general population. In Washington State, formerly incarcerated individuals accounted for 8% of all overdose deaths in the state from 2000 to 2009.[10] Among youth, the proportions are even higher. In Victoria, Australia, young males released from juvenile detention accounted for 23% of drug-related deaths among all males in the state aged 15 to 19.[19] These findings suggest that people released from prison should be included in broader public health approaches to reducing overdose.

Health Behaviors and Self-Management

In contrast to the direct toxic effects of substances, health conditions and poor health outcomes may be due to *health behaviors associated with using or acquiring substances or under the influence of substances*. Injecting drugs with needles and syringes previously used by someone else can lead to blood-borne infections (eg, HIV, hepatitis B, and hepatitis C). Trading sex for drugs or money to purchase drugs may lead to sexually transmitted infections (STIs), including gonorrhea, chlamydia, trichomoniasis, syphilis, HPV, and HIV. STIs are prevalent among people who move through custodial settings; these infections are significant public health concerns because of their potential for transmission to sexual partners, particularly when the person released from prison is unaware of his or her infection and/or engages in high-risk sexual behavior. Among 402 prisoners in Ukraine scheduled for release from custody within 6 months, 19% were HIV infected, but half of these were unaware of their HIV status.[20] In a study of 245 women in Rhode Island who transitioned from prison to the community, an incidence rate of new STI (trichomoniasis, chlamydia, or gonorrhea) of 36.2 new infections per 100 person-years, calculated using non-incarceration days, was observed.[21] In a study of 200 people recently released from prison in Colorado, 22% of men and 41% of women reported having unprotected vaginal sex, while 5% of men and 8% of women reported having unprotected anal sex in the 7 days before the interview.[22] Engaging in sexual risk behaviors after release from prison may increase the risk of HIV transmission, particularly because lapses in medication or poor adherence to treatment increases viral load[23] (see chapter 7). The post-release social, legal, and economic context may make it particularly difficult for people to engage in optimal health behaviors.

HPV is an STI that has garnered less attention than HIV or hepatitis C, but it is common among women in prison, especially those with a history of drug use. Among female prisoners in Ananindeua, Brazil, the prevalence of HPV was 10.5%.[24] In female prisoners in Taiwan who were incarcerated for drug use, 63.9% of women with HIV and 47.4% of women who did not have HIV were infected with HPV.[25] In addition to the risk of transmission, HPV can cause long-term adverse health consequences, such as cervical cancer in women and head and neck cancers in men. A nationally representative study in the United States suggests that women in prison have a high prevalence of cervical cancer.[26]

Additionally, substance use and the post-release context can negatively influence *chronic disease self-management*. People in prisons have a high prevalence of a number of chronic medical and mental health conditions.[26] In a nationally representative sample, US jail and prison inmates had higher odds of asthma, arthritis, hypertension, and hepatitis compared with the general US population, even after adjusting for demographic factors and alcohol consumption.[26] A third of people in Australian prisons have ever been told that they have a chronic condition, the most common being asthma (24%), arthritis (7%), and cardiovascular disease (5%).[27] Managing chronic health conditions requires seeking (and paying for) healthcare, adhering to potentially complex medication regimens, and engaging in healthy behaviors, such as eating fruits and vegetables. Limited access to healthcare and housing, limited income, and transitional challenges after release may contribute to suboptimal chronic disease self-management, which may be exacerbated by drug use and hazardous drinking.[28]

Consequences of Addiction

Among people released from prison who meet criteria for substance use disorders, poor health outcomes can result from conditions that are *acquired, exacerbated, or progress as a result of the "downstream" social, behavioral, occupational, and economic consequences of addiction*. These consequences are generally worsened by the additional disruption of an incarceration or a criminal record. Individuals who have difficulty maintaining employment due to an untreated, severe substance use disorder and a prior felony conviction may have trouble finding safe and appropriate housing. Low income can result in the loss of access to healthcare or medications. Such downstream effects have a negative influence on public health.

Relationship dissolution from addiction or incarceration (or both) may also signal the loss of important social support that may be critical during the transition back into the community. Along with an increased risk for divorce or separation, the well-being of partners and children suffers and family resources diminish due to reduced income during incarceration.[29,30] In the United States, incarceration is disproportionately concentrated among men from poor and minority communities[31,32]; thus, families with the least resources often bear this burden. This is also the case in Australia,[33] Canada,[34] and other countries,[35] where Indigenous people and other minority groups are disproportionately incarcerated.

Institutional, Policy, Environmental, and Social Contexts

The *institutional, policy, environmental, and social context* can influence the risk of poor substance use–related outcomes during the transition from prison to the community. Transitions of care between correctional institutions and the community, or between different types of facilities, can lead to decompensation or worsening of chronic conditions, such as asthma. This risk may be aggravated by fragmented care, poor communication of health information between care settings, interruptions in pharmacotherapy, and inadequate access to evidence-based care in correctional facilities and the community, particularly for substance use disorders.[23,28]

The health policy context is also an important factor in health outcomes for this population. In the United States, people leaving jails and prisons typically have limited health insurance and access to care.[36] Furthermore, they may have lost public health insurance (eg, Medicaid) during incarceration, which may result in less access to or use of preventive health services, including primary care, and an increase in untreated health problems. This can impact the use of high-cost and high-acuity healthcare. In a study of 110,419 Medicare beneficiaries recently released from incarceration in the United States, the risk of hospitalization for ambulatory care–sensitive conditions was higher than among matched controls, particularly in the days and weeks immediately following release.[37] In a study of emergency department visits in Rhode Island, 1,434 people who had been incarcerated had significantly higher odds of emergency department visits for mental health conditions, substance use disorders, and ambulatory care–sensitive conditions, compared with the general population in that state.[38]

The environmental context may also influence the health of people soon after release. In the United States, rates of homelessness and housing insecurity are high among criminal justice populations. An estimated 9% to 12% of people in prison in the United States were homeless in the year prior to their arrest, with rates substantially higher among those with drug use disorders or those who live in urban areas.[39] Congregate living conditions of prisons and jails as well as the halfway houses, shelters, and other group settings many people live in after release can lead to exposure to infectious diseases. Bacterial infections, such as soft-tissue infections due to methicillin-resistant *Staphylococcus aureus* (MRSA), are prevalent among people who use injection drugs,[40] many of whom experience incarceration. Similarly, tuberculosis is a concern for people who use drugs in many countries, particularly when these individuals are incarcerated (see chapter 8). Tuberculosis outbreaks in prisons have been extensively documented[41] and can put public health at risk.

Criminal justice transitions affect not only the individuals leaving prison but also their families and communities.[42] These transitions can subsequently negatively impact community health. Incarceration can be difficult on intimate partners of people in prison and can strain relationships. In a sample of 229 men with a history of incarceration and 144 women with partners who had a history of incarceration in North Carolina, 40% of primary intimate relationships dissolved during incarceration.[43] Ending a partnership during incarceration was associated with higher prevalence ratios of having two or more new sexual partners after release or having transactional sex (giving or receiving money for sex), behaviors that may increase a person's risk for STIs.

The reintegration period can be stressful both for individuals leaving prisons and for their family members, often related to substance use. In 2001, a qualitative study of ex-prisoners in Israel who used drugs found that their families brought additional stress when the study participants were released from prison because family members could not relate to the drug use and criminal activity and were not involved in their treatment. Drug use was reported as a way to cope with stress.[44] In a sample of people recently released from prison in Chicago in 2003, family members also reported stress related to a return to substance use and/or re-arrests, which were often related to substance use.[45] Preparing family members for reintegration and engaging them in the former prisoner's treatment may help to maintain these crucial social supports and ease the transition to the community.[44,45] Support from family and friends to stay away from drugs has been linked with a higher likelihood of successfully transitioning back into the community after prison[46]; thus, bolstering these social relationships may yield public health benefits.

In the United States, approximately 7% of all African American children had a parent in prison in the late 1990s.[47] Many families are deeply affected by prisoner re-entry, and the effects of poor health and high-risk behavior may impact future generations.[48] Romantic partners, parents, and children of incarcerated adults may experience mental health problems related to incarceration, including shame from having an incarcerated partner, psychological stress from having an incarcerated child, or post-traumatic stress disorder among children from losing a parental figure to prison. Social relationships are also disrupted during this time, such as when children are placed in the foster care system while the custodial parent is in prison. Incarceration can thus impact the social support system for children and partners, and reduce the social network of the person in prison if his or her relationships dissolve. Changes in living arrangements and care arrangements for a child may further contribute to the mental and physical health problems that family members experience.

In addition to more proximal impacts on people leaving prison and their families, some studies have suggested that broader community health may be impacted by incarceration. For instance, Thomas and colleagues examined incarceration as "forced migration," in which males are removed from their social, family, and sexual networks, resulting in reduced stability of these networks. The result may be increasing rates of STIs and teenage pregnancies in communities with high incarceration rates.[49]

TRANSITION NEEDS AND PROMISING STRATEGIES

People reintegrating from the highly structured prison setting to the community often have extensive transitional assistance needs, including substance use disorder treatment, housing, employment, mental health counseling, job training, education, parenting assistance, and family support.[50,51] Transition support can range from pharmacological treatment to address substance use disorders, to comprehensive transition assistance programs specifically geared toward people leaving prisons who use drugs, and housing and healthcare programs. Given that health conditions and outcomes may be due to exposures that occurred many years prior to incarceration, during a recent incarceration, and/or shortly after release, prevention efforts should not be restricted to the weeks immediately following release.

Treatment for Substance Use Disorders

Enhancing access to evidence-based treatments for substance use disorders, such as cognitive and motivational therapies and medications (eg, methadone and buprenorphine), is crucial to improving health outcomes for criminal justice populations (see chapter 16).[52] Further, there is evidence that *in-prison* treatment, particularly if *continued after release*, may reduce mortality after release.[53,54] Medication-supported treatment during the transition from prison to the community is an important strategy to reduce the health risks faced by people who have been incarcerated. In a study of 181 people on probation participating in opioid agonist maintenance in Baltimore, participants' drug use was lower at 2, 6, and 12 months than at baseline.[55] In Taiwan, among people who had been incarcerated with a history of opioid injecting, the 700 participants who enrolled and continued participation in methadone maintenance treatment had substantially lower mortality compared with the 2,375 people who did not enroll or the 1,982 people who enrolled and dropped out.[56]

Overdose Education and Naloxone Distribution

Another pharmacological treatment, naloxone, has prevented overdose deaths in Europe and the United States among people who use heroin.[57,58] Given the high risk for drug-related mortality during the first few weeks after release, programs in Scotland and Wales distribute naloxone to people coming out of prison,[59,60] and the World Health Organization recommends giving naloxone to people being released from prison.[61] Family members and other individuals in the social support system of people leaving jails and prisons may be ideal recipients of education and naloxone.[62]

However, significant gaps remain in understanding how to implement overdose education and naloxone in the large number of diverse jails and prisons in the United States.

Transition Assistance Programs

Transition assistance programs tailored to people with drug use disorders have addressed some post-release challenges. Among 16- to 18-year-old males leaving jails in New York City, people who were assigned to a jail/community-based intervention program (n = 277) were less likely to report past-year alcohol or drug dependence (based on the *DSM-IV*) after release compared with those who were not part of the intervention program (n = 275).[63] In Massachusetts, among 1,285 people with co-occurring mental illness and substance use disorders recently released to the community, those under probation or parole were more likely to utilize substance use disorder treatment than those not under correctional supervision.[64]

Housing Programs

A variety of housing programs exist for people exiting incarceration.[65] For example, a randomized trial of a transition assistance program for chronically ill recently released adults in San Francisco, 58% of whom were homeless or living in transitional housing, found that treatment program participants (n = 98) were less likely to have an emergency department visit compared with control group participants (n = 102), but there was no difference in primary care utilization between the two groups.[66] In Toronto, Canada, 301 participants in a supportive housing intervention for homeless adults had more reductions in alcohol problems compared with 274 participants in the treatment-as-usual group, but there was no difference between groups in drug problems.[67] Other benefits of the program included housing stability and community functioning.[68] More evaluation work is needed to understand whether these programs are able to address the substance use issues of people recently released from prison, but they hold promise for improving outcomes during the transition back to the community.

Enhancing Access to Health Care

People with a history of criminal justice involvement and substance use have historically faced challenges accessing healthcare. Some of these challenges may be addressed through changes in national and regional healthcare policy. In 2013, healthcare policy reform was introduced in the United States with the Affordable Care Act (ACA), designed to provide more US citizens with access to commercial and public health insurance. The ACA was thought to be likely to improve access to coverage during the transition from prison to the community.[69] Among adults with justice involvement (defined as being arrested and booked, on probation, or paroled in the last 12 months), key provisions of the ACA were associated with lower rates of being uninsured.[70] Prior to these healthcare reforms, health insurance was tied to employment. Thus, for adults who lost jobs due to substance use, they may also have lost their health insurance and access to treatment for substance use disorders. By early 2017, the direction of health policy reform in the United States is yet to be determined, along with any resulting impact on people with a history of incarceration. Other barriers to healthcare access may be addressed with individualized interventions. In Colorado, a patient navigation intervention to help people with chronic conditions and a history of drug involvement access appropriate outpatient health services resulted in reduced rates of inpatient hospitalization compared with a control intervention.[71]

Public Health Approaches

Traditional public health interventions that focus on the environment, such as reducing exposure to second-hand smoke in homeless shelters or other transitional housing,[72] may be effective in reducing the direct toxic effects of these substances. Evidence-based smoking cessation programs reduce the risk of cardiovascular and pulmonary disease and lung cancer among smokers, and limit the effects of second-hand smoke among individuals who share their living quarters.

Facilitating the use of sterile needles and syringes may prevent HIV transmission among people in prison[73] and after release. For instance, automated dispensers for syringe exchange offer promise for prison environments.[73] Vaccination programs in juvenile detention, jails, and prisons may help reduce transmission of infectious diseases, such as HPV, after release.[74] Public health strategies must include attention to infection control in jails and prisons[75] and the congregate settings to which people return in the community, such as homeless shelters, halfway houses, and drug treatment settings.

Public health interventions conducted in prisons have the potential to improve community health outcomes. A study on a chlamydia screening and treatment program for men in prisons in Philadelphia found that positive chlamydia tests among women in the community decreased after men in the same area were treated through the prison program, although there was no evidence of a direct link to the prison program.[76] Smoke-free prisons are associated with a reduced risk of tobacco-related death in prison,[77] but less is known about whether such policies reduce tobacco-related death after release.

OPPORTUNITIES TO DEVELOP FURTHER KNOWLEDGE

Important knowledge gaps remain related to the public health consequences of alcohol, tobacco, and other drug use among people who have been released from jail or prison. Most important, the bulk of related scientific publications are from high-income countries. There is limited knowledge about drug use patterns in low-income countries, despite their importance in terms of burden of disease. Patterns of substance use and consequent public health impacts likely vary by country, due to differing enforcement patterns directed at people who use drugs, access to substances, culturally specific norms and attitudes toward people who use substances, access to healthcare or other transition supports, and broader public health interventions offered. For example, countries where there is more opium use or limited access to syringe exchange programs may have increased risk of HIV transmission.

Furthermore, there are gaps in research on technologically supported interventions, tailored or patient-centered approaches, and implementation approaches. Implementation studies are particularly needed because of the challenges in translating evidence-based practices into the large numbers of geographically dispersed jails, prisons, and post-release settings. Implementation has also been challenged by a range of factors, including the complexity of the issues faced by populations leaving prisons, strong biases against opioid agonist treatment in jails and prisons, separate funding streams for correctional and community health services, misalignment of the public health and custody missions of prisons and jails, and scientific disagreements over the level of evidence needed to implement promising interventions.[78,79] Finally, there are few studies on the effects of incarceration policies on the long-term health of people who have been released.

RECOMMENDATIONS AND CONCLUSIONS

Among people transitioning out of prison, substance use can have serious consequences for individual health, the health of families, and the communities to which individuals return, but many of the risks can be addressed. At the individual level, improved access to evidence-based treatments to reduce risky substance use behaviors and treat substance use disorders is critical, both in prisons/jails and in the community. Wider distribution of naloxone could also reduce some of the mortality risk from the toxic effects of substances after release.

Access to affordable health insurance that covers evidence-based substance use treatment and ensures continuity of healthcare during the transition from prison to the community is also critical. To address these issues, institutional, regional, and national policy action may be needed.

Interventions that may improve the health of both people released from prison and family and community members include the implementation of behavioral and education programs to improve health behavior (eg, HIV medication adherence, condom use) and programs that facilitate the use of sterile needles and syringes. Infection control interventions are needed in prisons, as well as in the community settings that house individuals after release, such as halfway houses and homeless shelters.

Given the importance of social relationships during the transition back to the community, family-level interventions may also yield public health benefits. Educating family members about the challenges people face upon returning home and engaging them in the treatment process may decrease some of the stress family members experience and strengthen their coping mechanisms, and consequently their capacity to support the ex-prisoner during re-entry.

In addition to helping family members, transitional assistance while reintegrating into the community will likely result in public health benefits. Medical clinics that focus on providing culturally appropriate care for people leaving prisons and jails are one form of assistance that directly addresses some of the health needs of this population. However, there are a multitude of interconnected challenges faced by people who have been incarcerated that need to be addressed in holistic and integrated programs, including housing, job training, employment, education, and parenting/family support. Although promising programs are on the horizon, more work is needed to understand the optimal combination of transition assistance needed for this population, as well as the public health benefits and cost-effectiveness of such comprehensive support.

REFERENCES

1. Binswanger IA, Mueller S, Clark CB, Cropsey KL. Risk factors for cervical cancer in criminal justice settings. *J Womens Health*. 2011;20(12):1839–1845.
2. Friedman H, Pross S, Klein TW. Addictive drugs and their relationship with infectious diseases. *FEMS Immunol Med Microbiol*. 2006;47(3):330–342.
3. van Dooren K, Kinner SA, Forsyth S. Risk of death for young ex-prisoners in the year following release from adult prison. *Aust N Z J Public Health*. 2013;37(4):377–382.
4. Kariminia A, Law MG, Butler TG, et al. Factors associated with mortality in a cohort of Australian prisoners. *Eur J Epidemiol*. 2007;22(7):417–428.
5. Andrews JY, Kinner SA. Understanding drug-related mortality in released prisoners: a review of national coronial records. *BMC Public Health*. 2012;12:270.
6. Joukamaa M. The mortality of released Finnish prisoners; a 7 year follow-up study of the WATTU project. *Forensic Sci Int*. 1998;96(1):11–19.
7. Hakansson A, Berglund M. All-cause mortality in criminal justice clients with substance use problems—a prospective follow-up study. *Drug Alcohol Depend*. 2013;132(3):499–504.
8. Bird SM, Hutchinson SJ. Male drugs-related deaths in the fortnight after release from prison: Scotland, 1996–99. *Addiction*. 2003;98(2):185–190.
9. Farrell M, Marsden J. Acute risk of drug-related death among newly released prisoners in England and Wales. *Addiction*. 2008;103(2):251–255.
10. Binswanger IA, Blatchford PJ, Mueller SR, Stern MF. Mortality after prison release: opioid overdose and other causes of death, risk factors, and time trends from 1999 to 2009. *Ann Intern Med*. 2013;159(9):592–600.
11. Merrall EL, Kariminia A, Binswanger IA, et al. Meta-analysis of drug-related deaths soon after release from prison. *Addiction*. 2010;105(9):1545–1554.
12. Forsyth SJ, Alati R, Ober C, Williams GM, Kinner SA. Striking subgroup differences in substance-related mortality after release from prison. *Addiction*. 2014;109(10):1676–1683.
13. Binswanger IA, Stern MF, Deyo RA, et al. Release from prison—a high risk of death for former inmates. *N Engl J Med*. 2007;356(2):157–165.
14. Stewart LM, Henderson CJ, Hobbs MS, Ridout SC, Knuiman MW. Risk of death in prisoners after release from jail. *Aust N Z J Public Health*. 2004;28(1):32–36.
15. Moore E, Winter R, Indig D, Greenberg D, Kinner SA. Non-fatal overdose among adult prisoners with a history of injecting drug use in two Australian states. *Drug Alcohol Depend*. 2013;133(1):45–51.
16. Winter R, Stoové M, Degenhardt L, et al. Incidence and predictors of non-fatal drug overdose after release from prison among people who inject drugs in Queensland, Australia. *Drug Alcohol Depend*. 2015;153:43–49.

17. Kinner SA, Milloy MJ, Wood E, Qi J, Zhang R, Kerr T. Incidence and risk factors for non-fatal overdose among a cohort of recently incarcerated illicit drug users. *Addict Behav.* 2012;37(6):691–696.
18. Seal KH, Kral AH, Gee L, et al. Predictors and prevention of nonfatal overdose among street-recruited injection heroin users in the San Francisco Bay Area, 1998–1999. *Am J Public Health.* 2001;91(11):1842–1846.
19. Coffey C, Veit F, Wolfe R, Cini E, Patton GC. Mortality in young offenders: retrospective cohort study. *BMJ.* 2003;326(1064):1–4.
20. Azbel L, Wickersham JA, Grishaev Y, Dvoryak S, Altice FL. Burden of infectious diseases, substance use disorders, and mental illness among Ukrainian prisoners transitioning to the community. *PLoS One.* 2013;8(3):e59643.
21. Stein MD, Caviness CM, Anderson BJ. Incidence of sexually transmitted infections among hazardously drinking women after incarceration. *Women's Health Issues.* 2012;22(1):e1–7.
22. Binswanger IA, Mueller SR, Beaty BL, Min SJ, Corsi KF. Gender and risk behaviors for HIV and sexually transmitted infections among recently released inmates: a prospective cohort study. *AIDS Care.* 2014;26(7):872–881.
23. Baillargeon J, Giordano TP, Rich JD, et al. Accessing antiretroviral therapy following release from prison. *JAMA.* 2009;301(8):848–857.
24. de Aguiar SR, Villanova FE, Martins LC, et al. Human papillomavirus: prevalence and factors associated in women prisoners population from the eastern Brazilian Amazon. *J Med Virol.* 2014;86(9):1528–1533.
25. Chu FY, Lin YS, Cheng SH. Human papillomavirus infection in human immunodeficiency virus-positive Taiwanese women incarcerated for illicit drug usage. *J Microbiol Immunol Infect.* 2013;46(4):282–287.
26. Binswanger IA, Krueger PM, Steiner JF. Prevalence of chronic medical conditions among jail and prison inmates in the USA compared with the general population. *J Epidemiol Community Health.* 2009;63(11):912–919.
27. Australian Institute of Health and Welfare. *The Health of Australia's Prisoners 2012.* Canberra, Australia: AIHW; 2013.
28. Binswanger IA, Nowels C, Corsi KF, et al. "From the prison door right to the sidewalk, everything went downhill," a qualitative study of the health experiences of recently released inmates. *Int J Law Psychiatry.* 2011;34(4):249–255.
29. Wildeman C, Western B. Incarceration in fragile families. *Future Children.* 2010;20(2):157–177.
30. Murray J. The cycle of punishment: social exclusion of prisoners and their children. *Criminol Crim Just.* 2007;7(1):55–81.
31. Williams NH. Prison health and the health of the public: ties that bind. *J Correct Health Care.* 2007;13(2):80–92.
32. Western B, Pettit B. Incarceration and social inequality. *Daedalus.* 2010;139(3):8–19.
33. Krieg AS. Aboriginal incarceration: health and social impacts. *Med J Aust.* 2006;184(10):534–536.
34. Monchalin L. Canadian Aboriginal peoples victimization, offending and its prevention: gathering the evidence. *Crime Prev Comm Safety.* 2010;12(2):119–132.
35. Townes O'Brien M. Criminal law's tribalism. *Connecticut Public Interest Law Journal.* 2011;11(1):31–49.
36. Somers SA, Nicolella E, Hamblin A, McMahon SM, Heiss C, Brockmann BW. Medicaid expansion: considerations for states regarding newly eligible jail-involved individuals. *Health Aff.* 2014;33(3):455–461.
37. Wang EA, Wang Y, Krumholz HM. A high risk of hospitalization following release from correctional facilities in Medicare beneficiaries: a retrospective matched cohort study, 2002 to 2010. *JAMA Int Med.* 2013;173(17):1621–1628.
38. Frank JW, Andrews CM, Green TC, Samuels AM, Trinh TT, Friedmann PD. Emergency department utilization among recently released prisoners: a retrospective cohort study. *BMC Emerg Med.* 2013;13:16.

39. Metraux S, Caterina R, Cho R. *Incarceration and Homelessness*. National Symposium on Homelessness Research; 2007; Washington, DC.
40. Gordon RJ, Lowy FD. Bacterial infections in drug users. *N Engl J Med*. 2005;353(18):1945–1954.
41. Kendig N. Tuberculosis control in prisons. *Int J Tuberc Lung Dis*. 1998;2(9) (suppl 1):S57–63.
42. Binswanger IA, Redmond N, Steiner JF, Hicks LS. Health disparities and the criminal justice system: an agenda for further research and action. *J Urban Health*. 2012;89(1):98–107.
43. Khan MR, Behrend L, Adimora AA, Weir SS, Tisdale C, Wohl DA. Dissolution of primary intimate relationships during incarceration and associations with post-release STI/HIV risk behavior in a southeastern city. *Sex Transm Dis*. 2011;38(1):43–47.
44. Gideon L. Family role in the reintegration process of recovering drug addicts: a qualitative review of Israeli offenders. *Int J Offender Ther Comp Criminol*. 2007;51(2):212–226.
45. Naser RL, Visher CA. Family members' experiences with incarceration and reentry. *West Crim Rev*. 2006;7(2):20–31.
46. Bahr SJ, Harris L, Fisher JK, Armstrong AH. Successful reentry: what differentiates successful and unsuccessful parolees? *Int J Offender Ther Comp Criminol*. 2010;54(5):667–692.
47. Mumola C. Bureau of Justice Statistics Special Report: Incarcerated Parents and Their Children. Washington, DC: US Department of Justice; 2000.
48. Comfort M. Punishment beyond the legal offender. *Annu Rev Law Soc Sci*. 2007;3:271–296.
49. Thomas JC, Torrone E. Incarceration as forced migration: effects on selected community health outcomes. *Am J Public Health*. 2008;96(10):1762–1765.
50. Alemagno S. Women in jail: is substance abuse treatment enough? *Am J Public Health*. 2001;91(5):798–800.
51. van Olphen J, Freudenberg N, Fortin P, Galea S. Community reentry: perceptions of people with substance use problems returning home from New York City jails. *J Urban Health*. 2006;83(3):372–381.
52. Chandler RK, Fletcher BW, Volkow ND. Treating drug abuse and addiction in the criminal justice system: improving public health and safety. *JAMA*. 2009;301(2):183–190.
53. Binswanger IA, Stern MF, Yamashita TE, Mueller SR, Baggett TP, Blatchford PJ. Clinical risk factors for death after release from prison in Washington State: a nested case control study. *Addiction*. 2016;111(3):499–510.
54. Degenhardt L, Larney S, Kimber J, et al. The impact of opioid substitution therapy on mortality post-release from prison: retrospective data linkage study. *Addiction*. 2014;109(8):1306–1317.
55. Gryczynski J, Kinlock TW, Kelly SM, O'Grady KE, Gordon MS, Schwartz RP. Opioid agonist maintenance for probationers: patient-level predictors of treatment retention, drug use, and crime. *Subst Abuse*. 2012;33(1):30–39.
56. Huang YF, Kuo HS, Lew-Ting CY, et al. Mortality among a cohort of drug users after their release from prison: an evaluation of the effectiveness of a harm reduction program in Taiwan. *Addiction*. 2011;106(8):1437–1445.
57. Wheeler E, Davidson P, Jones T, Irwin K. Community-based opioid overdose prevention programs providing naloxone—United States, 2010. *MMWR Morb Mortal Wkly Rep*. 2012;61(6):101–105.
58. Dettmer K, Saunders B, Strang J. Take home naloxone and the prevention of deaths from opiate overdose: two pilot schemes. *BMJ*. 2001;322(7291):895–896.
59. McAuley A, Best D, Taylor A, Hunter C, Robertson R. From evidence to policy: the Scottish national naloxone programme. *Drugs-Educ Prev Polic*. 2012;19(4):309–319.
60. Bird SM, McAuley A, Perry S, Hunter C. Effectiveness of Scotland's national naloxone programme for reducing opioid-related deaths: a before (2006–10) versus after (2011–13) comparison. *Addiction*. 2016;111(5):883–891.

61. World Health Organization. *Prevention of Acute Drug-Related Mortality in Prison Populations During the Immediate Post-Release period.* Copenhagen, Denmark: WHO; 2010.
62. Walley AY, Xuan Z, Hackman HH, et al. Opioid overdose rates and implementation of overdose education and nasal naloxone distribution in Massachusetts: interrupted time series analysis. *BMJ.* 2013;346:f174.
63. Freudenberg N, Ramaswamy M, Daniels J, Crum M, Ompad DC, Vlahov D. Reducing drug use, human immunodeficiency virus risk, and recidivism among young men leaving jail: evaluation of the REAL MEN re-entry program. *J Adolesc Health.* 2010;47(5):448–455.
64. Hartwell SW, Deng X, Fisher W, et al. Predictors of accessing substance abuse services among individuals with mental disorders released from correctional custody. *J Dual Diagn.* 2013;9(1):11–22.
65. Roman CG, Travis J. *Taking Stock: Housing, Homelessness, and Prisoner Reentry.* Washington, DC: Urban Institute; 2004.
66. Wang EA, Hong CS, Shavit S, Sanders R, Kessell E, Kushel MB. Engaging individuals recently released from prison into primary care: a randomized trial. *Am J Public Health.* 2012;102(9):e22–29.
67. Kirst M, Zerger S, Misir V, Hwang S, Stergiopoulos V. The impact of a Housing First randomized controlled trial on substance use problems among homeless individuals with mental illness. *Drug Alcohol Depend.* 2015;146:24–29.
68. Aubry T, Tsemberis S, Adair CE, et al. One-year outcomes of a randomized controlled trial of Housing First with ACT in five Canadian cities. *Psychiatr Serv.* 2015;66(5):463–469.
69. Cuellar AE, Cheema J. As roughly 700,000 prisoners are released annually, about half will gain health coverage and care under federal laws. *Health Affairs.* 2012;31(5):931–938.
70. Winkelman TN, Kieffer EC, Goold SD, Morenoff JD, Cross K, Ayanian JZ. Health insurance trends and access to behavioral healthcare among justice-involved individuals—United States, 2008–2014. *J Gen Int Med.* 2016;31(12):1523–1529.
71. Binswanger IA, Whitley E, Haffey PR, Mueller SR, Min SJ. A patient navigation intervention for drug-involved former prison inmates. *Subst Abuse.* 2015;36(1):34–41.
72. Arangua L, McCarthy WJ, Moskowitz R, Gelberg L, Kuo T. Are homeless transitional shelters receptive to environmental tobacco control interventions? *Tob Control.* 2007;16(2):143–144.
73. Jurgens R, Ball A, Verster A. Interventions to reduce HIV transmission related to injecting drug use in prison. *Lancet Infect Dis.* 2009;9(1):57–66.
74. Gaskin GL, Glanz JM, Binswanger IA, Anoshiravani A. Immunization coverage among juvenile justice detainees. *J Correct Health Care.* 2015;21(3):265–275.
75. Bick JA. Infection control in jails and prisons. *Clin Infect Dis.* 2007;45(8):1047–1055.
76. Peterman TA, Newman DR, Goldberg M, et al. Screening male prisoners for *Chlamydia trachomatis*: impact on test positivity among women from their neighborhoods who were tested in family planning clinics. *Sex Transm Dis.* 2009;36(7):425–429.
77. Binswanger IA, Carson EA, Krueger PM, Mueller SR, Steiner JF, Sabol WJ. Prison tobacco control policies and deaths from smoking in United States prisons: population based retrospective analysis. *BMJ.* 2014;349:g4542.
78. Lenton SR, Dietze PM, Degenhardt L, Darke S, Butler TG. Naloxone for administration by peers in cases of heroin overdose. *Med J Aust.* 2009;191(8):469.
79. Strang J, Bird SM, Parmar MK. Take-home emergency naloxone to prevent heroin overdose deaths after prison release: rationale and practicalities for the N-ALIVE randomized trial. *J Urban Health.* 2013;90(5):983–996.

CHAPTER 15

Supply Reduction in Prison

The Evidence

ROBERT L. TRESTMAN, MD AND ASHBEL T. WALL, JD

INTRODUCTION

Illicit drug use has long been a feature of correctional institutions. The literature is replete with examples. In Glenochil prison, a Scottish facility, a 1993 outbreak of HIV and hepatitis B was directly linked to injection drug use during incarceration.[1] In a Finnish prison in 1995, 28% of inmates anonymously reported illicit drug use during their present incarceration.[2] In 1999, the Correctional Services of Canada found evidence of illicit substances in 25% of 8,606 urine samples of incarcerated individuals.[3] The California Department of Corrections and Rehabilitation found illicit drugs in urine samples of nearly 23% of inmates tested in 2013.[4] Although no credible practitioner openly condoned the use of illegal addictive substances in correctional facilities, there tended to be a certain resignation about the problem, evidenced by the belief that drugs were an inevitable part of prison life and that interdiction was unlikely to eliminate them. Thankfully, the attitude of those who work in prisons, or who run correctional systems, toward drugs of abuse has evolved over the past several years. Greater efforts are now placed on keeping illicit substances out of prisons, more effectively managing the prisons, and implementing more extensive treatment programs for substance use disorders.

This shift has occurred in the thinking of both administrators and uniformed personnel, due to multiple factors. It has taken place in response to a surge in the number of prisoners incarcerated for drug-related crimes, the percentage (upwards of 70% in many prison or jail populations)[5] who report use of drugs or alcohol, and a greater appreciation for the impact of narcotics on institutional operations and culture. Correctional staff have approached this concern in a host of ways, including a substantial focus on preventing illicit substances from entering the facility in the first place: interdiction. This interdiction effort requires a wide array of interventions, including the monitoring of phone calls and mail, the structuring and oversight of the visitation process, the use of trained canines, and intrusive searches any time a prisoner leaves the facility and returns. These efforts interface with an ongoing process to monitor prison activities for the presence of drugs that get past screening efforts.[6] Random drug testing, canine tours of the facility, and an intricate system of informants are elements of effective monitoring activities.[7] The effectiveness of such interventions and their cost-effectiveness will be reviewed in this chapter, along with the consequences of failure.

THE IMPERATIVE OF INTERDICTION

All correctional staff know that the maintenance of security inside the prison is at the core of their responsibilities. Unless inmates and employees feel safe, nothing good can happen there. Failure to provide safety and order can lead to very serious consequences for correctional officers, their peers, and the inmates they are sworn to safeguard. The introduction of narcotics into this environment sets the stage for significant security breaches and destabilizes institutional operations. In this respect, drug contraband can be as much of a threat as weapons or a handcuff key.

In view of the manifold consequences that can flow from the prison drug trade, correctional administrators cannot afford to be indifferent. Inmates who are able to have drugs brought into the facility hold rank and power, particularly among those whose dependence on narcotics renders them desperate to get a fix. Of relevance in jurisdictions where gangs are prevalent, one of the hallmarks of gang leadership is control of the prison drug trade. The gangs compete with one another for dominance of the prison marketplace.[8] Some inmates will hurt and kill other inmates over drugs.

The effects of illicit drugs on the institution's climate are wide-ranging. Controlled substances can be bartered for valuable commodities such as cell phones or escape-related paraphernalia. Extortion for sex as well as other services or goods is intertwined with drug deals and debts. There may be threats to family and friends in the community. Apart from these scenarios, the possibility of overdoses and the liability that accompanies them exists. In short, the presence of narcotics gives inmates power while staff lose control. In view of the stakes, correctional administrators pay a great deal of attention to the problem of illicit drugs coming into prisons and the subsequent management and safety concerns such drugs present. The current attitude in the correctional systems of most developed countries and many developing countries can be characterized, in the authors' opinion, by determination: a belief that the conveyance of narcotics occurs only to the degree that the correctional authorities let it happen. There are limited avenues for the introduction of contraband, drugs included, into correctional institutions. One is via civilians through contact visits or the mail (including the backs of stamps or the seals of envelopes). Another is through staff in ways that range from breakdowns in policy or practice (inadequate searches, for example) to outright complicity. A third method, somewhat less common, is literally "over the wall," through the use of, for example, tennis balls[9] or more recently drones.[10,11] Given the reality of a prison drug economy (whether small or substantial) in most prisons, effective interdiction is a priority in every well-run facility.

STOPPING THE ENTRY OF DRUGS INTO THE FACILITY
Entry and Re-entry of the Prisoner

Each time a prisoner enters a facility, there is an opportunity to introduce contra-band material.[12] Following arrest, return from a hospital visit, or return from a court hearing, each entry into the facility is a new challenge. A variety of standard inter-ventions are typically employed in most correctional facilities for prisoner entry and re-entry. Metal detection is nearly universal. Canines may be present for their ability to detect drugs by smell. Clothing is removed and searched. The person is usually strip-searched. Some facilities will make use of visual body cavity inspections; a few will use electronic devices such as ion mobility spectrometry to detect trace amounts of drugs on skin or clothing.[13] New clothing is issued. This procedure is typically followed by well-run facilities dedicated to drug interdiction every time a prisoner enters the facility. It is surprisingly common to find drugs hidden in shoes, under-wear, or body cavities.

Entry of Staff

A well-run facility will have routine inspection of all staff that enter the facility. While the level of detail varies, it may be as exhaustive as that used for prisoners in certain maximum security settings on a routine or random basis. Consistent searches of staff, whether random or routine, when combined with similarly appro-priate searches of entering inmates, will reduce the entry of drugs through this com-mon mechanism.

Phone Calls and Mail

Phone communication is a very significant way in which drug smuggling is coordi-nated. Most telephone systems in correctional facilities are regulated, and calls are recorded for monitoring. Limiting who the inmate may call or receive calls from is standard. That said, once the call is made, someone else may be handed the phone. Knowing that calls are recorded and may be reviewed immediately or subsequently is an important element of deterrence. Further, individuals attempting to organize drug transactions may speak in a coded form. Correctional intelligence officers must therefore stay current with the latest "code" jargon to be effectively able to decipher the messages and take appropriate action.

With the exception of legal communications, mail in jails and prisons is not subject to the confidentiality regulations standard in most communities. Any outgoing or incoming letters (except those between client and attorney) may be reviewed for content. Not only is the wording reviewed for evidence of drug-trafficking activity, but the incoming mail may actually contain drugs. Sometimes pills are crushed into a powder or dissolved in liquid, and the paper is soaked in that liquid.[14] Some medications are now formulated as dissolving films; these may easily be hidden beneath a stamp.[15]

Mobile Phones

Mobile phones are highly prized by inmates in jails and prisons because calls from them are not monitored. Cell phones, particularly those that are Internet enabled, have been used by prisoners to coordinate drug deals and smuggling networks.[16] The Arizona prison system in the United States reported finding 283 cell phones in its facilities in 2011.[17] All facilities ban such devices; given the small size, and the correctional black-market value of a basic cell phone (many hundreds of dollars), keeping them out has been a challenge for many facilities. While some systems have contemplated jamming cell phone frequencies, the cost of jamming equipment is high, and the legality and impact on surrounding areas have prevented implementation. Interestingly, canines can be trained to recognize the smell of ferric chloride (circuit board etching), rosin (from soldering), epoxy (circuit board fabrication), and lithium ion (battery off-gassing).[17] Appropriately trained canines are now in use in many jurisdictions to significant benefit.

Visitation

Visitation by family and friends is of enormous value in maintaining a social support network for inmates. There is growing evidence that such visits, particularly contact visits (where there is no glass barrier between the inmate and the visitor), reduce and delay reoffending and reincarceration.[18,19] Sadly, such contact visits also allow for exchange of contraband. To prevent contraband from being exchanged at visits, visitors go through a multi-stage process. First, people being proposed for the approved visitor list are screened through review of law enforcement databases. Once approved, they arrive at the correctional center and check any coats, bags, or packages. Visiting rooms are now routinely equipped with quite visible video monitoring and recording equipment. The equipment is intended to provide both deterrence and detection of any potential contraband.

Over the Wall

Many facilities in the United States are located in rural settings, with broad open perimeters. Many are in urban settings close to adjoining properties. The latter provide opportunities for launching tennis balls or similar objects over the fence to selected inmates. Such objects can contain substantial amounts of drugs. The example of Kingston Prison in Portsmouth, England, will serve. In 2006, enough drugs inside tennis balls came over the wall into the exercise yard at Kingston Prison that 35% of the facility's inmates tested positive for illicit drugs: a rate more than three times greater than England's national prison average.[9] Once this method was interdicted, the prison's drug abuse rate rapidly fell to 12.9%.[9] Other approaches, aided by modern technology, have been used in the more open settings of rural prisons. Remote-controlled quadcopters (drones) have reached the US consumer market in growing numbers and are making their way to rural prison exercise yards.[10,11,20] The Mansfield Correctional Institution in Ohio was the site of one such incursion. A fight erupted in the exercise yard among 75 inmates struggling to get at a package containing tobacco, marijuana, and heroin. A review of surveillance tapes discovered that the package had been dropped by a drone.[10]

Staff Corruption

The single most common mechanism by which illicit drugs enter correctional facilities is through correctional staff. Corruption of correctional staff is a substantial challenge, especially given the relatively modest pay scale compared with the money available from drug distribution. Bribery is sadly not uncommon; a recent case included six Pennsylvania correctional officers paid to smuggle prescription opiate pills into the facility.[21] Correctional staff may also become extortionists, as well as succumb to bribery. A recent example is an indictment in the state of Georgia in which the US Attorney's Office charged a correctional officer and a correctional kitchen worker with extortion and conspiracy to distribute illicit drugs.[16] The standard approach to reducing such corruption includes the creation of strong and clear policy; the use of fair, firm, and consistent supervision; and a well-structured and empowered investigative unit.

FACILITY MONITORING
Mandatory (Targeted) and Random Drug Testing

Urinalysis for drugs is a standard procedure in most correctional facilities, certainly for prisoners and commonly for correctional staff as well. The degree to which such testing is carefully monitored to prevent faked samples is an important element in interdiction protocols. As a typical management protocol, any time someone refuses to be tested, there is the presumption of a positive test.

Under any scenario, one of the factors needed to succeed in the effort to interdict controlled substances is the extensive use of drug testing. Tests may be administered randomly, for cause, or in relation to participation in or graduation from a substance abuse treatment program. It is of course important to recognize that appropriately prescribed medications may lead to falsely positive urine drug screens.[22] Therefore, positive urine drug screens need to be reviewed to assure that medication is not the cause of the positive test result. Further, urine drug screens are not perfect; some require subsequent confirmatory analyses.[23] Every inmate who tests positive must be interviewed by investigative staff. The goal is to gather intelligence that can be used to shut off a source of supply. While most inmates refuse to cooperate, some will provide information. Their motives for doing so may vary, but they are rarely altruistic. They may have been threatened by the dealer for failure to pay up or may be looking to eliminate a competitor in the prison drug marketplace. Similarly, even inmates who are not involved in this drug trade may want to use information in pursuit of other objectives such as transfer to another facility. Steps must be taken to protect the informant. If information comes via a confidential source, the source must be included in the subsequent shakedown of persons and cells. Numerous interviews with a variety of inmates must be conducted in all instances. They should be of approximately the same duration regardless of their productivity so that no single inmate can be identified as the one who broke ranks.

Facility-wide monitoring can be approached from a different, less intrusive perspective, through wastewater analysis.[24,25] One such study quantitatively examined drugs in the wastewater of a prison in Catalan, Spain, using combined liquid chromatography and mass spectrometry. Among the illicit substances tested, cannabis, heroin, cocaine, and multiple amphetamine derivatives were found.[25] While somewhat costly, this method could provide useful monitoring data for correctional administrators. Standards for using wastewater analysis[26] and ethical concerns in its use[27] are currently being explored.

A challenge for such testing is whether the right drugs are being screened for. With the evolution in and range of drugs of abuse, knowing what street and prescription drugs to test for should be determined on a thoughtful basis and regularly reviewed for need to update.

Random Searches

Searching for contraband is a critical component of security and safety in all jails and prisons. How, when, and how often to search inmate cells and common spaces are important questions to answer. Unannounced searches produce the best results and have a deterrent effect as well. Searches are disruptive to routine operations, so a balance between routine function and effective contraband interdiction must be sought.

Use of Canines

Canine units are able to go into relatively small spaces and can scan a large area efficiently. They do have limitations, though, including initial training costs, need for dedicated staff, and working hour limits due to exhaustion.

Ion Spectrometry

Similar to the way a dog can smell drugs, ion spectrometry offers a reliable way to detect even trace amounts of drug materials. Disadvantages include a substantial expense, both in initial equipment and in staffing to implement its use,[28] although newer equipment is less costly to purchase and use.[13] Further, current equipment is stationary, limiting its use to entry screening of inmates, staff, and visitors, and to mail room screening.

Informants

Much like law enforcement agencies in the community, most correctional systems make use of some type of informant system. Such information is important for safety and security in general. Informants (internal facility inmates and community-based individuals) can provide both general and detailed information about drug smuggling, location of drug caches, and distribution rings.

Effectiveness and Costs

In one of the few projects of its kind, the US National Institute of Corrections funded eight different drug interdiction initiatives in the Drug Free Prison Zone project.[29] Each state awardee implemented and evaluated drug interdiction strategies. One comprehensive initiative was undertaken in the state of Maryland and included a formal investigations unit; narcotic detection dogs; ion spectrometry scanning; mail inspection; restriction of inmate telephone calls to approved numbers; and interagency cooperation with state, regional, and national organized crime units. Evaluation data for the canine unit found the cost during the 28-month study was $87,000. Compared with the baseline, at the conclusion of the trial there was a 50% reduction in alerts and a complete elimination of confirmed contraband. The investigations unit expenditures totaled $66,000 over the same 28-month period. Incidents were reduced by more than 80% during this time frame, from 103 in 1999 to 16 in 2001. Despite the ambitious nature of this intervention, this was not a randomized trial, and causal linkages are therefore weak. The overall result does, however, suggest that vigorous interventions can indeed reduce illicit substance abuse in prisons.

The California experience included ion detection equipment and canine teams. The experience with the ion detection equipment was very limited, as it was used in selected prisons, screened only incoming inmates, and did not screen visitors. Canine teams conducted cell searches in conjunction with intelligence reports early in the intervention and were successful in locating contraband. However, canine drug detection teams yielded many false positive results, with only 10% of their alerts resulting in discovery of actual illicit substances. Despite that, tests of inmates identified by the canine drug detection team alerts yielded a 23% positive-plus-refusal rate, suggesting that even if no drugs were present at the time of the search, they were recently used. This reflects the utility of coordinating canine teams with intelligence gathered from informants or other sources.

Sanctions

In most systems worldwide, conveyance of drugs to the inmate trafficker and any confederates, whether by civilians or staff, leads to the pursuit of criminal charges. In virtually all instances, a positive urine sample is treated as a rule violation. It results in removal from the general population and placement in a punitive status, known as disciplinary confinement or disciplinary segregation, for a set period of time. While the conditions in this setting vary, they almost always include restrictions on out-of-cell time to an hour or two a day. Additional deprivations may involve the prohibition of televisions and radios, denial of visits and telephone privileges, or limitations on programmatic opportunities and interaction with other inmates. Other consequences can also ensue, either in tandem with or above and beyond the immediate sanction of disciplinary confinement. Examples are prolonged suspension of visiting privileges, reclassification to a higher level of security, notification to the parole board, or increased drug testing at the inmate's expense. One assumption that drives the use of sanctions is simply that punishment will reduce the likelihood of repeated misbehavior. Sadly, the evidence that punishment such as restricted housing or solitary confinement works to reduce future misbehavior is quite limited despite its widespread use in US facilities.[30] There is growing and substantial evidence, however, of the harm caused through such deprivation.[31]

Some jurisdictions employ graduated sanctions for the repeat usage of illicit drugs. For instance, a first offense may yield 20 days of segregation and a month of suspended visiting privileges following release, while second or third violations entail increasing amounts of both segregation time and prohibitions on visitation. A carrot-and-stick approach is used by some corrections departments in an effort to provide incentives for desistance from drug use. Should an inmate agree to enter and then comply with the terms of an authorized institutional substance abuse treatment program, a portion of the disciplinary time may be suspended. Similarly, he or she may be permitted to remain at the same level of custody following release from segregation. These measures are not so much predicated on the assumption that treatment will yield a reduction in demand sufficient to drive down supply as they are recognition that drug use presents challenges to both safety and health. From this perspective, treatment is consistent with institutional and societal goals.

WHERE OUR THINKING IS NOW

But what about the reaction of correctional staff who see the number of drug-dependent inmates who not only churn in and out of our institutions due to drug-related recidivism but repeatedly revolve through disciplinary confinement for drug use while they are inside? In many ways the feelings of correctional personnel, including uniformed officers, mirrors the divergent points of view in the larger community from which our staff are drawn. Some members of the public favor harsh sanctions for crime in general, including offenses related to drugs. Others argue that punishment alone is unrealistic as a crime prevention strategy and emphasize instead the importance of prevention, intervention, and treatment. The same is true of correctional employees. It is also true, however, that many have come to better understand the nature of drug abuse through their work in prison settings. They may also know family and friends who are drug-dependent. They sometimes recognize the symptoms of drug dependence in their own colleagues. Comments such as "once an addict always an addict" or "what do you expect—he's just a druggie" are heard less often. There is certainly cynicism when staff perceive that some drug users are "gaming the system" by entering treatment programs for no purpose other than to earn sentence reduction credits or buff up their credentials for the parole board. Yet as programs have proliferated in jails and prisons, personnel have had greater exposure to them and become more knowledgeable about the treatment and recovery process. They increasingly recognize that relapse can be part and parcel of recovery, and that punitive measures alone are unlikely to produce sustained change in drug-dependent prisoners. Evidence continues to mount that treatment, including medication-assisted therapy,[32,33] during incarceration leads to reduced drug abuse and reduced reoffending.[34-36]

Correctional practitioners know that a frequent conduit for the introduction of drug contraband is contact visiting, where touching, embracing, and brief kissing are permitted (albeit under the watchful eyes of officers and cameras). This long-standing practice, prevalent in all but the highest-security institutions, nevertheless represents a tacit acknowledgment that security should sometimes accommodate other important objectives such as preparation for re-entry into the larger society following release. Institutional safety and rehabilitation are both paramount concerns for the corrections profession. We cannot raise the white flag on either.

CONCLUSION

In recent decades, given the surge in prisoners incarcerated for drug-related crimes or who abuse drugs, the impact of narcotics on institutional operations and culture is starting to receive much-needed attention. Correctional staff have approached this concern in a host of ways, including a substantial focus on preventing illicit substances from entering the facility (eg, through the monitoring of phone calls and mail, closer oversight of the visitation process, the use of trained canines, and intrusive searches any time a prisoner leaves the facility and returns). These efforts interface with an ongoing process to monitor prison activities for the presence of drugs that get past screening efforts. Random drug testing, canine tours of the facility, and an intricate system of informants are elements of effective monitoring activities. Coupled with an increased emphasis on treatment of substance use disorders, these efforts have yielded institutions that are safer, more secure, healthier working environments for staff, and more effective rehabilitation settings for inmates.

REFERENCES

1. Gore SM, Bird AG, Burns SM, Goldberg DJ, Ross AJ, Macgregor J. Drug injection and HIV prevalence in inmates of Glenochil prison. *BMJ*. 1995;310(6975):293–296.
2. Korte T, Pykalainen J, Seppala T. Drug abuse of Finnish male prisoners in 1995. *Forensic Sci Int*. 1998;97(2–3):171–183.
3. Fraser AD, Zamecnik J, Keravel J, McGrath L, Wells J. Experience with urine drug testing by the Correctional Service of Canada. *Forensic Sci Int*. 2001;121(1–2):16–22.
4. California Department of Corrections and Rehabilitation. *Division of Adult Institutions Urinalysis Baseline Testing*. Sacramento: California Department of Corrections and Rehabilitation; 2014.
5. Mumola C, Karberg J. *Drug Use and Dependence, State and Federal Prisoners, 2004*. Washington, DC: US Department of Justice; 2006.
6. Feucht TE, Keyser A. Reducing drug use in prisons: Pennsylvania's approach. *National Institute of Justice Journal*. 1999;241:10–15.
7. Blakey D. *Disrupting the Supply of Illicit Drugs Into Prisons: A Report for the Director General of National Offender Management*. London, England: Ministry of Justice; 2008.
8. Skarbek D. *The Social Order of the Underworld*. New York, NY: Oxford University Press; 2014.
9. Payne S. Is that a tennis ball? no it's a drugs racket. *The Telegraph*. Published June 21, 2006. Accessed December 11, 2015.
10. Ferrigno L. Ohio prison yard free-for-all after drone drops drugs. *CNN*. Published August 5, 2015. Accessed December 11, 2015.
11. Fieldstadt E. Drone carrying package with drugs and blades found in Oklahoma prison yard. *NBC News*. Published October 27. 2015. Accessed December 11, 2015.
12. George S, Clayton S, Namboodiri V, Boulay S. "Up yours": smuggling illicit drugs into prison. *BMJ Case Rep*. 2009. http://casereports.bmj.com/content/2009/bcr.06.2009.1935.full
13. Johnson S, Dastouri S. *Use of Ion Scanners in Correctional Facilities: An International Review*. Montreal, ON: Correctional Service Canada; 2011.
14. Goodnough A, Zezima K. When children's scribbles hide a prison drug. *New York Times*. Published May 26, 2011. Accessed December 12, 2015.
15. Warner D. Drugs hidden under postage stamps in prison smuggling scheme. *Reuters*. Published March 22, 2011. Accessed December 12, 2015.
16. Adams D. Georgia inmates and prison guards face drugs and bribery charges. *Reuters*. Published September 24, 2015. Accessed December 11, 2015
17. Associated Press. Dogs trained to detect hidden cell phones in Arizona prisons. *Fox News*. Published May 29, 2012. Accessed January 2, 2014.
18. Bales WD, Mears DP. Inmate social ties and the transition to society: does visitation reduce recidivism? *J Res Crime Delinq*.2008;45(3):287–321.
19. Duwe G, Clark V. Blessed be the social tie that binds: the effects of prison sisitation on offender recidivism. *Crim Justice Pol Rev*. 2011;24(3):271–296.
20. Ernst D. Special delivery: drone drops contraband into Georgia prison yard. *Washington Times*. Published November 27, 2013. Accessed December 12, 2015.
21. Roebuck J. Prison guard caught in FBI sting pleads guilty. *The Inquirer*. Published December 10, 2015. Accessed December 11, 2015.
22. Brahm NC, Yeager LL, Fox MD, Farmer KC, Palmer TA. Commonly prescribed medications and potential false-positive urine drug screens. *Am J Health Syst Pharm*. 2010;67(16):1344–1350.
23. Moeller KE, Lee KC, Kissack JC. Urine drug screening: practical guide for clinicians. *Mayo Clin Proc*. 2008;83(1):66–76.
24. van Dyken E, Thai P, Lai FY, et al. Monitoring substance use in prisons: assessing the potential value of wastewater analysis. *Sci Justice*. 2014;54(5):338–345.

25. Postigo C, de Alda ML, Barcelo D. Evaluation of drugs of abuse use and trends in a prison through wastewater analysis. *Environ Int.* 2011;37(1):49–55.
26. Castiglioni S, Thomas KV, Kasprzyk-Hordern B, Vandam L, Griffiths P. Testing wastewater to detect illicit drugs: state of the art, potential and research needs. *Sci Total Environ.* 2014;487:613–620.
27. Hall W, Prichard J, Kirkbride P, et al. An analysis of ethical issues in using wastewater analysis to monitor illicit drug use. *Addiction.* 2012;107(10):1767–1773.
28. Whitworth A. Detecting contraband: current and emerging technologies and limitations. *Corr Today.* 2010(October):105–107.
29. Holsinger A. *National Institute of Corrections' Drug-Free Prison Zone Project, Evaluation Component for Each of Eight State Sites: Final Report.* Washington, DC: National Institute of Corrections; 2002.
30. Trestman RL. Ethics, the law, and prisoners: protecting society, changing human behavior, and protecting human rights. *J Bioeth Inq.* 2014;11(3):311–318.
31. Shames A, Wilcox J, Subramanian R. *Solitary Confinement: Common Misconceptions and Emerging Safe Alternatives.* New York, NY: Vera Institute; 2015.
32. Stallwitz A, Stöver H. The impact of substitution treatment in prisons—a literature review. *Int J Drug Policy.* 2007;18(6):464–474.
33. Stöver H, Michels I. Drug use and opioid substitution treatment for prisoners. *Harm Reduct J.* 2010;7(17):1–7.
34. Hser YI, Li MD, Normand J, Tai B, Chen Z, Chang L. Promoting global health—treatment and prevention of substance abuse and HIV in Asia. *J Neuroimmune Pharmacol.* 2015;10(suppl 1):S1–S55.
35. Olson DE, Lurigio AJ. The long-term effects of prison-based erug treatment and aftercare services on recidivism. *J Offender Rehabil.* 2014;53(8):600–619.
36. Rich JD, McKenzie M, Larney S, et al. Methadone continuation versus forced withdrawal on incarceration in a combined US prison and jail: a randomised, open-label trial. *Lancet.* 2015;386(9991):350–359.

CHAPTER 16

Drug Treatment for Prisoners

Opioid Substitution Treatment, Therapeutic Communities, and Cognitive Behavioral Therapy

KATE DOLAN, PhD, ZAHRA ALAM-MEHRJERDI, PhD,
AND BABAK MOAZEN, MSc

THE RATIONALE FOR DRUG TREATMENT PROGRAMS IN PRISON

There are good reasons for providing drug treatment to prisoners. These relate to (1) the preponderance of people who use or inject drugs in prisons, (2) high rates of drug-related harm in prison and after release, and (3) the high level of re-incarceration among drug users after release from custody. Drug-using inmates are at elevated risk of HIV, hepatitis C, and hepatitis B transmission during imprisonment, and of fatal drug overdose both during imprisonment and soon after release.

Preponderance of Drug Users Including Injectors in Prison Populations

In 2013, there were more than 10.2 million people in prison on any given day.[1] Over the last 15 years the world imprisonment rate has risen from 136 per 100,000 to the current rate of 144 per 100,000.[1] Internationally, the prevalence estimates of drug abuse and dependence in prison vary from 10% to 48% in male and 30% to 60% in female prisoners.[2]

Drug dependence is the key factor in the continuous growth of prison populations. From 1996 to 2006, the US population rose by 13% and the incarcerated population rose by 33%, while the proportion of prisoners with a drug problem rose by 43%.[3] Of 2.3 million prison and jail inmates in the United States in 2011, 65%

met *DSM-IV* criteria for alcohol or other drug abuse and dependence, but only 11% received treatment for their addictions, with less than 1% of prison budgets spent on treatment.[3] In the United States, between 24% and 36% of all persons dependent on heroin pass through the correctional system each year, representing more than 200,000 individuals.[4] Similarly, approximately 40% of prisoners in a large survey in Australia reported a history of heroin use,[5] in sharp contrast with the general community, where less than 1% had recently used heroin.[6]

HIV Transmission and Fatal Overdose

Prison populations have a very high prevalence and incidence of blood-borne viral infections (see chapters 7 and 9). For example, in 2000, 28% of general prisoners in Vietnam were HIV-positive.[7] In Estonia, up to 90% of inmates were HIV-positive in 2004.[8] Lithuania and Russia suffered major outbreaks of HIV in particular prisons. In Lithuania, the outbreak in Alytus prison resulted in at least 284 inmates being infected within a 6-month period. These new infections doubled the total number of HIV cases in the country.[9,10] Meanwhile, the outbreak in a Russian prison in Nizhnekamsk resulted in more than 400 inmates in a population of 1,824 acquiring HIV, again within a brief period.[11]

Fatal overdose can occur during imprisonment[12] or after release.[13] A large retrospective study of 48,771 prisoners released in England and Wales between 1998 and 2000 identified 442 deaths.[14] In the first week after release, male and female prisoners were 29.4 and 68.9 times, respectively, more likely to die than their counterparts in the community. People recently released from prison are also at markedly increased risk of non-fatal overdose[15] (see chapter 18).

High Rates of Re-incarceration of Drug-Using Inmates

Rates of re-incarceration are especially high for ex-inmates with a drug problem. In the United States, 50.2% of drug-dependent inmates have a previous incarceration, compared with 31.2% of other inmates.[3] In New South Wales, Australia, 84% of heroin-dependent inmates were re-incarcerated within 2 years of release,[16] compared with 44% of all prisoners.[17] People who inject drugs experience multiple incarcerations: one study in Australia found that they reported an average of five imprisonments during their drug-using careers.[18] These high rates of incarceration indicate that drug offenders are not receiving effective treatment for their substance use while in prison.

Given all these factors relating to drug use and harms among inmates, it is clear that the prison setting is a logical point to provide drug treatment. In the next section, three different treatment modalities are reviewed. These were chosen to cover the range of treatments available in most prison systems, such as a medical model (opioid substitution treatment), a self-help model (therapeutic communities and drug-free units), and a psychologically based treatment (cognitive behavioral therapy).

OPIOID SUBSTITUTION TREATMENT

In some countries, methadone patients are allowed to continue treatment when they enter prison, while other countries allow for commencement of treatment on prison entry. In most jurisdictions, however, prison authorities discontinue methadone treatment for patients when they enter prison. The dispensing of opioid substitution treatment (OST) in the prison setting requires more stringent monitoring than in the community setting. The extra precautions are necessary to prevent diversion. Inmates are often detained in a holding cell after being dosed to ensure that the medicine has been digested.[19]

The first study of methadone maintenance treatment in custody was in New York City's Rikers Island Jail in 1968. Thirty-two inmates who were about to be released from prison were randomly allocated either to a control condition (n = 16) or to receive treatment (n = 16). At the 6-month follow-up, 15 of the 16 inmates in the control condition had become dependent on heroin and had been re-incarcerated. In comparison, none of the treated inmates had become dependent, and just 3 had been re-incarcerated.[20]

Reduction of Injecting and Sharing in Prison

One reason for providing drug treatment to prisoners is to reduce injecting-related harm in prison. A systematic review found that when inmates were in OST, their risk of injecting and sharing were reduced by 55% to 75% and 47% to 73%, respectively, compared with those who went untreated.[21] A recent "natural experiment" in Australia has provided further support for these findings.[22]

Hepatitis C Transmission and Fatal Overdose

Several studies have identified a protective effect of OST on hepatitis C infection.[13,23] In an Australian study of ex-prisoners in OST, no deaths were recorded while subjects were enrolled in OST, but 17 subjects died when not in OST. This represented an untreated mortality rate of 2.0 per 100 person-years.[13]

Reduction of Re-incarceration and the Cost of Imprisonment

Another reason for providing treatment to inmates is to reduce their risk of re-incarceration. Prison-based OST has been shown to reduce re-incarceration among inmates. In one Australian study, being on OST when released from prison and continuing treatment after release reduced the risk of re-incarceration by an average of 20% among a group with a heightened rate of re-incarceration compared with non-drug-using inmates.[16] Another Australian study estimated that the average cost of prison OST was AU$3,234 per prisoner per year,[24] and that only 20 days of re-incarceration need to be avoided to offset the annual cost of methadone treatment in prison.

In the United States, inmates in Baltimore who received OST and counseling were significantly more likely than others to be retained in drug treatment and to test negative for opioids and cocaine on urinalysis.[25] Magura et al. found that the Rikers Island Jail methadone program facilitated entry into community-based treatment (85%) and retention at 6 months (27%) compared with prisoners enrolled in detoxification programs (37% entry, 9% retained).[26] Kinlock and colleagues found that a high proportion of prisoners who commenced OST in prison continued it in the community; they concluded that OST may be effective in engaging a sizable number of inmates who are dependent on opioids during and after incarceration.[25]

Barriers to and Coverage of OST in Prison

For OST to have an impact, there needs to be a reasonable level of coverage, yet places are very limited in many prison systems. In the United States, 43% of medical directors in prisons and jails report that they do not believe or do not know whether methadone is appropriate for treating inmates with drug dependence. The medical directors cite preferences for drug-free detoxification, security concerns, administrative opposition, and prohibitive cost as the primary reasons for not providing OST.[3] Senior correctional administrators in Australia reported that methadone places were limited because of inmates' security classification, the unavailability of community placements for inmates to transfer to once released, and the cost of providing OST in prison.[27]

Internationally, OST provision to inmates is growing, albeit slowly. In 1996, 5 countries provided OST to prisoners[28]; this number increased to 29 countries in 2009,[29] 43 countries in 2014, and 52 countries in 2016.[30] However, a review found that the proportion of inmates who received treatment in most systems was exceptionally low.[29] The proportion of all prisoners who were receiving OST could be calculated in 20 countries, and in 17 countries fewer than 10% of inmates were in treatment.

Conclusion

Cycles of drug use, crime, arrest, imprisonment, release, and return to drug use plague the lives of many people who inject drugs (PWID). The concentration of PWID in prisons means that targeting this population for treatment is likely to be cost-effective. International organizations have called for the implementation of OST in the prison setting.[31,32]

For the last four decades, the evidence has been mounting that OST reduces mortality,[20] heroin consumption,[20] criminality,[33] and HIV infection.[34] Yet prison authorities remain unconvinced of the benefits of providing this treatment modality. As recently as 2013, prison authorities tried unsuccessfully to stop methadone treatment in an Albuquerque jail.[35] A concerted effort at persuading policymakers of the evidence is required if OST implementation is to be accepted in the prison setting.

THERAPEUTIC COMMUNITIES AND DRUG-FREE UNITS

A therapeutic community (TC) is a drug-free treatment approach in which drug- or alcohol-dependent individuals live in small and highly structured communities.[36] The self-help treatment approach of TC is enhanced by additional services related to clients' physical and mental well-being and their relationships with their family. The TC model is appropriate for a wide range of clients, including those with a history of poly-drug use and those with complex social and psychological disorders.[37] As an important element, TC participants are encouraged to be curious about themselves, other clients, the staff, the group process, and other circumstances related to their recovery.[38] TCs in the broader community have been shown to be an effective treatment option for some clients.[39]

Numerous factors might influence the effectiveness of TC treatment programs. In this regard a study on polysubstance users receiving TC treatment showed that mindfulness meditation and goal management training might have a positive impact on performance of the target population in laboratory tasks of basic and complex executive functions, as well as ecological tasks of goal-directed behavior.[40]

TC Programs in Prison

In-prison drug treatment approaches were evaluated and discussed in a comprehensive report published by the Center for Substance Abuse Treatment in 2005.[41] According to the report, TCs are among the most successful programs to treat substance use and dependence in prison and are preferable due to the intensity of treatment. Reviewing the evidence, the report suggested that in-prison TCs might provide the best outcome for those with 9- to 12-month length of residency in prison, although the effectiveness is highly dependent on the "community-building capabilities" of the participants and service providers.

Many prison authorities find the abstinence-orientation approach of TCs attractive. A study of inmates in TC compared with other inmates found that participation in treatment was the strongest predictor of abstinence from illicit drug use at a 5-year follow-up. Participants were more than three times more likely than nonparticipants to be drug-free.[42]

Impacts on Recidivism

There is good evidence that TCs reduce recidivism, although this may be mediated by engagement in treatment after release from prison, and the effects may be greater if the program is gender-sensitive, at least for women. One evaluation of a TC for women incarcerated in Washington State, USA found that while 30% of women in the control group were convicted of another offense following release, only 13% of those who completed the treatment program were reconvicted. Even some exposure to treatment resulted in a reduced level of conviction (22%).[43]

A systematic review of the effectiveness of therapeutic communities examined the outcomes of post-release re-arrest, re-incarceration, or drug use in studies published between 2007 and 2014.[44] According to that review, 75% of the studies demonstrated the effectiveness of TC in reducing re-incarceration rates, about 70% showed a reduction of drug use among inmates in TC, and 55% showed a reduction in re-arrest among TC participants. This review also suggested more effectiveness of short-term TC on reducing re-incarceration rates and, to a lesser extent, drug use relapse, compared with long-term intervention.

The effect of TC treatment on criminal recidivism is maximized when participants leave prison and directly enter a community-based treatment. After a 2-year follow-up of 396 previously incarcerated drug users in Texas, 36% of treated inmates had been re-arrested, compared with 42% of a matched, untreated group. However, among inmates who attended TC in prison and in the community, only 30% were re-arrested. Compared with the untreated group, the risk of re-arrest was halved when inmates completed both treatment programs.[45] A study evaluating the 36-month recidivism outcome of a prison-based TC with aftercare among 478 participants in San Diego revealed a 27% recidivism rate after completing both in-prison and aftercare programs, compared with 75% in those who had not received both TC and aftercare.[46] That study also found a significant association between duration in treatment and time until return for recidivist felons.[46] Two randomized controlled trials evaluating the effectiveness of TC programs in US prisons found significantly fewer re-incarcerations and significantly fewer alcohol and drug offenses among those treated.[47,48]

Another evaluation of a TC for US inmates showed significant reductions in alcohol and other drug use among TC group participants compared with a comparison group at 12 months after release.[49] Another study compared the effectiveness of a gender-responsive treatment (GRT) and standard prison-based TC among women in a US prison. The study found that despite improved psychological well-being in both groups, participants in GRT showed more reduction in substance use and had longer residential aftercare and lower re-incarceration at 12 months after release.[50] It has been suggested that factors associated with completion of a TC program in prison are age, race, motivation and participation in the program.[51] Therefore, attention to these variables seems to be necessary to maximize the benefits of treatment.

Drug-Free Units

Voluntary drug-free units are a type of residential program within a prison. The main aim is to rehabilitate prisoners with drug problems. Residents of drug-free units are separated from the general prison population and pledge to refrain from drug use, usually in return for increased privileges such as access to recreational facilities or improved accommodation. Inmates are subjected to urinalysis and can be punished for a positive result, including through loss of privileges or expulsion from the program.[52]

Positive outcomes were reported from an Australian study of a drug-free unit. Thirty-one inmates in the general prison population were compared with 31 inmates in a drug-free unit. The majority (84%) of the general population inmates reported using drugs, compared with one-third (32%) of those in the drug-free unit. Urinalysis confirmed a significant difference in drug use between the two groups, with half (49%) of the general population inmates returning positive samples, compared with 6% of those in the drug-free unit.[52]

In a Dutch study, inmates in a drug-free unit were compared with the general prison population.[53] There were no differences between groups at 1-year follow-up on drug use, recidivism, social functioning, or physical functioning. However, compared with the comparison group, more inmates in the drug-free unit were referred to drug treatment after release (64% vs. 26%) and contacted a treatment agency (42% vs. 8%). However, it should be noted that most research has not evaluated the effectiveness of TCs specifically on drug use in prisons. Furthermore, most studies have been conducted in developed countries and the findings may not be transferable to prisons in developing countries.

Drug-free units are used in prisons across Europe[54] and Australia,[55] yet little is known about their long-term effectiveness because few have been rigorously evaluated. Because programs offered in drug-free units also vary widely, the precise factors that contribute to a positive rehabilitative environment are unclear.

COGNITIVE BEHAVIORAL THERAPY

Cognitive behavioral therapy (CBT) is one of the most common methods of drug use treatment in prison settings. CBT refers to a structured and client-centered model of intervention that encourages, teaches, and supports individuals to stop and then change their irrational beliefs and behaviors.[56-58] CBT is based on the assumption that irrational beliefs, attitudes, and behaviors of prisoners in regard to illicit drug use can be learned and then changed.[59]

Goals of CBT in the Treatment of Drug Use in Prison Settings

The main goals of CBT in prison settings include reducing the rates of illicit drug use problems and recidivism. CBT aims to teach self-control, which helps prisoners identify and modify their beliefs and behaviors and reduce or cease illicit drug use. To achieve these goals, CBT in prison settings attempts to promote motivations to change, relapse prevention, and behavior modifications that can also result in improved health. For example, two recent studies of CBT for incarcerated people found that CBT was effective in reducing relapse and improving health among the participants.[59,60]

CBT-Based Methods for Prisoners Who Use Illicit Drugs

CBT for illicit drug problems among prisoners can be provided through four main methods:

1. Strategies for Self-Improvement and Change
2. Getting Smart Recovery Program
3. Motivational Interviewing
4. Relapse Prevention[61]

Strategies for Self-Improvement and Change (SSC), which was first established in the United States, is a well-structured treatment for prisoners who report illicit drug use problems. SSC is a long-term (9 to 12 months), extensive CBT for prisoners to change their beliefs and behaviors, with 12 treatment modules. Although only a few studies have been conducted on SSC in prison settings, the current evidence suggests that the treatment is effective in reducing illicit drug use among prisoners. For example, in a study in the United States, prisoners were encouraged to complete 12 treatment modules, as well as some homework assignments. The study found that SSC significantly contributed to reducing illicit drug use among the participants after 12 months.[61]

In Australia, the CBT-based method known as Getting Smart Recovery Program (GSRP) has recently been provided for prisoners with illicit drug use problems. The program is based on CBT and has a strong focus on increasing motivations to change and problem-solving skills. GSRP is a psycho-educational program of 12 sessions (totaling 18 to 24 hours) designed for group delivery, complemented by homework assignments. The aims of the program are to reduce the risk of recidivism, treat alcohol and illicit drug use, and motivate prisoners to contunie participating in the GSRP recovery program. In a study in Australia, 355 prisoners participated in the program from six custody-based sites over 18 months. The study included only male prisoners, with an average age of 33 years. The study found that the overall rate of program completion was 83%. Among 288 prisoners who completed the program, 99% reported that the program was effective in reducing drug and alcohol use problems.[62]

Motivational Interviewing (MI) is a frequently used CBT-based method. Increasing prisoners' readiness to engage in change can have a positive effect on reducing illicit drug use problems because responsivity can increase the effectiveness of CBT treatment.[62,63] In prison settings, MI is widely implemented using the Stages of Change Model, which is based on Prochaska and DiClemente's model and consists of five stages. These stages—precontemplation, contemplation, preparation, action, and maintenance—have proven useful in the treatment of problematic beliefs and behaviors in regard to illicit drug use.[62,63]

Prisoners may not be motivated to change illicit drug use behaviors at precontemplation and contemplation stages. Therefore, CBT providers in prison settings provide MI at this stage. To resolve their ambivalence to change at the contemplation stage, prisoners are helped to choose positive changes over their current situations. Prisoners at the preparation stage may require assistance in identifying potential change strategies and selecting the most appropriate ones. At the action stage, CBT therapists also provide MI and help prisoners comply with the change strategies. At the maintenance stage, prisoners may become more confident that they are highly motivated to continue their changes.[62,63]

MI has been shown to be effective in the reduction of illicit drug use problems among prisoners. For example, in a study in the United States, Taxman and Belenko[64] found that using MI in a group of prisoners increased participation in continued drug treatment. MI has also been shown to be useful to increase treatment engagement among prisoners with illicit drug use problems. For example, in a study in the United States, McMurran and Ward found that MI increased treatment readiness among a group of prisoners, which acted as an effective factor in treatment engagement.[65]

Finally, Relapse Prevention (RP) is frequently used in prison settings to teach prisoners how to anticipate and cope with drug relapse. RP rejects the use of labels such as drug-dependent and encourages prisoners to take full responsibility for their addictive behaviors. RP has been found to be an effective program that helps prisoners to maintain positive changes in their behaviors and deal with relapse. For example, a meta-analysis of RP studies in the United States found that the treatment significantly increased psychosocial functioning and reduced illicit drug use.[66]

It should be noted that prisoners' illicit drug use may cause multiple problems for the prison setting, when treatment is not provided.[61] CBT has emerging evidence for effectiveness in prison settings, having value in motivating prisoners to change behaviors and helping them reduce illicit drug use. Some CBT-based methods such as SSC and GSRP still suffer from a paucity of rigorous research in prison settings.[61,63] However, there is strong evidence that MI is effective for those prisoners who are resistant to or ambivalent about change. The model of change advocated by Prochaska and DiClemente (1986) confirms that MI can help those who are not motivated to change and increase the likelihood of effective thought and behavioral changes. Further studies are still required to evaluate CBT for prisoners with drug use problems.

CONCLUSION AND RECOMMENDATIONS

This chapter reviewed three treatments for drug-dependent prisoners: opioid substitution treatment, therapeutic communities and drug-free units, and cognitive behavioral therapy. Based on current evidence, OST is the most effective treatment for heroin users in reducing their drug use and recidivism. However, this treatment is suitable only for opioid-dependent populations; users of psychostimulants and other non-opioid drugs remain poorly served by current treatment approaches in prison.

Prison authorities in countries where OST is available in the community should introduce OST programs urgently and expand implementation to scale as soon as possible. It is important that prisoners on OST prior to imprisonment can continue treatment upon imprisonment, and after release from prison, without interruption.[67]

Prison authorities should also provide a range of other treatment options for prisoners who are dependent on other substances such as cocaine and amphetamines.

Treatments such as therapeutic communities and cognitive behavioral therapy should be offered.

Drug treatment should be freely available to all inmates who wish to receive it; treatment needs to be based on sound evidence. Evidence-based treatments involve screening and assessment, the development of individual treatment plans, and referral to community programs on release.

REFERENCES

1. Walmsley R. *World Prison Population List.* 10th ed. London, England: International Centre for Prison Studies; 2013.
2. Fazel S, Bains P, Doll H. Substance abuse and dependence in prisoners: a systematic review. *Addiction.* 2006;101(2):181–191.
3. CASA. *Behind Bars II: Substance Abuse and America's Prison Population.* New York, NY: National Center on Addiction and Substance Abuse at Columbia University; 2010.
4. Boutwell AE, Nijhawan A, Zaller N, Rich J. Arrested on heroin: a national opportunity. *J Opioid Manag.* 2006;3(6):328–332.
5. Butler T, Lim D, Callander D. *National Prison Entrants' Bloodborne Virus and Risk Behaviour Survey 2004, 2007, and 2010.* Sydney, Australia: Kirby Institute; 2011.
6. Australian Institute of Health and Welfare. *National Drug Strategy Household Survey Detailed Report: 2013.* Canberra, Australia: AIHW; 2014.
7. Anonymous. *Vietnam: Increasing Number of HIV Cases in Prison. HEPP Report.* 2000;3:8.
8. Tsereteli Z. Situation with HIV in Estonian prison system. *Baltic Health.* 2004. http://web.archive.org/web/20041019071822/www.baltichealth.org/cparticle77892-7717a.html
9. Caplinskiene I, Caplinskas S, Griskevicius A. Narcotic abuse and HIV infection in prisons. *Medicina.* 2002;39(8):797–803.
10. Dolan K, Kite B, Black E, Aceijas C, Stimson GV. HIV in prison in low-income and middle-income countries. *Lancet Infect Dis.* 2007;7(1):32–41.
11. Nikolayev Y. HIV on plank prison beds: immunodeficiency virus outbreak registered in Nizhnekamsk colony. 2014. http://www.thelancet.com/journals/laninf/article/PIIS1473-3099(06)70685-5/references
12. Larney S, Gisev N, Farrell M, et al. Opioid substitution therapy as a strategy to reduce deaths in prison: retrospective cohort study. *BMJ Open.* 2014;4(4):e004666.
13. Dolan KA, Shearer J, White B, Zhou J, Kaldor J, Wodak AD. Four-year follow-up of imprisoned male heroin users and methadone treatment: mortality, re-incarceration and hepatitis C infection. *Addiction.* 2005;100(6):820–828.
14. Farrell M, Marsden J. Acute risk of drug-related death among newly released prisoners in England and Wales. *Addiction.* 2008;103(2):251–255.
15. Kinner SA, Milloy M, Wood E, Qi J, Zhang R, Kerr T. Incidence and risk factors for non-fatal overdose among a cohort of recently incarcerated illicit drug users. *Addict Behav.* 2012;37(6):691–696.
16. Larney S, Toson B, Burns L, Dolan K. Effect of prison-based opioid substitution treatment and post-release retention in treatment on risk of re-incarceration. *Addiction.* 2012;107(2):372–380.
17. Steering Committee for the Review of Government Service Provision. *Report on Government Services 2010.* Canberra, Australia: SCRGSP; 2010.
18. Dolan K, Wodak A, Wayne H. HIV risk behaviour and prevention in prison: a bleach programme for inmates in NSW. *Drug Alcohol Rev.* 1999;18(2):139–143.
19. World Health Organization, Western Pacific Region. *Clinical Guidelines for Withdrawal Management and Treatment of Drug Dependence in Closed Settings.* Geneva, Switzerland: WHO; 2009.

20. Dole VP, Robinson JW, Orraca J, Towns E, Searcy P, Caine E. Methadone treatment of randomly selected criminal addicts. *N Engl J Med*. 1969;280(25):1372–1375.
21. Larney S. Does opioid substitution treatment in prisons reduce injecting-related HIV risk behaviours? a systematic review. *Addiction*. 2010;105(2):216–223.
22. Kinner SA, Moore E, Spittal MJ, Indig D. Opiate substitution treatment to reduce in-prison drug injection: a natural experiment. *Int J Drug Policy*. 2013;24(5):460–463.
23. Marco A, Gallego C, Cayla JA. Incidence of hepatitis C infection among prisoners by routine laboratory values during a 20-year period. *PloS One*. 2014;9(2):e90560.
24. Warren E, Viney R, Shearer J, Shanahan M, Wodak A, Dolan K. Value for money in drug treatment: economic evaluation of prison methadone. *Drug Alcohol Depend*. 2006;84(2):160–166.
25. Kinlock TW, Gordon MS, Schwartz RP, Fitzgerald TT, O'Grady KE. A randomized clinical trial of methadone maintenance for prisoners: results at 12 months postrelease. *J Subst Abuse Treat*. 2009;37(3):277–285.
26. Magura S, Rosenblum A, Lewis C, Joseph H. The effectiveness of in-jail methadone maintenance. *J Drug Issues*. 1993;23(1):75–99.
27. Rodas A, Bode A, Dolan KA. *Supply, Demand and Harm Reduction Strategies in Australian Prisons: An Update*. Sydney, Australia: National Drug and Alcohol Research Centre; 2011.
28. Dolan K, Wodak A. An international review of methadone provision in prisons. *Addict Res*. 1996;4(1):85–97.
29. Larney S, Dolan K. A literature review of international implementation of opioid substitution treatment in prisons: equivalence of care? *Eur Addict Res*. 2009;15(2):107–112.
30. Stone K. *The Global State of Harm Reduction 2014*. London, England: Harm Reduction International; 2014.
31. United Nations Office on Drugs and Crime, International Labour Organization, United Nations Development Program, World Health Organization, UNAIDS. *HIV Prevention, Treatment and Care in Prisons and Other Closed Settings: A Comprehensive Package of Interventions*. Vienna, Austria: United Nations Office of Drugs and Crime; 2013.
32. Stöver H. *HIV/AIDS Prevention, Care, Treatment and Support in Prison Settings: A Framework for an Effective National Response*. Vienna, Austria: United Nations Office on Drugs and Crime; 2006.
33. Newman RG, Bashkow S, Cates M. Arrest histories before and after admission to a methadone maintenance treatment program. *Contemp Drug Probs*. 1973;2(3):417–430.
34. Novick DM, Joseph H, Croxson TS, et al. Absence of antibody to human immunodeficiency virus in long-term, socially rehabilitated methadone maintenance patients. *Archives Int Med*. 1990;150(1):97–99.
35. Frosch D. Plan to end methadone use at Albuquerque jail prompts alarm. *New York Times*. January 6, 2013.
36. Dolan K, Larney S, Wodak A. The integration of harm reduction into abstinence-based therapeutic communities: a case study of We Help Ourselves. *Asian J Counsel*. 2007;14:1–19.
37. De Leon G. *The Therapeutic Community: Theory, Model, and Method*. New York, NY: Springer; 2000.
38. Campling P. Therapeutic communities. *Adv Psychiatr Treat*. 2001;7(5):365–372.
39. Gowing L, Cooke R, Biven A, Watts D. *Towards Better Practice in Therapeutic Communities*. Bangalow, Australia: Australasian Therapeutic Communities Association; 2002.
40. Valls-Serrano C, Caracuel A, Verdejo-Garcia A. Goal Management Training and Mindfulness Meditation improveexecutive functions and transfers to ecological tasks of daily life in polysubstance users enrolled in therapeutic community treatment. *Drug Alcohol Depend*. 2016;1(165):9–14.

41. Center for Substance Abuse Treatment. *Substance Abuse Treatment for Adults in the Criminal Justice System.* Rockville, MD: Center for Substance Abuse Treatment; 2005.
42. Inciardi JA, Martin SS, Butzin CA. Five-year outcomes of therapeutic community treatment of drug-involved offenders after release from prison. *Crime Delinq.* 2004;50(1):88–107.
43. Mosher C, Phillips D. The dynamics of a prison-based therapeutic community for women offenders: retention, completion, and outcomes. *Prison J.* 2006;86(1):6–31.
44. Galassi A, Mpofu E, Athanasou J. Therapeutic community treatment of an inmate population with substance use disorders: post-release trends in re-arrest, re-incarceration, and drug misuse relapse. *Int J Environ Res Public Health.* 2015;12(6):7059–7072.
45. Hiller ML, Knight K, Simpson DD. Prison-based substance abuse treatment, residential aftercare and recidivism. *Addiction.* 1999;94(6):833–842.
46. Wexler HK, Melnick G, Lowe L, Peters J. Three-year reincarceration outcomes for Amity in-prison therapeutic community and aftercare in California. *Prison J.* 1999;79(3):321–336.
47. Wexler HK, De Leon G, Thomas G, Kressel D, Peters J. The Amity prison TC evaluation reincarceration outcomes. *Crim Just Behav.* 1999;26(2):147–167.
48. Sacks S, Sacks JY, McKendrick K, Banks S, Stommel J. Modified TC for MICA offenders: crime outcomes. *Behav Sci Law.* 2004;22(4):477–501.
49. Sullivan CJ, McKendrick K, Sacks S, Banks S. Modified therapeutic community treatment for offenders with MICA disorders: substance use outcomes. *Am J Drug Alcohol Abuse.* 2007;33(6):823–832.
50. Messina N, Grella CE, Cartier J, Torres S. A randomized experimental study of gender-responsive substance abuse treatment for women in prison. *J Subst Abuse Treat.* 2010;38(2):97–107.
51. Larney S, Mathers B, Dolan KA. *Illicit Drug Treatment in Prison: Detoxification, Drug-Free Units, Therapeutic Communities, and Opioid Substitution Treatment.* Sydney, Australia: National Drug and Alcohol Research Centre, University of New South Wales; 2007.
52. Incorvaia D, Kirby N. A formative evaluation of a drug-free unit in a correctional services setting. *Int J Offender Ther and Comp Criminol.* 1997;41(3):231–249.
53. Schippers GM, Hurk AAvd, Breteler MH, Meerkerk G-J. Effectiveness of a drug-free detention treatment program in a Dutch prison. *Subst Use Misuse.* 1998;33(4):1027–1046.
54. Zurhold H, Stöver H, Haasen C. *Female Drug Users in European Prisons—Best Practice for Relapse Prevention and Reintegration.* Hamburg, Germany: Centre for Interdisciplinary Addiction Research, University of Hamburg; 2004.
55. Black E, Wodak A, Dolan KA. *Supply, Demand and Harm Reduction Strategies in Australian Prisons: Implementation, Cost and Evaluation.* Canberra, Australia: Australian National Council on Drugs; 2004.
56. Sanders D, Bennett-Levy J. When therapists have problems: what can CBT do for us? In: Mueller M, Kennerley H, McManus F, Westbrook D, eds. *The Oxford Guide to Surviving as a CBT Therapist.* Oxford, England: Oxford University Press; 2010:457–480.
57. Bennett-Levy J, Richards DA, Farrand P. Low intensity CBT interventions: a revolution in mental health care. In: Bennett-Levy J, Richards DA, Farrand P, et al., eds. *Oxford Guide to Low Intensity CBT Interventions.* London, England: Oxford University Press; 2010:3–18.
58. Baker A, Kay-Lambkin F, Lee NK, Claire M, Jenner L. *A Brief Cognitive Behavioural Intervention for Regular Amphetamine Users.* Canberra, Australia: Australian Government Department of Health and Ageing; 2003.
59. Lanza PV, Garcia PF, Lamelas FR, González-Menéndez A. Acceptance and commitment therapy versus cognitive behavioral therapy in the treatment of substance use disorder with incarcerated women. *J Clin Pych.* 2014;70(7):644–657.

60. Shirazi M, Lachinnani F, Joubari FY, Halajian Z, Sarabi SD, Khan MA. The effectiveness of cognitive-behavioral training on increasing self-concept's measure and the attitude style toward narcotic drugs in Tonekabon addicted prisoners. *Int J High Risk Behav Addict*. 2013;2(1):39–42.
61. Milkman HB, Wanberg KW. *Cognitive-Behavioral Treatment: A Review and Discussion for Corrections Professionals*. Washington, DC: US Department of Justice, National Institute of Corrections; 2007.
62. Aydin E, Kevin M, Xie Z, Perry V. *Evaluation of the Getting SMART Program*. Sydney, Australia: NSW Justice Corrective Services; 2013.
63. Prochaska JO, Velicer WF, Rossi JS, et al. Stages of change and decisional balance for 12 problem behaviors. *Health Psych*. 1994;13(1):39–46.
64. Taxman FS, Belenko S. Organizational change—technology transfer processes: a review of the literature. In: Taxman FS, Belenko S, eds. *Implementing Evidence-Based Practices in Community Corrections and Addiction Treatment*. New York, NY: Springer New York; 2012:91–128.
65. McMurran M, Ward T. Treatment readiness, treatment engagement and behaviour change. *Crim Behav Mental Health*. 2010;20(2):75–85.
66. Irvin JE, Bowers CA, Dunn ME, Wang MC. Efficacy of relapse prevention: a meta-analytic review. *J Consult Clin Psychol*. 1999;67(4):563–570.
67. Jürgens R, World Health Organization. *Interventions to Address HIV in Prisons: Drug Dependence Treatments*. Vienna, Austria: United Nations Office on Drugs and Crime; 2007.

CHAPTER 17

Harm Reduction in Prisons

KATHRYN SNOW, MSc AND MICHAEL LEVY, MPH

INTRODUCTION

The criminalization of drug use directly results in the mass incarceration of people who use drugs. The use of incarceration against people who use drugs restricts their individual freedoms, including their capacity to make decisions regarding their own health, and thus potentially compounds the harms associated with drug use. The prison environment may be both directly and indirectly deleterious to health, frequently subjecting prisoners to overcrowding, poor nutrition, chronic stress, preventable exposure to communicable diseases, and restricted access to health services.[1] Prisoners have limited opportunities to protect their own health while incarcerated, with the result that responsibility for their health rests largely with correctional authorities and with the state. While this provides some prisoners with improved access to health services for some conditions, it may also remove access to health services that are available in the community—in particular, harm reduction services for injecting drug use.

People who use drugs commonly enter prison with complex health needs, which may be the result of poor engagement with the health system, drug dependence, poorly managed mental illness, or other chronic medical conditions. The prevalence of communicable diseases such as tuberculosis, viral hepatitis, and human immunodeficiency virus (HIV) infections, when measured, is often found to be substantially higher within prisons than in the surrounding community.[2,3] Some individuals enter prison with these infections, while others become infected while incarcerated.

Although prisons are frequently conceptualized and referred to as "closed environments," their walls are in fact semi-permeable, since both inmates and staff move between prison and the surrounding community. Communicable diseases not only circulate within prisons but also are imported and exported from and to the community. Thus, transmission of infection in prison potentiates epidemics in the surrounding community, which ultimately contributes new cases to the prison system.

Although prisoners may have a history of several forms of drug use, including heavy alcohol use (commonly involved in assaults and reckless driving charges) and misuse of prescribed medications (eg, benzodiazepines, opiate analgesics), the harms related to injecting drug use in particular are common, serious, well understood, and amenable to intervention. That many people continue to inject drugs in prison has been conclusively demonstrated in a variety of settings, as has the transmission of blood-borne viruses within prisons.[2,4] Indeed, the less detectable and more efficient nature of injecting drug use relative to other methods of drug administration (eg, smoking) may push prisoners toward injecting, at least when detection of either form of drug use is known to attract equivalent punitive sanctions.

The modes of transmission of viral hepatitis and HIV have been known for decades, and exposure to these diseases is not, or at least should not be, an accepted aspect of the prison experience. Many of the control measures that might be implemented to reduce the risks that prisoners face while incarcerated are well understood, and among these measures, harm reduction programs remain neglected in the overwhelming majority of settings.[1] In addition to blood-borne virus transmission, the transition to or continuation of injecting drug use puts prisoners at risk of other drug-related harms, including abscesses and vein damage, drug-drug interactions, and overdoses.

Harm reduction approaches to drug use are those that seek to minimize the risks associated with drug use rather than to simply minimize or prevent the actual use of drugs.[5] Harm reduction programs are incorporated into national public health systems to varying degrees in different countries, and many harm reduction interventions can also be implemented in prison settings.

The underlying principle of the United Nations (UN) Nelson Mandela Rules is that prison authorities have a responsibility to respect the inherent human dignity of all prisoners.[6] The first rule that specifically addresses health services (Rule 24) states that:

> The provision of health care for prisoners is a State responsibility. Prisoners should enjoy the same standards of health care that are available in the community, and should have access to necessary health-care services free of charge without discrimination on the grounds of their legal status. Health-care services should be organized in close relationship to the general public health administration and in a way that ensures continuity of treatment and care, including for HIV, tuberculosis and other infectious diseases, as well as for drug dependence.[6]

As such, in jurisdictions that make harm reduction measures available to people who use drugs in the community, the decision to deny equivalent services to prisoners constitutes a breach of their human rights. This alone provides a strong argument for instituting harm reduction measures in prisons, even under circumstances where the impact that they may have on disease transmission in a particular setting is difficult to prove.

The World Health Organization (WHO), the United Nations Office on Drugs and Crime (UNODC), and the Joint United Nations Program on HIV/AIDS have called repeatedly for the implementation of comprehensive harm reduction programs in prisons.[7,8] The specific measures that can and, per the Mandela Rules, should be implemented in prisons around the world are many and varied, and the success of each measure frequently depends on the effective implementation of others.

Effective health programming requires that we recognize that prisons are a part of broader society, and that prisoners are not in quarantine. Prisoners are drawn from the wider community, and almost all of them will eventually return to it. If the global epidemics of HIV and hepatitis C are to be effectively controlled, interventions to protect the health of prisoners are critical. Likewise, if we are committed to reducing the broader negative impacts of drug use on public health, the risk of incarceration exacerbating drug-related harms must be acknowledged and addressed.

HARM REDUCTION IN PRISONS

Because many prisoners experience multiple transitions between prison and the community, a comprehensive harm reduction approach to drug use in prisons must interface with measures taken in the community.[1] People who use drugs are often incarcerated repeatedly for short periods, and as such, ensuring continuity of care through harm reduction initiatives is critical. Small-scale programs focused on single interventions during incarceration are inadequate to address the drug-related harms to which prisoners and ex-prisoners are exposed. The elements that might be included in a comprehensive, prison-based harm reduction policy are listed in Table 17.1.

Core Harm Reduction Strategies Relevant to Prisoners

Insofar as incarceration can be understood as a harm of injecting drug use, or at least insofar as it may compound other harms, decriminalization and diversion may be considered harm reduction strategies. Incarceration is a cause of profound disruption to normal life. Family and other close relationships may be strained, and connections to community-based health services may be broken. Furthermore, fear of prosecution and harassment by police (eg, arrests on the basis of possession of injecting paraphernalia, including clean syringes) may substantially restrict access to harm reduction services in the community.[1] For people who are taking steps to address their drug dependence in the community, the interruption to psychosocial support and health services access that arrest and incarceration frequently entail may undermine their efforts.

After incarceration, reintegration into the community is notoriously difficult, with many ex-prisoners experiencing homelessness, unemployment, and life-threatening health complications in the months after release.[9-12] Common causes of post-release mortality include suicide and drug overdoses, with prisoners who use drugs at particularly high risk of death shortly after release. By implication, reducing the excessive incarceration of people who use drugs is a vital first step in mitigating drug-related harms.[13]

Table 17.1. ELEMENTS OF A COMPREHENSIVE HARM REDUCTION PROGRAM IN PRISON SETTINGS

Throughcare: Continuous, uninterrupted access to health services for the prevention and management of blood borne virus infections, problematic substance use, mental illness, and other chronic or acute conditions

At entry into prison	During incarceration	Upon release from prison
Universal health assessment that provides the opportunity for each of the following, subject to the consent of the individual prisoner:	Uninterrupted access to OST and antiviral therapy (UNODC,[34] WHO[32])	Referral to community-based health services to ensure continuity of care for those on, or in need, of antiviral therapy or treatment for drug or alcohol dependence (UNODC,[34] WHO[32])
1. Counseling and testing for HIV, hepatitis B, and hepatitis C, with access to appropriate preventative and treatment services as needed (WHO[32,33])	Access to clean injecting equipment (WHO,[32] UNODC[16])	Provision of naloxone and training of the released prisoner in its use (not yet an official UN recommendation; evidence to date reviewed by Strang et al.,[30] UNODC[34])
2. Provisions of vaccination for hepatitis B, ideally with an accelerated schedule (WHO[32,33])	Access to naloxone as a first-line response to opioid overdose, and amnesties for prisoners alerting staff to drug-related medical emergencies (UNODC[34])	
3. A mechanism by which opioid dependent prisoners can identify themselves and access timely opioid substitution treatment (UNODC,[34] WHO[32])	Health services that support disclosure of current drug use and that people who use drugs can access without discrimination or fear of repercussions, in particular vein care, treatment for abscesses, and safe prescribing in order to avoid drug-drug interactions (Mandela Rule 31c[6])	
	Minimal-barrier access to mental health services and treatment for drug and alcohol dependence (Mandela Rule 25[6])	

However, decriminalization and diversion alone would not prevent people who use drugs being incarcerated for other crimes, and prison-based measures to protect their health would still be necessary. States have a minimum obligation to provide prisoners with access to the WHO essential medicines, which include methadone and buprenorphine.[14] The denial of these drugs to prisoners who would otherwise experience the adverse effects of opiate withdrawal can be characterized as cruel, inhumane, or degrading treatment. Where these drugs are available to people who inject drugs in the community, the refusal to provide them to prisoners violates the principle of equivalence embodied in the Mandela Rules.

Furthermore, because the risk of fatal overdose in the weeks after release from prison is dramatically elevated (partly as a result of lowered tolerance following limited access to opioids in prison),[9] the refusal to provide opioid substitution therapy (OST) to prisoners may contribute to avoidable deaths after release. If such deaths are to be prevented, prison-based OST programs must include strong referral mechanisms to ensure continuity of care during the high-risk period immediately after return to the community. Release onto OST in the community has been shown to be a highly cost-effective way of reducing post-release mortality among opioid-dependent ex-prisoners in Australia,[15] and it seems likely that the same would be true elsewhere. Prison-based OST programs and other demand reduction measures are described in detail in chapter 16.

For those who do continue to inject drugs in prison, adequate infection control measures must be implemented to prevent, or at least minimize, the risk of exposure to blood-borne viruses. At the time of writing, needle and syringe programs (NSPs) have been implemented in at least 60 prisons in 11 countries.[4] Various approaches to distribution have been trialed, including vending machines, dispensing by prison health service staff, and peer-led initiatives.[16] These programs have been shown to decrease risky injecting behavior and virus transmission without leading to increases in injecting drug use[17]; however, such programs remain unavailable in the overwhelming majority of prisons worldwide, due in part to continued political opposition in many settings.

For opioid-dependent prisoners who continue to inject, incarceration in a setting without needle and syringe exchange facilities may require higher-risk injecting behavior than they would otherwise engage in. For those who are hepatitis C- or HIV-naive, sharing injecting equipment in prison presents a very high risk of exposure. Outbreaks of HIV, hepatitis B, and hepatitis C have been described in several prisons,[18-20] and the high viral load experienced shortly after seroconversion to HIV may facilitate especially rapid transmission through prison injecting networks. Treatment of HIV, hepatitis B, and hepatitis C suppresses viremia, reducing the risk of transmission to others. The provision of treatment for viral hepatitis and for HIV, then, may be considered an ecological harm reduction measure, complementing individual measures such as NSP access and OST provision. The management of HIV and hepatitis C in prisons is discussed in chapters 7 and 9, respectively.

A second intervention targeted toward individuals that may also protect those around them is the provision of the opioid antagonist naloxone, both in prison and upon release. Naloxone, which is a first-line treatment for opioid overdose that is administered via intramuscular injection or intranasal spray,[21] can be carried by people who are likely to be in attendance prior to the arrival of emergency medical personnel. The effects of opioid overdose make self-administration difficult; however, naloxone can be administered either by its owner to a "buddy" experiencing an overdose, or by the buddy to the owner, provided appropriate instructions are given ahead of time. Naloxone may be provided to prisoners as an in-prison harm reduction measure; it should also be provided upon release to mitigate the substantial risks of fatal overdose after return to the community.[22]

EVALUATING THE EVIDENCE FOR HARM REDUCTION INTERVENTIONS IN PRISONS

Evidence regarding the implementation of harm reduction interventions in community settings is abundant; however, research focused specifically on implementation in prisons is sparser, with the majority of studies focused on reducing recidivism rather than improving health. Attempts at rigorous evaluation of harm reduction interventions in prison settings are complicated by a variety of factors, some specific to the prison health field, and some common to many population health interventions. Selecting an appropriate "control" or comparator against which to measure the impact of a given harm reduction intervention is challenging. Several of the interventions described here have been (or could be) adopted at the level of individual prisons, within state or provincial prison systems, or at the national level. Before-and-after comparisons in the same setting may be confounded by changes in other relevant factors over time, and comparisons between different prisons, prison systems, or countries may be confounded by other important differences between them. Unfortunately, although programs in real-world settings may be evaluated using observational and sometimes even randomized approaches, producing "gold standard" evidence on the impact of harm reduction interventions in prisons is not always possible.

Measuring the impact of a given harm reduction intervention requires reliable ascertainment of drug-related harms among prisoners and ex-prisoners, for instance, by accurately measuring the incidence of overdoses (both fatal and nonfatal) and seroconversions after exposure to blood-borne viruses. Ascertaining such events requires repeated contact with individuals both in prison and after release, something that is notoriously challenging in many longitudinal studies, especially in this population.[23] Even if perfect ascertainment of these types of events were feasible, without high-quality randomized controlled trials it would be difficult to determine whether any positive changes in the incidence of these events were due to the intervention or to other factors such as concurrent changes in patterns of drug use, changes in legislation and policing, or improvements to community-based health services.

Given the highly politicized nature of the problem of drug-related harms in society, and of many of the solutions at hand, debate over the efficacy of specific interventions is often protracted and sometimes irresolvable. Perfect epidemiological rigor in the assessment of some harm reduction interventions for incarcerated drug users may be impossible; however, several of the interventions described in this chapter are supported by those evaluations that have been undertaken in prisons, as well as extensive evaluation of their impacts when implemented in the broader community. The case for their implementation is further strengthened by the demands of international human rights law.[1]

In the absence of evidence that they cause substantial harms of their own, arguments against implementing harm reduction measures consistent with the human rights of incarcerated people who use drugs are weak. The histories of the implementation of two core interventions not discussed in detail elsewhere in this book are detailed in the following, along with what evidence is currently available regarding their impacts.

Case Study 1: Needle and Syringe Programs in Switzerland and Germany

In the early 1990s the world's first prison-based NSPs were implemented in Switzerland.[16] Two decades later, at least 60 NSPs have been implemented in prisons in 11 countries, using a variety of distribution methods, including dispensing machines, provision by prison health staff or non-governmental organizations, and peer-led delivery programs.[4] The most extensive programs have been implemented in Spain and Kyrgyzstan; however, the programs in Switzerland and Germany have been subjected to the most comprehensive evaluations.[17] The majority of these evaluations have been published in German. The following information is drawn predominantly from a book chapter[24] and two review articles,[4,17] all published in English, as well as several additional journal articles.

Of seven evaluated prison-based NSPs in Germany, all observed substantial decreases in self-reported sharing of injecting equipment, and none observed an increase in injecting drug use. There were no reported incidents in which a syringe was used as a weapon in any of the prisons with an NSP in place. Staff, including prison officers, expressed support for programs in several evaluations; in particular, NSPs were perceived by prison staff to contribute to their safety by reducing the risk of needle-stick injuries from concealed injecting equipment.[17,24] They were also perceived to facilitate the enrolment of PWID into treatment for drug dependence. None of the three evaluations that assessed blood-borne virus transmission observed any cases of seroconversion for HIV while the programs were in place.[17]

After the implementation of NSPs in two Berlin prisons, four hepatitis C seroconversions were reported among 124 prisoners over a 32-month period.[25] The baseline prevalence of hepatitis C antibodies among participants with a history of injecting drug use in this study was 71%, and given the natural history of the disease, approximately three-quarters of these inmates would have had active (and therefore infectious) hepatitis C. Hepatitis C is substantially more infectious than HIV; as a consequence, sharing injecting equipment on even a few occasions presents a high risk of infection to hepatitis C–naive prisoners. Given the very high prevalence of infection in the prisons at that time, the apparently low incidence of transmission after the implementation of the NSP is striking.

However, the seroconversions in this example show that NSPs alone are not sufficient to reduce hepatitis C transmission in prisons to zero, and as such they highlight the need for additional hepatitis C prevention measures alongside NSPs. As long as PWID are incarcerated in large numbers, the background prevalence of active hepatitis C infection in prisons will remain high, unless hepatitis C prevalence among PWID in the community is lowered very substantially. Treatment as prevention may help to reduce the risks to hepatitis C–naive prisoners, particularly as direct-acting antivirals become more widely available.[26] Hepatitis C infection control and treatment programs must be implemented simultaneously in order to be effective at lowering transmission within prisons; the risk of reinfection to those who are cured but continue to inject will remain high unless these individuals can protect themselves against re-exposure by using only sterile injecting equipment (or abstaining from injecting entirely).

In spite of their apparent effectiveness at reducing risky injecting behaviors, attempts to implement or expand prison-based NSPs around the world have met with substantial resistance. Notably, prison officers in several German states opposed the introduction of NSPs, although they later came to support them after implementation.[17] Programs in several prisons around Germany have been closed after changes in state governments, often against the express wishes of prison staff. At the time of writing, despite protracted efforts in several countries and repeated recommendations from the WHO and other UN agencies, there are no prison-based NSPs anywhere in the English-speaking world.

Case Study 2: Post-Release Naloxone in the United Kingdom

The risk of death after release from prison has been documented through multiple data linkage studies in Europe, Australia, North America, and Asia.[12] The crude rate of mortality among released prisoners across these settings was 38 per 1,000 persons in the year after release (95% confidence interval 23-64), although these rates vary markedly by study and setting. Within the first year after release, ex-prisoners are at an estimated 20-fold higher risk of death than members of the general public. Many studies find that a high proportion of deaths shortly after release from prison are drug related, and that ex-prisoners with a history of drug use are at higher risk of death than those without such a history.[9,12]

In 2011, Scotland instituted its National Naloxone Program, with the aim of reducing opioid-related deaths through the provision of naloxone to people at risk of overdose, including those being released from prison.[27] This occurred in the context of a broader policy debate over how, when, and to whom naloxone should be provided in the United Kingdom. This debate was sparked, in part, by the development of and planning for a large randomized controlled trial of take-home naloxone for heroin users leaving prison, the N-ALIVE trial.[22] Prior to the beginning of recruitment for the trial, Scotland's Department of Health decided to pre-emptively implement take-home naloxone as official policy, based on the strength of existing observational evidence for its benefits.

At the time of implementation, Scotland's rate of drug-related death was 11 per 100,000 population per year, around five times the UK average.[28] The average age of those who died was 37 years, compared with the national life expectancy of 78 years. Opioids were the class of drugs most commonly implicated in drug-related deaths, often in combination with benzodiazepines and/or alcohol. Prior to implementation, an average of 10% of opioid-related deaths annually occurred within 4 weeks of release from prison; after implementation, this proportion decreased steadily to 3.8% in 2014,[29] suggesting that the program reduced the danger faced by released prisoners in this high-risk period.

Although the trend after implementation is striking, conclusively demonstrating the impacts of take-home naloxone for prisoners on mortality in Scotland is complicated by the same factors that complicate all evaluations of national health policy. However, other opportunities for evaluation exist, since the United Kingdom as a whole is currently at a transitional stage with regard to naloxone provision. Although Scotland and Wales have adopted naloxone provision as official health policy and developed programs for its delivery, England has refrained, and the randomized controlled trial is now underway there.[22]

The N-ALIVE trial, originally planned to cover all three jurisdictions, is now recruiting in England only, with a planned sample size of 56,000 released prisoners who are to be randomized to receive either take-home naloxone or standard care.[30] This will allow a direct, robust assessment of the impact of take-home naloxone on post-release mortality without confounding by national or historical factors that complicate the evaluation of the Scottish program, and should provide high-quality evidence to guide implementation in other jurisdictions around the world.

CONCLUSION

Although harm reduction programs have a long history of implementation in community settings, their implementation in prisons has lagged behind substantially, undermining broader efforts to mitigate drug-related harms. If prisons are to play a meaningful role in broader harm reduction efforts, prison authorities will need to come to terms with a shift away from an emphasis on the control and prohibition of drugs, toward a focus on the health and welfare of prisoners—including those who continue to use drugs while incarcerated.

Additional evidence from both community and prison settings is needed to identify the optimal ways of implementing some harm reduction measures during and around incarceration, and to build the evidence base required to overcome sometimes substantial political opposition to particular interventions. There is a need to establish the impact of decriminalization and diversion on drug-related harms, interventions that have not yet been subject to extensive evaluation even observationally. There is abundant evidence from Germany and Switzerland regarding the impact of in-prison NSPs, and from other settings regarding the impact of in-prison

OST as described in chapter 16. High-quality evidence on the impact of take-home naloxone is expected to emerge from the United Kingdom in the coming years, both from implementation in Scotland and Wales and from the randomized controlled trial currently underway in England.

In addition to current and developing evidence regarding in-prison implementation, a compelling case for implementing harm reduction strategies in prison settings is provided by evidence of successful implementation in community settings, as well as by international human rights law as described in chapter 12. Although much of society may not condone recreational illicit drug use, it must be acknowledged that incarceration does not in itself stop the harmful use of substances, and that the state has a responsibility to protect the health of those it incarcerates. Prisoners and prison staff are entitled to the same level of health protection as those living and working in the broader community. Combined political will and advocacy around the implementation of harm reduction strategies with a single focus—the minimization of drug-related harms, rather than the cessation of illicit drug use—is necessary.

The major achievement of this endeavor would be the long-overdue recognition and protection of the rights of prisoners. This would, in turn, have benefits for the health and welfare of their loved ones and the wider community. There would of course also be benefits to governments, prison authorities, and prison staff: the financial costs associated with the criminalization of drug use and our collective failure to mitigate its harms are massive, and the work of prison staff who witness repeated returns to custody after relapses into drug dependence is often unfulfilling. The comparative financial cost of harm reduction measures is trivial,[31] and their benefits can be profound. While some of the changes required are radical, their introduction can be incremental. Ultimately, though, nothing less than total implementation will effectively address the harms that prisoners endure, and in which prison staff are complicit.

REFERENCES

1. Jürgens R, Csete J, Amon JJ, Baral S, Beyrer C. People who use drugs, HIV, and human rights. *Lancet*. 2010;376(9739):475–485.
2. Larney S, Kopinski H, Beckwith CG, et al. Incidence and prevalence of hepatitis C in prisons and other closed settings: results of a systematic review and meta-analysis. *Hepatology*. 2013;58(4):1215–1224.
3. Gough E, Kempf M, Graham L, et al. HIV and hepatitis B and C incidence rates in US correctional populations and high risk groups: a systematic review and meta-analysis. *BMC Public Health*. 2010;10(777):1–14.
4. Jürgens R, Nowak M, Day M. HIV and incarceration: prisons and detention. *J Int AIDS Soc*. 2011;14(26):1–17.
5. Hunt N, Ashton M, Lenton S, Mitcheson L, Nelles B, Stimson G. *A Review of the Evidence-Base for Harm Reduction Approaches to Drug Use*. London, England: Forward Thinking on Drugs: A Release Initiative; 2010.
6. United Nations General Assembly. *United Nations Standard Minimum Rules for the Treatment of Prisoners (the Nelson Mandela Rules)*. Vienna, Austria: UNODC; 2015.

7. UNAIDS. *Guidance Note: Services for People in Prisons and Other Closed Settings.* Geneva, Switzerland: UNAIDS; 2014.
8. UNODC. *Policy Brief. HIV Prevention, Treatment and Care in Prisons and Other Closed Settings: A Comprehensive Package of Interventions.* Vienna, Austria: UNODC; 2012.
9. Merrall EL, Kariminia A, Binswanger IA, et al. Meta-analysis of drug-related deaths soon after release from prison. *Addiction.* 2010;105(9):1545–1554.
10. Chang Z, Lichtenstein P, Larsson H, Fazel S. Substance use disorders, psychiatric disorders, and mortality after release from prison: a nationwide longitudinal cohort study. *Lancet Psychiat.* 2015;2(5):422–430.
11. Jama-Alol KA, Malacova E, Ferrante A, Alan J, Stewart L, Preen D. Influence of offence type and prior imprisonment on risk of death following release from prison: a whole-population linked data study. *Int J Prison Health.* 2015;11(2):108–118.
12. Kinner SA, Forsyth S, Williams G. Systematic review of record linkage studies of mortality in ex-prisoners: why (good) methods matter. *Addiction.* 2013;108(1):38–49.
13. Csete J, Kamarulzaman A, Kazatchkine M, et al. Public health and international drug policy. *Lancet.* 2016;387(10026):1427–1480.
14. Hogerzeil HV. Essential medicines and human rights: what can they learn from each other? *Bull World Health Organ.* 2006;84(5):371–375.
15. Gisev N, Shanahan M, Weatherburn DJ, et al. A cost-effectiveness analysis of opioid substitution therapy upon prison release in reducing mortality among people with a history of opioid dependence. *Addiction.* 2015;110(12):1975–1984.
16. UNODC. *A Handbook for Starting and Managing Needle and Syringe Programmes in Prisons and Other Closed Settings.* Vienna, Austria: UNODC;2014.
17. Jürgens R, Ball A, Verster A. Interventions to reduce HIV transmission related to injecting drug use in prison. *Lancet Infect Dis.* 2009;9(1):57–66.
18. Centers for Disease Control Prevention. Hepatitis B outbreak in a state correctional facility, 2000. *MMWR Morb Mortal Wkly Rep.* 2001;50(25):529–532.
19. Hutchinson S, Goldberg D, Gore S, et al. Hepatitis B outbreak at Glenochil prison during January to June 1993. *Epidemiol Infect.*1998;121(1):185–191.
20. Taylor A, Goldberg D, Emslie J, et al. Outbreak of HIV infection in a Scottish prison. *BMJ.* 1995;310(6975):289–292.
21. Kerr D, Kelly AM, Dietze P, Jolley D, Barger B. Randomized controlled trial comparing the effectiveness and safety of intranasal and intramuscular naloxone for the treatment of suspected heroin overdose. *Addiction.* 2009;104(12):2067–2074.
22. Strang J, Bird SM, Dietze P, Gerra G, McLellan AT. Take-home emergency naloxone to prevent deaths from heroin overdose. *BMJ.* 2014;349:g6580.
23. David MC, Alati R, Ware RS, Kinner SA. Attrition in a longitudinal study with hard-to-reach participants was reduced by ongoing contact. *J Clin Epidemiol.* 2013;66(5):575–581.
24. Stöver H, Kastelic A. *Drug Treatment and Harm Reduction in Prisons.* In: Enggist S, Møller L, Galea G, Udesen C, eds. Prisons and Health. Copenhangen, Denmark: World Health Organization; 2014;113–133.
25. Stark K, Herrmann U, Ehrhardt S, Bienzle U. A syringe exchange programme in prison as prevention strategy against HIV infection and hepatitis B and C in Berlin, Germany. *Epidemiol Infect.* 2006;134(4):814–819.
26. Hellard M, Doyle JS, Sacks-Davis R, Thompson AJ, McBryde E. Eradication of hepatitis C infection: the importance of targeting people who inject drugs. *Hepatology.* 2014;59(2):366–369.
27. Information Services Division Scotland. *National Naloxone Programme Scotland— Naloxone Kits Issued in 2013/14 and Trends in Opioid-Related Deaths.* Edinburgh, Scotland: Information Services Division; 2014.
28. UK Focal Point on Drugs. *United Kingdom Drug Situation.* London, England: UK Focal Point on Drugs; 2013.

29. Information Services Division Scotland. *National Naloxone Programme Scotland: Monitoring Report 2014/15*. Edinburgh, Scotland: Information Services Division; 2015.

30. Strang J, Bird SM, Parmar MK. Take-home emergency naloxone to prevent heroin overdose deaths after prison release: rationale and practicalities for the N-ALIVE randomized trial. *J Urban Health*. 2013;90(5):983–996.

31. Harm Reduction International. *Global State of Harm Reduction 2014*. London, England: Harm Reduction International; 2014.

CHAPTER 18

Preventing Drug-Related Death in Recently Released Prisoners

JULIE BRUMMER, MPH, LARS MØLLER, MD, AND
STEFAN ENGGIST, MA

INTRODUCTION

Findings from a broad range of studies consistently demonstrate increased drug-related mortality rates among ex-prisoners, compared with the general population.[1-13] Most drug-related deaths among ex-prisoners, especially in the period immediate following release, are due to overdose, and opioid overdose in particular. The concurrent use of multiple drugs[14] and decreased tolerance resulting from a period of abstinence or diminished drug use during incarceration are thought to contribute to these incidents.

Table 18.1 summarizes results from selected studies in Australia, Denmark, the United Kingdom, France, Switzerland, the United States, and Taiwan comparing drug-related standardized mortality ratios (SMRs) of ex-prisoners to a reference population. Although there is considerable variability in the extent to which the rate of death is elevated compared with matched members of the wider community, the data consistently show that post-release drug-related mortality rates greatly surpass the adjusted rates of the general population.

Table 18.2 presents findings from studies examining the relative risk of drug-related mortality among ex-prisoners in the first 2 weeks after release against a specified period thereafter. The data illustrate that, in all studies, the prospect of ex-prisoners dying from drugs in the first 2 weeks after discharge exceeds that of drug-related death during a subsequent post-release period.

In sum, the findings presented in Tables 18.1 and 18.2 highlight the alarmingly high rate of drug-related death risk among ex-prisoners both in the immediate post-release period and in the long term.

Table 18.1. STANDARDIZED MORTALITY RATIO (SMR) FOR DRUG-RELATED DEATH IN EX-PRISONERS (SELECTED STUDIES)

Study	SMR (95% CI) for post-release drug-related mortality	Time frame (post-release)	Reference population	SMR adjustments (original study)
Binswanger et al. (2007)[9]	Males and females = 129.0	First 2 weeks	Residents of Washington State, USA	Age, sex, and race
Binswanger et al. (2013)[13, a]	Males and females = 10.3	Not time limited (median = 4.4 years)	Residents of Washington State, USA	Age, sex, and race
Chen et al. (2010)[12, b]	Total = 29.3 Schedule I users = 76.3 Schedule II users = 16.4	3 years	General population of Taiwan	Age and sex
Christensen et al. (2006)[4]	Males and females = 61.9[c]	First 2 weeks	General population of Denmark	Age and sex
Farrell and Marsden (2008)[6]	Males, first week after release = 28.3 Males, second week after release = 15.8 Females, first week after release = 68.9 Females, second week after release = 56.3	First and second weeks (calculated separately)	General population of England and Wales	Age and sex
Harding-Pink (1990)[8]	Males and females = 50.0[c]	First 45 days	Population of Geneva, Switzerland	Age and sex
Kariminia et al. (2007a)[2]	Males = 14.5 Females = 50.3	Not time limited, follow-up ranged from 1 day to 15 years (median = 7.7 years)	Population of New South Wales, Australia	Age and sex
Lim et al. (2012)[11, d]	8.0 2.2	First 2 weeks Follow-up ranged during study period of 2001–2004	General population of New York City	Age, sex, race, and neighborhood
Singleton et al. (2003)[5]	First week after release = 37.1 Second week after release = 12.4 (male and female combined)[e]	First and second weeks (calculated separately)	General population of England and Wales	Age and sex

Table 18.1. CONTINUED

Study	SMR (95% CI) for post-release drug-related mortality	Time frame (post-release)	Reference population	SMR adjustments (original study)
Spaulding et al. (2011)[10]	3.5[f]	Up to 15.5 years	General population of New York City	Age, sex, race, educational level
Stewart et al. (2004)[1]	Female Aboriginal = 3.3 Female non-Aboriginal = 115.9 Male Aboriginal = 2.9 Male non-Aboriginal = 20.1	Not time limited, follow-up ranged from 0–2,160 days (median = 1,223 days)	Aboriginal and non-Aboriginal populations of Western Australia aged 20–40 years	Ethnicity, age, and sex
Verger et al. (2003)[7]	15–34 years = 124.1 35–54 years = 274.2 (male only)	First year	General population of France	Age and sex

[a] Participants included the cohort studied by Binswanger et al. (2007), with additional follow-up time through 2009, as well as participants released from 2004 to 2009.
[b] Study participants: first-time drug offenders.
[c] Authors' calculations: the estimate was based on deaths per 1,000 person-years of reference population and discharged prisoners. No confidence interval (CI) was obtained.
[d] Studied people released from New York City jails.
[e] The CI was not specified by Singleton et al. (2003).
[f] Accidental poisoning.

THE RISKS

Overdose is the principle cause of drug-related death among ex-prisoners immediately after release. Although a number of factors contribute to these deaths, the decreased tolerance resulting from a period of abstinence or reduced drug use during incarceration, followed by concurrent use of multiple drugs, are believed to be especially important. By the same process of lowered tolerance, acute drug-related mortality is disproportionately high among ex-prisoners who relapse subsequent to prison methadone detoxification.[8,15] Indeed, having undertaken methadone detoxification within the past year is positively correlated with overdose, whereas the inverse is true of methadone maintenance.[16] Thus, as noted in chapter 16, retention in prison and community methadone maintenance therapy is associated with a decline in mortality among ex-prisoners.[17,18] This may be understood by acknowledging that opioid dependence is a chronic disorder that disposes sufferers to high relapse rates and often requires long-term continuous treatment. Substance dependence is overrepresented among both prison populations[19,20] and drug-related fatalities in ex-prisoners.[5,8,21]

Table 18.2. TEMPORAL MATCHING IN STUDIES ASSESSING THE RELATIVE
RISK (RR) OF DRUG-RELATED DEATH IN THE FIRST 2 WEEKS AFTER RELEASE,
COMPARED WITH OTHER TIMES AFTERWARD

Study	Country	RR (temporal matching)	Temporal comparison
Bird and Hutchinson (2003)[79]	Scotland	7.4	Subsequent 10 weeks (3–12 weeks)
Christensen et al. (2006)[4]	Denmark	4.6[a]	Subsequent 10 weeks (3–12 weeks)
Farrell and Marsden (2008)[6]	England and Wales	Male = 8.3 Female = 10.6	52 weeks
Kariminia et al. (2007b)[34]	Australia (New South Wales)	Male = 9.3 Female = 6.4	26 weeks
Lim et al. (2012)[11]	United States	3.8	5 weeks or more since release
Ødegård et al. (2010)[80]	Norway	10.2[b]	Up to 52 weeks
Seaman, Brettle, and Gore (1998)[81]	Scotland (Edinburgh)	7.7[c]	Subsequent 10 weeks (3–12 weeks)
Singleton et al. (2003)[5]	England and Wales	First week = 12.5 Second week = 4.2	13–52 weeks

[a] Study participants: drug users.
[b] Adjusted for gender, age at first imprisonment, age at first illicit drug use, years of drug abuse, and daily use of opioids the year before admission.
[c] Study participants: injecting drug users infected with HIV.

A significant percentage of post-release drug-related deaths result from the concurrent use of multiple psychoactive substances.[5,8,9,13,14,21–24] The respiratory depressive effects of opioids are enhanced by concurrent administration of other drugs, especially central nervous system depressants such as alcohol, benzodiazepines, and tricyclic antidepressants.[25,26] Gossop et al.[27] established that, for every supplementary illicit drug administered in conjunction with an opioid, the risk of death from opioids nearly doubles. McGregor et al.[28] reported that co-administration of heroin and psychotropic substances occurred in three quarters of fatal overdoses among ex-prisoners in the month after release. The authors reflected on the inherent difficulties in determining the relative effects of diminished tolerance versus the use of multiple psychoactive drugs in contributing to death. The cumulative effect of these distinct processes, however, places ex-prisoners at a significantly elevated risk of acute drug-related mortality in the immediate post-release period, compared with other periods after release. Prisoners are often insufficiently aware of the risks posed by either decreased tolerance or the concomitant use of multiple psychoactive substances after release from custody. It is the responsibility of pre-release prison programs to educate prisoners adequately about the nature and extent of these risks.

Tied to the processes just discussed are risk factors, including chronic disease progression and socio-demographic determinants. According to non-prisoner-specific studies,[29] drug-related deaths among ex-prisoners typically occur in people older than 25 years of age,[5,7,9,22,30] suggesting extended careers of substance use. Using a retrospective cohort study design, Binswanger et al.[31] investigated the association between inmate characteristics and risk of death in the post-release period. The cohort was investigated in a previous study assessing the risk of death compared with a general population.[9] Binswanger et al.[31] found that, for participants under age 50, each additional 10 years of age was significantly associated with an increased risk of all-cause mortality, overdose death, and death within 30 days of liberation. However, for participants over 50, there was a significant relationship only between increasing age and all-cause mortality. In a study focusing on risk of death among young adult ex-prisoners, van Dooren et al.[32] found that the SMR for all-cause mortality decreased with age. In other words, the elevated risk of all-cause death compared with the general population was higher among those under 25 than among older ex-prisoners. Nearly half of the deaths among the young ex-prisoners were due to drug-related causes. Looking at risk of death among different age groups at the time of release from prison, Singleton et al.[5] found that in all age groups, there was a higher number of deaths compared with what would be expected of matched groups in the general population, but the risk was highest among 25- to 39-year-olds. Furthermore, approximately two thirds of the higher risk in this age group was attributable to drug-related causes. Singleton et al.[5] determined that, of the subset of prisoners who subsequently died of drug-related causes (as compared with the whole sample), 72% were assessed as being drug-dependent within the year of interview, with 40% dependent on opiates and stimulants; 85% used drugs in the month before their prison term, and 54% had abstained from drugs while in prison. Both drug use in the month before incarceration and in-prison drug abstinence were found to be independently associated with post-release drug-related mortality.

There is also evidence that individuals who experience multiple imprisonments are at an increased risk of post-release death,[8,33,34] which implies a cumulative detrimental effect of periods of reduced tolerance due to disruption to drug use or treatment.

There is evidence that drug-related deaths in female ex-prisoners on average occur at a younger age than among males. Farrell and Marsden[21] found that more than two thirds of excess drug-related mortality in a cohort of ex-prisoners occurred in men aged 25 to 39 years and women aged 20 to 29 years. Similarly, Kariminia et al.[34] found that the age distribution of deaths in a cohort of ex-prisoners in Australia differed by gender, such that drug-related SMRs among women showed a decreasing trend with increasing age, while drug-related mortality among men was prominent among the youngest and oldest age groups.

Consistent with the fact that the vast majority of prisoners in most countries are male, the majority of drug-related deaths in ex-prisoners are among men. However, studies in a number of countries have found that the elevation in risk of drug-related death (the SMR) is greater for female ex-prisoners.[1,2,6,13,35] Studies from Australia, England and Wales, and Switzerland have shown that for both men and women, most post-release substance-related deaths involved opioids,[5,8,21,22] although recent research from Australia suggests that such findings may not capture differences in patterns of substance use among subgroups in a population.[36]

Besides age and sex, a number of sociodemographic characteristics are associated with an increased risk of post-release drug-related mortality. Studies from Australia, England and Wales, and the United States have indicated that inmates from the dominant ethnic background are at a relatively heightened risk of drug-related mortality[1,5,11,13,21,34]; however, such results should be considered in light of recent research examining differences in patterns of use among subgroups, and implications for substance-related causes of death.[36] As regards mental health factors, studies employing a multivariate statistical analysis have found that in-prison psychiatric hospital admission,[34] suicidality, in-prison victimization, and taking medication that acted on the central nervous system[5] are independent predictors of drug-related mortality. However, similar analyses of criminological risk factors have not shown a consistent association between offense type (eg, imprisonment for a sex-related crime or a property crime) and drug-related death.[5,34] Additional independent risk factors for post-release drug-related mortality include living off crime before the current prison term and having a primary support network of fewer than four people.[5] These findings emphasize that many ex-prisoners lack formal and informal psychosocial support structures.

Comparing Australian ex-prisoners who died from accidental drug-related causes with those who died from all other causes, Andrews and Kinner[14] found that those who died from drug-related causes were significantly younger (median age of 30 vs. 36), less likely to be Indigenous, Australian-born, married, or living alone and were less likely to have had a mental health condition or a risk of self-harm noted in the coronial record. Drug-related mortality was also associated with recent injecting drug use, history of heroin use, and drug withdrawal/detox in the past 6 months.

Several recent studies have investigated the relationship between duration of imprisonment and risk of premature mortality, but a clear trend has not emerged as to whether longer prison stays are protective or hazardous. Using administrative records of former inmates who had served no more than 10 years in prison and were released to parole in New York from 1989 to 1993 and followed through 2003, Patterson[37] found that time in prison had a negative dose-response relationship with life span. Controlling for time spent on parole and other demographic and criminal justice–related variables, Patterson[37] found that for each year that the individual was incarcerated, the odds of all-cause death during the post-release period increased by 15.6%. The risk was most elevated immediately following release and subsequently declined so that each month that an individual was on parole decreased the odds of all-cause death by 2.0%. For every year spent in prison, the expected life span of an ex-prisoner was reduced by approximately 2 years. The expected life span of ex-prisoners was found to return to pre-prison levels after they had been on parole for the equivalent of two thirds of the time they were in prison. Furthermore, Lim et al.[11] found that longer jail sentences were associated with a shorter duration between release and drug-related death, and van Dooren et al.[32] found that longer duration of incarceration (measured in 1-year increments) was associated with an increased hazard for post-release death. However, Binswanger et al.[31] found that, among former inmates, increased duration of incarceration (assessed in 1-year increments) had a significant protective effect for all-cause mortality and overdose deaths in particular, after adjustment for other covariates, including age. This protective effect was also found in a subsequent study of this cohort, which included additional follow-up time and analysis of inmates released in the subsequent 6 years.[13]

The settings in which drug-related deaths in ex-prisoners occur highlight the social obstacles and marginalization encountered by ex-prisoners on release—in particular, the difficulty of procuring permanent housing.[22] Looking at a particularly vulnerable sub-group, formerly-incarcerated individuals who used a homeless shelter, Lim et al.[11] found that these individuals had a significantly increased rate of drug-related mortality compared with former inmates who had not spent at least one night in a shelter. However, these findings provide insight into potential target areas for programs that might reduce drug-related death in ex-prisoners, such as assistance in securing accommodation. Furthermore, because a significant proportion of drug-related deaths occur in residential settings, observers may be trained to recognize, intervene in, and seek medical assistance for an overdose.[5,14,21]

However, in a retrospective registry study of all drug-induced deaths occurring between January 1, 2006, and December 31, 2008, among individuals aged 15 to 65 in Oslo (a total of 231 deaths), Gjersing et al.[38] found that half of the 18 deceased former inmates were found outdoors or in public buildings; this contrasts with findings from other studies indicating that most post-release drug-related deaths occur in residential settings.[5,14,21] Eight of the deaths occurred in the first 2 weeks after release. The median time from release until death was 18 days. Toxicology reports showed that heroin overdose was the main cause of death in 83% of the cases.[38]

HUMAN RIGHTS CONTEXT

In accordance with international law and human rights instruments (see chapter 12), the effect of imprisonment on human rights is limited to the deprivation of liberty,[39] referred to as "limited exceptionalism."[40] As such, prisoners, like all people, are to be afforded the highest attainable standard of physical and mental health,[41–43] fulfilling the principle of "equivalence of care" between prison and community healthcare service provision.[39,44–48] Also, a consolidated system of healthcare in prisons is advocated, such that prison health systems interact or integrate with national public health systems.[47–50]

As expressed by the joint World Health Organization (WHO), United Nations Office on Drugs and Crime, and Joint United Nations Program on HIV/AIDS position paper on substitution maintenance therapy,[51] a flexible, needs-based, client-centered approach to opioid dependence is necessary to effectively address the individual needs of clients. Utilization of pharmacotherapy, of which substitution maintenance therapy is an "important component,"[51] psychotherapy, psychosocial rehabilitation, and risk reduction interventions are thus endorsed. With respect to prisons, harm reduction and prevention measures are recommended[46,52]; and in nations where methadone maintenance therapy is available in the community, this therapy is to be extended to prisoners, so that they may continue or initiate substitution therapy while in custody.[46,53] Failure to do so may constitute torture or cruel, inhumane, or degrading treatment or punishment, or a breach of the right to life.[54,55]

While regional and international instruments detail comprehensive recommendations on minimum standards of prisoner health, it is the responsibility of national authorities to determine how to best implement these principles.

MODELS AND PRACTICE IN COUNTRIES

Specific models and interventions to reduce drug-related deaths in ex-prisoners have been developed in many countries. Examples from Australia, Canada, England and Wales, and Spain are described here.

With reference to system-wide policy and practice modalities, a case in point is that of the framework for England and Wales, which delivers an integrated multi-entry-point throughcare model of drug treatment. This national framework, the Integrated Drug Treatment System in Prisons in partnership with the Drug Interventions Program, enlists the multidisciplinary collaboration of therapeutic jurisprudence structures. The provision of prison healthcare services, under the direction of the National Health Service since 2004, utilizes evidence-based therapy and, in so doing, has vastly expanded the prison-based methadone maintenance therapy program.[56,57] The objective of the Drug Interventions Program is to guide adult drug users into treatment and away from crime. The commitment of political and professional entities endorses the principle of equivalence of care with community-based interventions in terms of quality, coverage, and treatment alternatives. To this end, comprehensive training packages and guides[57,58] and protocols on modes of clinical management[59-61] have been developed for working with drug-using prisoners.

Additionally, judicial provisions—such as conditional cautioning, restrictions on bail, drug treatment and testing orders, and the drug rehabilitation requirement of community orders—redirect prisoners into treatment at the expense of the prison.[56,62] The national framework also documents end-to-end strategic guidelines for throughcare and aftercare, from a prisoner's first contact with the criminal justice system.[63] Indeed, team case management maintains continuity of care as individuals make the transition between prison (counseling, assessment, referral, advice, and throughcare services) and the community (criminal justice integrated teams), utilizing a common data-gathering instrument, the Drug Interventions Record.[56]

Best practice in system-wide service delivery for drug-dependent prisoners requires a range of treatment options founded on evidence-based practices. This requires that interventions incorporate flexible client-centered programs, utilizing a multiphase interdisciplinary approach of an equivalent standard to community interventions. The WHO Regional Office for Europe[52] has outlined harm reduction strategies of relevance to prison populations. These include needle and syringe exchange programs, educational measures in the form of overdose prevention programs, formalized information dissemination, outlining of treatment expectations and peer-based support, and pharmacotherapy. The Regional Office further advocates the inclusion of substitution therapy as a central component of prison pharmacotherapy interventions, in recognition of its currently being the most effective treatment to curb mortality among heroin-dependent injecting drug users.[64]

Psychotherapy and psychosocial interventions are fundamental components of drug therapy and necessitate program integrity, responsiveness to criminogenic and psychosocial needs, and aftercare.[65] Consolidating psychosocial support and pharmacotherapy is positively correlated with greater prisoner motivation to address drug-related problems.[66] Also, in recognition that the post-liberation transition represents a period of uncertainty for many ex-prisoners, pre- and post-release programs need to target the development of psychosocial skills and resilience as well as to provide the necessary practical support. Standardized risk assessments and screening are warranted to identify prisoners at a heightened risk of drug-related mortality. Thus, equality of care requires an integrated system-wide psychosocial and pharmacotherapeutic interface that addresses the specific post-release needs of ex-prisoners.

Spain has the most extensive and developed prison-based harm reduction measures in Europe.[52,67] More than one fifth (22%) of opioid substitution therapy in Spain is delivered in prisons, accounting for 19,010 opioid-dependent prisoners in 2005.[57] The health of prisoners in Spain is collaboratively administered by the Ministry of Health and the Ministry of Interior, which offer considerable service and treatment options. These include pre-release education[57] and post-release treatment referral to community services.[65] The utility of service delivery to drug-dependent prisoners in Spain is advanced by psychosocial interventions, which are viewed as indispensable to treatment. One criticism, however, is the restricted availability of psychosocial support[57,66,68] and of interventions delivered by external non-governmental organizations.[45] The latter, when present, assist post-release social reintegration.

Specific programs may be tailored to redress the dynamic adverse health risks encountered by drug-dependent prisoners after release by targeting the differential needs of this subpopulation. Interventions may be multimodal, incorporating such elements as skill development and problem-solving, deinstitutionalization, domestic and financial management, and counseling. In this manner, the drug problem may be put in context so as to develop an integrated care model and shift the focus from offending behavior to building capacity. Best practice in program development and delivery thus involves the creation of partnerships and effective working relationships with all stakeholders, including correctional and treatment staff, prisoners, and external service providers.

One such initiative is the Bolwara House Transitional Centre in New South Wales, Australia, an intensive community-based pre-release program for women with a history of drug addiction. This non-custodial therapeutic community provides structured transitional support that implements throughcare principles. It incorporates pharmacotherapy, psychosocial development, and family and community reintegration in a holistic, client-centered approach. The program consists of two phases, beginning with a 4-week in-house deinstitutionalization process, after which time women commence community programs based on their assessed needs.[69] Such programs include paid or voluntary employment, accommodation, parenting, and education. This fosters social inclusion and rehabilitation while strengthening competences, personal resources, and self-esteem.

Similarly, the Aboriginal Offender Substance Abuse Program in Canada is a national intervention that helps aboriginal men holistically address their drug dependence and offending behavior. This program includes opioid substitution therapy and examines substance use in terms of interpersonal and transgenerational trauma. Traditional techniques, such as cultural healing practices and re-establishing spiritual connectedness, are applied in conjunction with current therapeutic measures, including risk management and skill development.[70] In this way, the program confronts the causes of aboriginal drug addiction by implementing culturally appropriate strategies.

Naloxone, which binds preferentially to opioid receptors to counter the central nervous system and respiratory depression of an opioid overdose, has been recommended for released prisoners.[5,71,72] Considering the evidence indicating that many overdoses occur in the presence of others, particularly friends and partners,[71] and the ease with which naloxone can be administered by non-medical personnel, there has been interest in recent years in evaluating whether the peer administration of naloxone could be an effective means of reducing overdose mortality. Scotland implemented the National Naloxone Program and as of June 2011, all prisons in Scotland are taking part in the program to provide naloxone kits to at-risk individuals upon release.[73] Naloxone is also available to staff in all Australian prison jurisdictions[74] but is not yet provided to prisoners at release. Community pilot programs of take-home naloxone have had positive results[75,76] and have demonstrated preliminary support for the intervention in terms of feasibility and safety.

CONCLUSION AND GOOD PRACTICE

Custodial populations have markedly elevated rates of acute drug-related mortality in the period immediately after release. This is largely a consequence of diminished tolerance and use of multiple drugs. Nevertheless, these deaths are preventable. A number of prevention and harm reduction responses may be suitably applied at all levels of the criminal justice system. The best evidence from the literature suggests that the following should be implemented:

1. *Opioid substitution therapy*
   Opioid substitution therapy has been demonstrated to be the most effective treatment option for opioid-dependent persons and, among criminal justice populations, has been shown to reduce mortality during incarceration[77] and the immediate post-release period.[78] Opioid-dependent prisoners should be given the opportunity to commence or continue opioid substitution therapy if this is available in the community. Psychotherapeutic or psychosocial interventions and drug education should be available in prisons as essential components of drug treatment programs.
2. *Continuity of care and treatment stability*
   Due to the long persistence of substance use disorders and the severity associated with lack of treatment for this illness or therapeutic disruption, continuity of care and treatment stability are paramount. Comprehensive provision of healthcare

services for drug-dependent prisoners is necessary both throughout periods in the care of the criminal justice system and during subsequent community reintegration. Individuals should be linked to appropriate drug or support services on first contact with the criminal justice system or when targeted as being at risk of becoming a drug offender. The provision of services for drug-dependent people must be available while they are in police custody, pre-trial detention, and prison. Furthermore, pre-release drug services are to be coordinated with and linked to appropriate aftercare, to ensure uninterrupted service delivery.

3. *Building partnerships and networks*

Interagency partnerships between corrections-based and external service providers are essential to the establishment of effective and continuous services for prisoners. When correctly managed, the processes of government and nongovernmental agencies and community support can be integrated and coordinated, with appropriate referral systems. Formal and informal community interactions, especially social support structures, are of significant importance to prisoners and provide a post-release psychological buffer.

4. *At the prison level*

At the prison level, the service must include building healthy therapeutic relationships. This requires a range of needs-based, client-centered treatment modalities. Also, multi-faceted team case management partnerships are recommended. Treatment plans and service options need to be designed in consultation with service users to facilitate a culture of mutual respect, active participation, increased motivation, and empowerment.

5. *Education for all stakeholders*

Prison staff, prisoners, the people who support them, and external service providers (such as community care workers and non-governmental organizations) are to be made aware of the risks of acute, drug-related, post-release mortality. Prisoners and the people who support them are to receive pre-release public health education in areas of drug use prevention, risk behavior, and overdose prevention, including the emergency use of naloxone.

6. *At the national level*

At the national level, the provision of key structures and services must include the following:

- providing a comprehensive, countrywide framework of drug treatment;
- determining which service or agency must take responsibility;
- recognizing and addressing the specific needs of particular subgroups; and
- monitoring, risk assessment, and evaluation of interventions.

7. *Providing a comprehensive, countrywide framework of drug treatment*

A comprehensive, countrywide framework of drug treatment needs to be incorporated into all levels of the criminal justice system. The main principle is that, whenever possible, it is preferable for individuals with a substance use disorder to be diverted to an appropriate community treatment facility rather than be sent to prison. In cases where prison is deemed necessary, drug treatment should be provided, based on formalized end-to-end strategies of throughcare and aftercare.

8. *Determining which service or agency must take responsibility*
   Determining which service or agency must take responsibility for and address the needs of individuals at risk of acute drug-related mortality after release from prison requires conceptual reframing of prison health mandates to incorporate post-release well-being. This may necessitate:
   - evaluating data collection, to continually monitor post-release outcomes in prison health data and so adequately identify service gaps;
   - analyzing the legal frameworks and extent of duty of care and accountability for the health of people after their release from prison; and
   - including, under the jurisdiction of this national structure, individuals serving community sentences, those on home leave, and those on parole.

9. *Recognizing and addressing the specific needs of particular subgroups*
   Program design should target the assessed needs of vulnerable subgroups at increased risk, including women, sex workers, migrants, and foreign nationals. Also, standardized risk assessment and screening are useful in identifying individual prisoners who are at an increased risk of drug-related, post-release mortality and who would benefit from specialized programs and support.

10. *Monitoring, risk assessment, and evaluation of interventions*
    Monitoring, risk assessment, and evaluation of interventions include the implementation of a standardized monitoring protocol to:
    - determine baseline mortality rates;
    - assess prisoner needs, inside prison and upon release;
    - document implementation of interventions and the success of these measures; and
    - identify gaps in service provision.

REFERENCES

1. Stewart LM, Henderson CJ, Hobbs MST, Ridout SC, Knuiman MW. Risk of death in prisoners after release from jail. *Aust N Z J Public Health*. 2004;28(1):32–36.
2. Kariminia A, Butler T, Corben S, et al. Extreme cause-specific mortality in a cohort of adult prisoners—1988 to 2002: a data-linkage study. *Int J Epidemiol*. 2007;36(2):310–316.
3. Spittal MJ, Forsyth S, Pirkis J, Alati R, Kinner SA. Suicide in adults released from prison in Queensland, Australia: a cohort study. *J Epidemiol Community Health*. 2014;68(10):993–998.
4. Brehm Christensen P, Hammerby E, Smith E, Bird SM. Mortality among Danish drug users released from prison. *Int J Prison Health*. 2006;2(1):13–19.
5. Singleton N, Pendry E, Taylor C, Farrell M, Marsden J. *Drug-Related Mortality Among Newly-Released Offenders*. London, England: Home Office; 2003.
6. Farrell M, Marsden J. Acute risk of drug-related death among newly released prisoners in England and Wales. *Addiction*. 2008;103(2):251–255.
7. Verger P, Rotily M, Prudhomme J, Bird S. High mortality rates among inmates during the year following their discharge from a French prison. *J Forensic Sci*. 2003;48(3):614–616.
8. Harding-Pink D. Mortality following release from prison. *Med Sci Law*. 1990;30(1):12–16.
9. Binswanger IA. Release from prison—a high risk of death for former inmates. *N Eng J Med*. 2007;356(5):157–165.

10. Spaulding AC, Seals RM, McCallum VA, Perez SD, Brzozowski AK, Steenland NK. Prisoner survival inside and outside of the institution: implications for health-care planning. *Am J Epidemiol.* 2011;173(5):479–487.
11. Lim S, Seligson AL, Parvez FM, et al. Risks of drug-related death, suicide, and homicide during the immediate post-release period among people released From New York City jails, 2001–2005. *Am J Epidemiol.* 2012;175(6):519–526.
12. Chen C-Y, Wu P-N, Su L-W, Chou Y-J, Lin K-M. Three-year mortality and predictors after release: a longitudinal study of the first-time drug offenders in Taiwan. *Addiction.* 2010;105(5):920–927.
13. Binswanger IA. Mortality after prison release: opioid overdose and other causes of death, risk factors, and time trends from 1999 to 2009. *Ann Intern Med.* 2013;159(9):592–600.
14. Andrews JY, Kinner SA. Understanding drug-related mortality in released prisoners: a review of national coronial records. *BMC Public Health.* 2012;12(270:1–7.
15. Crowley D. The drug detox unit at Mountjoy Prison—a review. *J Health Gain.* 1999;3(3):17–19.
16. Seal KH, Kral AH, Gee L, et al. Predictors and prevention of nonfatal overdose among street-recruited injection heroin users in the San Francisco Bay Area, 1998–1999. *Am J Public Health.* 2001;91(11):1842–1846.
17. Dolan KA, Shearer J, White B, Zhou J, Kaldor J, Wodak AD. Four-year follow-up of imprisoned male heroin users and methadone treatment: mortality, re-incarceration and hepatitis C infection. *Addiction.* 2005;100(6):820–828.
18. Huang Y-F, Kuo H-S, Lew-Ting C-Y, et al. Mortality among a cohort of drug users after their release from prison: an evaluation of the effectiveness of a harm reduction program in Taiwan. *Addiction.* 2011;106(8):1437–1445.
19. Fazel S, Bains P, Doll H. Substance abuse and dependence in prisoners: a systematic review. *Addiction.* 2006;101(2):181–191.
20. Kastelic A, Pont J, Stover H. *Opioid Substitution Treatment in Custodial Settings: A Practical Guide.* Oldenburg, Germany: BIS-Verlag der Carl von Ossietzky Universität Oldenburg; 2008.
21. Farrell M, Marsden J. *Drug-Related Mortality Among Newly Released Offenders 1998 to 2000.* London, England: London Home Office; 2005.
22. Davies S, Cook S. Dying outside: women, imprisonment and post-release mortality. Paper presented at: Women in Corrections: Staff and Clients Conference; October 31, 2000; Adelaide, Australia.
23. Seymour A, Oliver JS, Black M. Drug-related deaths among recently released prisoners in the Strathclyde region of Scotland. *J Forensic Sci.* 2000;45(3):649–654.
24. Shewan D, Hammersley R, Oliver J, Macpherson S. Fatal drug overdose after liberation from prison: a retrospective study of female ex-prisoners from Strathclyde region (Scotland). *Addiction Res.* 2000;8(3):267–278.
25. Darke S, Zador D. Fatal heroin "overdose": a review. *Addiction.* 1996;91(12):1765–1772.
26. Darke S. Heroin overdose: research and evidence-based intervention. *J Urban Health.* 2003;80(2):189–200.
27. Gossop M, Stewart D, Treacy S, Marsden J. A prospective study of mortality among drug misusers during a 4-year period after seeking treatment. *Addiction.* 2002;97(1):39–47.
28. McGregor C, Hall K, Ali R, Christie P, Braithwaite R, Darke S. *It's Rarely Just the "h": Addressing Overdose Among South Australian Heroin Users Through a Process of Intersectoral Collaboration.* Parkside, Australia: Drug and Alcohol Services Council of South Australia; 1999.
29. Zador D, Sunjic D, Darke S. Heroin-related deaths in New South Wales, 1992: toxicological findings and circumstances. *Med J Aust.* 1996;164:204–207.
30. Sattar G. *Rates and Causes of Death Among Prisoners and Offenders Under Community Supervision: Home Office Research Study 231.* London, England: Home Office; 2001.

31. Binswanger IA, Blatchford PJ, Lindsay RG, Stern MF. Risk factors for all-cause, overdose and early deaths after release from prison in Washington State. *Drug Alcohol Depend*. 2011;117(1):1–6.
32. van Dooren K, Kinner SA, Forsyth S. Risk of death for young ex-prisoners in the year following release from adult prison. *Aust N Z J Public Health*. 2013;37(4):377–382.
33. Hobbs MST, Krazlan K, Ridout SC, Mai Q, Knuiman MW, Chapman R. *Mortality and Morbidity in Prisoners After Release From Prison in Western Australia 1995–2003*. Canberra, Australia: Australian Institute of Criminology; 2006.
34. Kariminia A, Law MG, Butler TG, et al. Factors associated with mortality in a cohort of Australian prisoners. *Eur J Epidemiol*. 2007;22(7):417–428.
35. Graham A. Post-prison mortality: unnatural death among people released from Victorian prisons between January 1990 and December 1999. *Aust N Z J Criminol*. 2003;36(1):94–108.
36. Forsyth SJ, Alati R, Ober C, Williams GM, Kinner SA. Striking subgroup differences in substance-related mortality after release from prison. *Addiction*. 2014;109(10):1676–1683.
37. Patterson EJ. The dose-response of time served in prison on mortality: New York State, 1989–2003. *Am J Public Health* 2013;103(3):523–528.
38. Gjersing L, Jonassen KV, Biong S, et al. Diversity in causes and characteristics of drug-induced deaths in an urban setting. *Scand J Public Health*. 2013;41(2):119–125.
39. United Nations. *Basic Principles for the Treatment of Prisoners: Annex*. New York, NY: United Nations; 1990.
40. Betteridge G. *Harm Reduction in Prisons and Jails: International Experience*. Toronto, Canada: Canadian HIV/AIDS Legal Network; 2005.
41. United Nations. *Constitution of the World Health Organization*. New York, NY: United Nations; 1946.
42. United Nations. *The Universal Declaration of Human Rights*. New York, NY: United Nations; 1948.
43. United Nations. *International Covenant on Economic, Social, and Cultural Rights*. Geneva, Switzerland: Office of the High Commissioner for Human Rights; 1976.
44. United Nations. *Principles of Medical Ethics*. New York, NY: United Nations; 1982.
45. UNODC, UNAIDS, WHO. *HIV/AIDS Prevention, Care, Treatment and Support in Prison Settings: A Framework for an Efficient National Response*. Vienna, Austria: United Nations Office on Drugs and Crime; 2006.
46. World Health Organization. *WHO Guidelines on HIV Infection and AIDS in Prisons*. Geneva, Switzerland: World Health Organization; 1993.
47. WHO Regional Office for Europe. *Good Governance for Prison Health in the 21st Century: A Policy Brief on the Organization of Prison Health*. Copenhagen, Denmark: WHO Regional Office for Europe; 2013.
48. Council of Europe Committee of Ministers. *Recommendation No. R 98(7) of the Committee of Ministers to Member States Concerning the Ethical and Organisational Aspects of Health Care in Prison*. Strasbourg, France: Committee of Ministers of the Council of Europe; 1998.
49. United Nations. *Standard Minimum Rules for the Treatment of Prisoners: Adopted by the First United Nations Congress on the Prevention of Crime and the Treatment of Offenders on 30 August 1955*. New York, NY: United Nations; 1955.
50. WHO Regional Office for Europe. *Declaration on Prison Health as Part of Public Health*. Copenhagen, Denmark: WHO Regional Office for Europe; 2002.
51. WHO, UNODC, UNAIDS. *Substitution Maintenance Therapy in the Management of Opioid Dependence and HIV/AIDS Prevention: Position Paper*. Geneva, Switzerland: World Health Organization; 2004.
52. WHO Regional Office for Europe. *Status Paper on Prisons, Drugs and Harm Reduction*. Copenhagen, Denmark: WHO Regional Office for Europe; 2005.

53. Lines R, Jurgens R, Stover H, et al. *Dublin Declaration on HIV/AIDS in Prisons in Europe and Central Asia: Good Prison Health Is Good Public Health*. Dublin, Ireland: Irish Penal Reform Trust; 2004.
54. United Nations. *International Covenant on Civil and Political Rights*. Geneva, Switzerland: Office of the High Commissioner for Human Rights; 1976.
55. United Nations. *Body of Principles for the Protection of All Persons Under Any Form of Detention or Imprisonment*. New York, NY: United Nations; 1988.
56. National Health Service. *Key messages for the Drug Interventions Programme—February 2007*. London, England: National Treatment Agency for Substance Misuse; 2007.
57. Weilandt C, Stover H, Eckert J, et al. *Reduction of Drug-Related Crime in Prison: The Impact of Opioid Substitution Treatment on the Manageability of Opioid Dependent Prisoners*. Bremen, Germany: BISDRO, University of Bremen WIAD—Scientific Institute of the German Medical Association, Bonn; 2008.
58. Jenkins R, Paton J, WHO Collaborating Centre for Research and Training in Mental Health, King's College London, University of London. *Mental Health Primary Care in Prison: A Guide to Mental Ill Health in Adults and Adolescents in Prison and Young Offender Institutions*. London, England: Royal Society of Medicine Press; 2002.
59. Department of Health (England). *Clinical Management of Drug Dependence in the Adult Prison Setting: Including Psychosocial Treatment as a Core Part*. London, England: Department of Health (England); 2006.
60. Department of Health (England). *Prisons Integrated Drug Treatment System: Continuity of Care Guidance*. London, England: Department of Health (England); 2007.
61. Department of Health (England), Scottish Office Department of Health, Welsh Office Department of Health, Department of Health and Social Services Northern Ireland. *Drug Misuse and Dependence—Guidelines on Clinical Management*. London, England: Her Majesty's Stationery Office; 1999.
62. Skodbo S, Brown G, Deacon S, et al. *The Drug Interventions Programme (DIP): Addressing Drug Use and Offending Through "Tough Choices."* London, England: Home Office; 2007.
63. Department of Health (England), Scottish Office Department of Health, Welsh Office Department of Health, Northern Ireland Executive. *Drug Misuse and Dependence—UK Guidelines on Clinical Management*. London, England: Department of Health (England); 2007.
64. WHO Regional Office for Europe. *Health in Prisons: A WHO Guide to the Essentials in Prison Health*. Copenhagen, Denmark: World Health Organization; 2007.
65. Stover H. *Assistance to Drug Users in European Union Prisons: An Overview Study*. London, England: European Network for Drug and HIV/AIDS Services in Prison and European Monitoring Centre for Drugs and Drug Addiction; 2001.
66. Stover H, Casselman J, Hennebel L. Substitution treatment in European prisons: a study of policies and practices in 18 European countries. *Int J Prison Health*. 2006;2(1):3–12.
67. Cook C, Kanaef N. *The Global State of Harm Reduction 2008: Mapping the Response to Drug-Related HIV and Hepatitis C Epidemics*. London, England: International Harm Reduction Association; 2008.
68. Stover H, Hennebel L, Casselman J. *Substitution Treatment in European Prisons: A Study of Policies and Practices in 18 European Countries*. London, England: European Network of Drug Services in Prison; 2004.
69. NSW Department of Corrective Services. *Inmate Classification and Placement Procedures Manual*. Sydney, Australia: NSW Department of Corrective Services; 2005.
70. Varis D, McGowan V, Mullins P. Development of an Aboriginal offender substance abuse program. *FORUM Corrections Res*. 2006;18:42–44.

71. Strang J, Darke S, Hall W, Farrell M, Ali R. Heroin overdose: the case for take-home naloxone. *BMJ*. 1996;312(7044):1435–1436.
72. Darke S. From the can to the coffin: deaths among recently released prisoners. *Addiction*. 2008;103(2):256–257.
73. Information Services Division Scotland. *National Naloxone Programme Scotland—Naloxone Kits Issued in 2012/ 13*. Edinburgh, Scotland: Information Services Division; 2013.
74. Black E, Dolan KA, Wodak AD. *Supply, Demand and Harm Reduction Strategies in Australian Prisons: Implementation, Cost and Evaluation*. Canberra, Australia: Australian National Council on Drugs; 2004.
75. Dettmer K. Take home naloxone and the prevention of deaths from opiate overdose: two pilot schemes. *BMJ*. 2001;322(7291):895–896.
76. Galea S, Worthington N, Piper TM, Nandi VV, Curtis M, Rosenthal DM. Provision of naloxone to injection drug users as an overdose prevention strategy: early evidence from a pilot study in New York City. *Addict Behav*. 2006;31(5):907–912.
77. Larney S, Gisev N, Farrell M, et al. Opioid substitution therapy as a strategy to reduce deaths in prison: retrospective cohort study. *BMJ Open*. 2014;4(4):e004666.
78. Degenhardt L, Larney S, Kimber J, et al. The impact of opioid substitution therapy on mortality post-release from prison: retrospective data linkage study. *Addiction*. 2014;109(8):1306–1317.
79. Bird SM, Hutchinson SJ. Male drugs-related deaths in the fortnight after release from prison: Scotland, 1996–1999. *Addiction*. 2003;98(2):185–190.
80. Ødegård E, Amundsen EJ, Kielland KB. Fatal overdoses and deaths by other causes in a cohort of Norwegian drug abusers—a competing risk approach. *Drug Alcohol Depend*. 2007;89(2-3):176–182.
81. Seaman SR, Brettle RP, Gore SM. Mortality from overdose among injecting drug users recently released from prison: database linkage study. *BMJ*. 1998;316:426–428.

CHAPTER 19

Drug Use in Prisoners

Epidemiology, Implications, and Policy Responses

STUART A. KINNER, PhD AND JOSIAH D. RICH, MD, MPH

THE EPIDEMIOLOGY OF DRUG USE IN PRISONERS

Drug use and prisons seem inextricably linked. International drug laws effectively criminalize people who use drugs, and individuals experiencing problems with substance use are often funneled into the criminal justice system rather than the health system.[1,2] People who are characterized by other risk factors for incarceration—such as homelessness and untreated, serious mental illness—are also more likely to engage in risky substance use, which further compounds their risk of incarceration and other adverse health and social outcomes.[3,4] The consequence is that prisons house a high concentration of marginalized individuals with a history of problematic substance use and complex, co-occurring health problems.[5] Given that many of these individuals have had limited engagement with appropriate treatment services in the community, prisons provide a rare—albeit regrettable—opportunity to identify these health problems and initiate appropriate care.

In Prison

The manner in which prison authorities respond to people who use drugs in their care varies enormously both within and between jurisdictions. Some jurisdictions invest heavily in evidence-based demand reduction programs such as opioid substitution treatment (OST), cognitive behavioral therapy, and/or therapeutic communities and drug-free units. However, in most settings these evidence-based responses are either absent or not to scale, such that the majority of incarcerated people who use drugs do not have access to evidence-based treatments. In a handful of settings, prison or prison health authorities have overcome political opposition to implement evidence-based harm reduction programs, such as prison needle exchange. Evaluations of such programs have been uniformly positive, yet their uptake in correctional settings remains poor.[6]

The overriding response to drugs in most correctional settings is supply reduction—that is, efforts to prevent drugs from entering prison—premised on a zero-tolerance approach to drug use. Despite this, drug use in prison is common and, in the absence of harm reduction services in most settings, particularly risky. For people who inject drugs, prisons represent a "perfect storm" of risk factors for the transmission of blood-borne viruses such as HIV and hepatitis C: the background prevalence of infection is high, demand for drugs is high, and users are typically deprived of the means to reduce their risk of infection through sharing of injecting equipment, even where such means are available in the surrounding community. Prisons are unique and challenging environments, and drug use in these settings poses significant challenges for both health and safety. Efforts to regulate the supply of drugs in these settings—as in the community—are appropriate but should be evidence-based and balanced by investment in demand reduction (ie, treatment) and harm reduction.[2] The overarching goal of responses to drug use in prisons should be to maximize public health, human rights, and civil society outcomes, not to punish people who use drugs. Responses based on stigma, ignorance, ingrained attitudes that are not supported by the evidence, or political expediency are likely to be counterproductive.

After Release From Prison

A large proportion of people who used drugs before prison relapse to the same behaviors soon after release from custody. This is equally true for illicit drugs and for legal substances such as alcohol and tobacco. As such, despite entrenched rhetoric that prisons are places of rehabilitation, there is mounting evidence that incarceration may be better conceived of as an interruption in drug use —at least for those who discontinue or reduce their use in prison.[7,8] To the extent that current correctional responses to drug use in prison are effective, the evidence suggests that these effects are rarely sustained beyond the prison walls.

Drug use after release from prison is common, often risky, and associated with a raft of poor health, social, and criminal justice outcomes. Release from prison precipitates a period of acutely elevated risk of fatal drug overdose[9]; this is presumed to be driven by reduced opioid tolerance, although increased risk-taking behavior and polydrug use likely play a role.[10] Although the risk of death is greatest in the weeks immediately following release from custody, ex-prisoners remain at elevated risk of death from drug-related causes, suicide, injury, and other preventable causes for years after they return to the community.[11] Recent studies have also documented high rates of nonfatal drug overdose and self-harm in ex-prisoners,[12-14] suggesting an unmet need for substance use and mental health treatment. Consistent with this, people released from prison present to emergency departments and are admitted to hospitals at a rate well above that of their community peers, often for reasons related to substance use or mental disorder, and at significant cost to the health system.[15-17] Individuals who relapse to substance use after release from prison are also at increased risk of reincarceration, such that effective responses to substance use in ex-prisoners are likely to yield benefits for both health and criminal justice systems.[18]

Reducing Drug-Related Harm

Effective responses to drug use in people who experience incarceration therefore require an investment in both prison-based treatment and harm reduction services, and post-release care and support. For those with a history of heroin use, there is good evidence that retention in OST throughout and beyond the prison walls reduces infection, overdose, and reincarceration.[19-21] For those who do overdose, evidence from observational studies suggests that take-home naloxone—an overdose reversal drug with no abuse potential—will save lives.[22] Prison authorities in Scotland and Wales now provide take-home naloxone kits to people at risk of opioid overdose at the point of release, and evaluation findings suggest a protective effect against overdose death.[23] Despite this, expansion of take-home naloxone programs to other prison settings has proven difficult, and preventable overdose deaths after release from prison remain tragically common.

For individuals dependent on other substances (such as alcohol, cannabis, methamphetamine, and cocaine), the evidence base is not as strong; more research regarding both the harms associated with use of these substances in ex-prisoners and the means to reduce these harms is urgently required. In addition to targeted harm reduction, broad-based transitional programs that support reintegration into the community and promote engagement with community health services are likely to contribute to improved health outcomes, including reduced drug-related harm.[24] Recent randomized trials have shown that even a low-cost intervention can increase engagement with primary care in people recently released from prison, and that this can both increase engagement with treatment services and reduce emergency department presentations.[25-27]

A WAY FORWARD

Weakening the links between drug use and prison, and improving outcomes for people who use drugs and experience incarceration, will require closing the gap between evidence and policy, and filling important gaps in the evidence base.

Policy Reform

The war on drugs has failed. Overwhelming evidence points to the health and social harms caused by criminalization of drug use and the criminogenic effects of incarceration.[1,28,29] The world prison population continues to grow at a rate in excess of population growth, substantially driven by punitive and largely ineffective responses to drug use.[2] Law enforcement agencies are increasingly recognizing that they cannot "arrest their way out of the problem" and that a different approach—a public health approach—is required.[1] Such an approach would be grounded in a human rights framework, informed by the evidence, and distinguished by a commitment to harm minimization—balancing supply, demand, and harm reduction.

Drug law reform is critical to weakening the links between drug use and prisons, but for those people who use drugs who are already caught in the revolving door of prison, reforms within the correctional system have the potential to meaningfully improve both health and criminal justice outcomes. Diversion programs for people whose offending is driven by drug use can reduce crime, reduce drug use, and save money by keeping people who use drugs out of prison.[30,31] Evidence-based drug treatment and harm reduction in prison settings reduce drug use, reduce the spread of infection, and prevent overdose. Effective drug treatment in prison can also reduce reincarceration, particularly when it is continued, as part of a coordinated transitional support program, after prisoners return to the community.[20]

Despite strong evidence for reform, closing the gap between evidence and correctional policy has proven to be a pernicious challenge. Prisons and prisoners are rarely the subject of informed public debate, such that there is comparatively little impediment to the adoption of punitive, populist policies. Conversely, adoption of humane, evidence-informed policies can attract criticism that the government has "gone soft on crime." Increased public awareness of the ways in which correctional policies and practices diverge from the evidence—and of the health, justice, and economic costs of this divergence—may increase public support for reform.[32]

Research Priorities

There is compelling evidence that OST is an effective treatment for heroin users, and that naloxone can reduce overdose deaths in these individuals both in and after release from prison. However, a large proportion of prisoners experiences problems with substances other than heroin, but neither these harms nor effective means to prevent them are well understood. Alcohol misuse is an important driver of incarceration in many countries and contributes to both preventable mortality and recidivism after release from prison.[33,34] Tobacco smoking is normative in most prisons, and despite adoption of prison smoking bans in some countries, smoking in prison persists, and relapse after release is typically rapid.[35] Use of methamphetamine is increasing at the global level,[36] with methamphetamine now the most common "drug of choice" among prison entrants in Australia.[37] There is an urgent need for further research on both the epidemiology of substance use in people who experience incarceration, and effective means of reducing the harms associated with this use.

Although it is now well established that drug use in prison is common, our understanding of how and why people use drugs in prison remains poor. Particularly for those who inject drugs in prison, a more nuanced understanding of perceptions of risk, and strategies for minimizing risk of blood-borne virus transmission, may inform more effective prevention strategies. Similarly, although it is clear that relapse to risky substance use soon after release from prison is common, we know remarkably little about precisely when, where, and why this occurs. A more detailed understanding of the epidemiology of substance use after release from prison would lay the groundwork for rigorous evaluation of prevention and harm reduction interventions.

In most correctional settings, the dominant response to drug use is supply control, yet the evidence to support many of these practices is weak. Rigorous evaluation of efforts to prevent drugs from entering prison facilities—including consideration of any collateral harms—would lead to more effective interdiction and improve alignment with a harm minimization framework.[38]

Despite the fact that prisoners are a "captive population," ethical considerations and restrictions on movement and access make research in correctional settings notoriously challenging. A sometimes one-eyed focus on maintaining prison "security and good order" at any price, coupled with an implicit view in some settings that people are sent to prison *for* punishment—rather than *as* punishment—can jeopardize independent scrutiny of the policies, practices, and outcomes engendered by these public institutions. Access to correctional populations requires the assent of prison authorities, with potential consequences for suppression of unwanted research findings. Despite the fact that prisons are a sentinel site for responding to important public health problems such as drug dependence, infectious disease, and mental disorders, obtaining funding for high-quality health and medical research in these settings can be difficult.[39] Reflecting this dearth of research, a recent systematic review identified only 95 studies globally that had evaluated any health intervention for prisoners using a randomized design. Of these, only 42 measured an outcome after release from prison.[40] Building the evidence base will require strong public investment in rigorous, independent research and fostering of a culture of evidence-based policy and practice in correctional settings.

Prisoner Health Is Public Health

Garnering support for investment in the well-being of drug-using prisoners can be challenging, despite a clear mandate to do so on human rights grounds.[41] Another argument for improving outcomes for people who use drugs and experience incarceration is that this is, in effect, an investment in public health. This argument is most pointed with respect to infectious disease. The prevalence of infectious diseases such as HIV, hepatitis C, and tuberculosis is markedly elevated in prisoners, and infection is concentrated in those who use and inject drugs.[42] In fact, in countries like the United States where the incarceration rate is high, a significant proportion of the infected population cycles through custodial settings each year.[42] Modeling studies suggest that effective treatment of these infections in prisoners—including through effective responses to drug dependence—can reduce the population prevalence of infection: so-called treatment as prevention.[42,44]

CONCLUSION

Punitive drug laws have resulted in the mass incarceration of people who use drugs, as well as a concentration of people with complex health and social needs in settings that are ill-equipped to respond. Correctional policies and practices with respect to drug use and related harms often diverge from the evidence. Where such responses are evidence-based, they are rarely delivered at scale. Health and justice outcomes for people who use drugs, after release from prison, are predictably poor, such that incarceration can at best be considered an interruption in drug use. Greater investment in independent, rigorous research and a renewed commitment to aligning correctional policy and practice with the evidence will have measurable benefits for public health, public safety, and the public purse.

REFERENCES

1. Csete J, Kamarulzaman A, Kazatchkine M, et al. Public health and international drug policy. *Lancet*. 2016;387(2):1427–1480.
2. Puras D, Hannah J. Reasons for drug policy reform: prohibition enables systemic human rights abuses and undermines public health. *BMJ*. 2017;356:i6586.
3. Chang Z, Larsson H, Lichtenstein P, Fazel S. Psychiatric disorders and violent reoffending: a national cohort study of convicted prisoners in Sweden. *Lancet Psychiatry*. 2015;2(10):891–900.
4. Saddichha S, Fliers JM, Frankish J, Somers J, Schuetz CG, Krausz MR. Homeless and incarcerated: an epidemiological study from Canada. *Int J Soc Psychiatry*. 2014;60(8):795–800.
5. van Dooren K, Richards A, Lennox N, et al. Complex health-related needs among young, soon-to-be released prisoners. *Health Justice*. 2013;1(1):1–8.
6. Jürgens R, Ball A, Verster A. Interventions to reduce HIV transmission related to injecting drug use in prison. *Lancet Infect Dis*. 2009;9(1):57–66.
7. Kinner SA. Continuity of health impairment and substance misuse among adult prisoners in Queensland, Australia. *Int J Prison Health*. 2006;2(2):101–113.
8. Thomas E, Degenhardt L, Alati R, Kinner SA. Predictive validity of the AUDIT for hazardous alcohol consumption in recently released prisoners. *Drug Alcohol Depend*. 2013;134:322–329.
9. Merrall ELC, Kariminia A, Binswanger IA, et al. Meta-analysis of drug-related deaths soon after release from prison. *Addiction*. 2010;105(9):1545–1554.
10. Andrews J, Kinner SA. Understanding drug-related mortality in released prisoners: a review of national coronial records. *BMC Public Health*. 2012;12(270):1–7.
11. Kinner SA, Forsyth S, Williams GM. Systematic review of record linkage studies of mortality in ex-prisoners: why (good) methods matter. *Addiction*. 2012;108(1):38–49.
12. Kinner SA, Milloy M-J, Wood E, Qi J, Zhang R, Kerr T. Incidence and risk factors for non-fatal overdose among a cohort of recently incarcerated illicit drug users. *Addict Behav*. 2012;37(6):691–696.
13. Winter R, Stoové M, Degenhardt L, et al. Incidence and predictors of non-fatal drug overdose after release from prison among people who inject drugs in Queensland, Australia. *Drug Alcohol Depend*. 2015;153:43–49.
14. Borschmann R, Thomas E, Moran P, et al. Self-harm following release from prison: a prospective data linkage study. *Aust N Z J Psychiatry*. 2017;51(3):250–259.
15. Erlyana E, Fisher DG, Reynolds GL. Emergency room use after being released from incarceration. *Health Justice*. 2014;2(5):1–7.

16. Frank JW, Andrews CM, Green TC, Samuels AM, Trinh TT, Friedmann PD. Emergency department utilization among recently released prisoners: a retrospective cohort study. *BMC Emerg Med*. 2013;13(16):1–8.
17. Alan J, Burmas M, Preen D, Pfaff J. Inpatient hospital use in the first year after release from prison: a Western Australian population-based record linkage study. *Aust N Z J Public Health*. 2011;35(3):264–269.
18. Kinner SA, Wang EA. The case for improving the health of ex-prisoners. *Am J Public Health*. 2014;104(8):1352–1355.
19. Larney S. Does opioid substitution treatment in prisons reduce injecting-related HIV risk behaviours? a systematic review. *Addiction*. 2010;105(2):216–223.
20. Larney S, Toson B, Burns L, Dolan K. Effect of prison-based opioid substitution treatment and post-release retention in treatment on risk of re-incarceration. *Addiction*. 2012;107(2):372–380.
21. Degenhardt L, Larney S, Kimber J, et al. The impact of opioid substitution therapy on mortality post-release from prison: retrospective data linkage study. *Addiction*. 2014;109(8):1306–1317.
22. Strang J, Bird S, Parmar MB. Take-home emergency naloxone to prevent heroin overdose deaths after prison release: rationale and practicalities for the N-ALIVE randomized trial. *J Urban Health*. 2013;90(5):983–996.
23. Bird SM, McAuley A, Perry S, Hunter C. Effectiveness of Scotland's National Naloxone Programme for reducing opioid-related deaths: a before (2006–10) versus after (2011–13) comparison. *Addiction*. 2016;111(5):883–891.
24. Kinner SA, Young JT, Carroll M. The pivotal role of primary care in meeting the health needs of people recently released from prison. *Australas Psychiatry*. 2015;23(6):650–653.
25. Kinner SA, Alati R, Longo M, et al. Low-intensity case management increases contact with primary care in recently released prisoners: a single-blinded, multisite, randomised controlled trial. *J Epidemiol Community Health*. 2016;70(7):683–688.
26. Wang EA, Hong CS, Shavit S, Sanders R, Kessell E, Kushel MB. Engaging individuals recently released from prison into primary care: a randomized trial. *Am J Public Health*. 2012;102(9):e22–e29.
27. Young JT, Arnold-Reed D, Preen D, Bulsara M, Lennox N, Kinner SA. Early primary care physician contact and health service utilisation in a large sample of recently released ex-prisoners in Australia: prospective cohort study. *BMJ Open*. 2015;5(e008021):1–12.
28. Vieraitis LM, Kovandzic TV, Marvell TB. The criminogenic effects of imprisonment: evidence from state panel data, 1974–2002. *Criminol Public Policy*. 2007;6(3):589–622.
29. Cullen FT, Jonson CL, Nagin DS. Prisons do not reduce recidivism. *Prison J*. 2011;91(3)(suppl):48S–65S.
30. ANCD. *Prison vs. Residential Treatment: An Economic Analysis for Aboriginal and Torres Strait Islander Offenders*. Canberra, Australia: Australian National Council on Drugs; 2013.
31. Wilson DB, Mitchell O, MacKenzie DL. A systematic review of drug court effects on recidivism. *J Exp Criminol*. 2006;2(4):459–487.
32. Simpson P, Guthrie J, Lovell M, Walsh C, Butler T. *Views on Alternatives to Imprisonment: A Citizens Jury Approach*. Melbourne: Lowitja Institute; 2014.
33. Weatherburn DJ. The role of drug and alcohol policy in reducing Indigenous over-representation in prison. *Drug Alcohol Rev*. 2008;27(1):91–94.
34. Forsyth SJ, Alati R, Ober C, Williams GM, Kinner SA. Striking subgroup differences in substance-related mortality after release from prison. *Addiction*. 2014;109(10):1676–1683.
35. de Andrade D, Kinner SA. A systematic review of health and behavioural outcomes of smoking cessation interventions in rrisons. *Tob Control*. 2016;0:1–7.
36. United Nations Office on Drugs and Crime. *World Drug Report 2016*. Vienna, Austria: United Nations Office on Drugs and Crime; 2016.

37. Australian Institute of Health and Welfare. *The health of Australia's Prisoners 2015.* Canberra, Australia: Australian Institute of Health and Welfare; 2015.
38. Watson TM. The elusive goal of drug-free prisons. *Subst Use Misuse.* 2016;51(1):91–103.
39. Kouyoumdjian FG, McIsaac KE, Foran JE, Matheson FI. Canadian Institutes of Health Research funding of prison health research: a descriptive study. *CMAJ Open.* 2017;5:E14–E18.
40. Kouyoumdjian FG, McIsaac KE, Liauw J, et al. A systematic review of randomized controlled trials of interventions to improve the health of persons during imprisonment and after release. *Am J Public Health.* 2015;105(4):e13–e33.
41. Lines R. From equivalence of standards to equivalence of objectives: the entitlement of prisoners to health care standards higher than those outside prisons. *Int J Prison Health.* 2006;2(4):269–280.
42. Dolan K, Wirtz A, Moazen B, et al. Global burden of HIV, viral hepatitis, and tuberculosis in prisoners and detainees. *Lancet.* 2016;388(10049):1089–1102.
43. Hammett TM, Harmon, Mary Patricia, Rhodes, William. The burden of infectious disease among inmates of and releasees from US correctional facilities, 1997. *Am J Public Health.* 2002;92(11):1789–1794.
44. Martin NK, Vickerman P, Goldberg D, Hickman M. HCV treatment as prevention in prison: key issues. *Hepatology.* 2015;61(1):402–403.

INDEX

Figures and tables are indicated by an italic *f* or *t* following the page number.